P9-DIY-245

THIS BOOK IS FOR SIMON,
AND FOR ALL NURSES:
THE TRUE GIVERS.

"DRAMATIC . . . RINGS TRUE . . . [A] GRIPPING ACCOUNT of training and ten years in the emergency and coronary care unit ... and her burnout from physical and emotional exhaustion."

Publishers Weekly

"More than graphic hospital war stories ... A HEARTFELT, GAMELY HUMOROUS NARRATIVE."

The Boston Phoenix

"Details the full range of emotions.... FAST-PACED, HUMOROUS, ENGROSSING."

Booklist

"RIVETING ... A first-person documentary that reads like a novel.... A winning combination of medical anecdotes and personal observations.... There's never a dull or preachy moment. *Intensive Care* could not be better reading."

Anniston Star

"A PASSIONATE AND PAINFUL LOOK AT NURSING by a woman who eloquently explains the good, the bad and the maddening about her profession. Heron makes the readers see why anyone would be drawn to the profession—and why anyone, even the most caring, would want to leave it."

The Kirkus Reviews

"Carries an emotional impact that will leave few readers unmoved.... FASCINATING READING."

John Barkham's Reviews

INTENSIVE CARE

The Story of a Nurse

Echo Heron

IVY BOOKS • NEW YORK

Ivy Books
Published by Ballantine Books
Copyright © 1987 by Echo Heron

All rights reserved under International and Pan-American Copyright
Conventions. Published in the United States by Ballantine Books, a
division of Random House, Inc., New York, and simultaneously in Canada by Random House of Canada Limited, Toronto.

The material used in the Prologue (pages 1 to 8) first appeared in
Reader's Digest, September 1983.

Library of Congress Catalog Card Number: 86-47940

ISBN-0-8041-0251-1

This edition published by arrangement with Atheneum Publishers, a
division of The Scribner Book Companies, Inc.

Manufactured in the United States of America

First Ballantine Books Edition: July 1988

Cover photo of Echo Heron © Henry Grossman

ACKNOWLEDGMENTS

I want to thank Norman L. Smith of *Reader's Digest* for giving me a place to begin and Richard S. Gebhardt for believing in me enough to push me to the mailbox with my first story.

Also, warm loving thanks to my friends: the people who've touched my life, helped me through the worst of times, and left the lasting impression that they are, by any measure, the very best kids on the block. Among them:

Mary C. Bianchi, Michael J. McClure, Janey O'Hara Justice, J. Patrick Heron, Harlan Cain, Colette Coutant Trembly, Ruah Cramer, and Martha Cramer Catricala.

Loving thanks to my father, Michael A. Salato, and to my siblings, Paul, Mari, Mikie, and Storm, for their love and understanding.

For their wonderful patience, enthusiasm, and hard work, I want to thank my agent, Dominick Abel, and my editor, Patricia Lande.

For their technical advice and personal support, I want to especially thank Thomas M. Meadoff, M.D. and Margie Dingfelder, MFCC.

Also, many thanks for their technical advice to Cathrine P. Murray, R.N.; Joel Sklar, M.D.; Gerald P. Wilner, M.D.; Peter Eisenberg, M.D.; James M. Kelly, M.D.; Susan Shapiro, R.N.; and Pamela Foley, M.D.

AUTHOR'S NOTE

This book, while based on true incidents, is not meant to betray medical or professional confidences or to single out any individual or group of individuals for criticism. It is meant only to portray my own experiences. Thus, I have taken the liberty of changing all names and identifying characteristics of people (with the exception of Jan Tobin, Janey Justice, my son, Simon, and me), hospitals, and schools in order to protect the rights of the people I have had as patients, their families, and the professionals I have learned from and worked with. In some cases, the people in this book are composites, and in a few instances the chronology has been altered. Accordingly, except as noted, any resemblance of the characters in this book to actual individuals is unintended and purely coincidental.

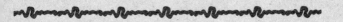

PROLOGUE

THE LARGE INSTITUTIONAL CLOCK read 2:50 P.M., and somewhere in the middle of the eight flights of stairs, I wondered what I would have to do for the next nine hours of my life.

What would they need? Would it be simply a matter of controlling the pain with a little morphine and oxygen, or would I constantly be on the run, checking vital signs every five minutes, suctioning secretions to keep an airway clear, calculating drug dosages, calibrating machines, and listening to my sixth sense—all while keeping one step ahead. And, of course, a portion of my attention was reserved for the one fear that loomed larger than the rest, the one always present: Would I make a fatal mistake?

I reached the last step and had to juggle my brown paper lunch bag, oversized purse, and umbrella to open the door to the green waiting room. As I walked under the ACUTE CORONARY CARE sign, I noticed a woman with white hair sitting on the couch, crying. A younger woman with red hair leaned over her, touching the woman's shoulder, saying nothing.

It could mean something critical; it could be overreaction. But there wasn't the usual hysteria that came with overreaction. This was the kind of sorrow and fear that came from something tragic.

I opened the door leading into the world of the four fishbowl rooms, each holding a single blue bed for the critically ill. The monitor banks stood directly in front of me. Only one scope was lighted and running: bed two.

Before taking another step, I named the rhythm and knew

what was wrong with the heart that generated it. Glancing at the assignment board, I saw bed two was mine.

I walked to my locker and took the blue cotton uniform from its hanger. As I slipped it over my head, I noticed an old bloodstain on the waistband that repeated laundering had not removed. I tried to remember the name of the patient who had contributed the small piece of color and felt guilty when I could not.

Next, my badge. I pinned the insignia of authority on the left shoulder seam of my uniform. RN, MICN, CCU, ER: Registered Nurse, Mobile Intensive Care Nurse, Coronary Care Unit, Emergency Room. How many years of school and hard work did those initials stand for? Ten?

Lacing the white shoes, I allowed my mind to drift toward work. Bed two. How old? Man? Woman? How bad was it? The grieving white-haired woman in a green waiting room hinted at the answer.

Glancing at myself in the mirror, I hastily repinned several wild strands of my chestnut hair back into the knot at the top of my head and picked up my tools: stethoscope, packaged ointments, germ-killing swabs, and blunted bandage scissors. I was ready to face the evening.

The familiar subtle thrill began to well up inside me as I walked to the nurse's station. I compared the feeling to what it must be like walking on stage. Even though I had memorized my lines for the scene, no one ever really knew what was going to happen.

The report from Kelly, the on-duty nurse, was tedious and uninformative. That was unusual. Kelly was one of the coronary unit's better nurses, but tonight she lacked her normal enthusiastic energy.

"The patient is a sixty-eight-year-old male, admitted in the wee hours this morning. The diagnosis: possible cerebral hemorrhage. He had a head scan this morning, and I haven't heard results as yet," said Kelly. She sighed and leaned forward. "I just couldn't get into doing the job today, I'm sorry. I didn't bathe him, and I turned him only a few times and . . ." She took in a deep breath, then hunched her shoulders even more. Exhaling, she looked directly at me. "Jesus, it just seems so pointless. I don't like taking care of corpses. I just want to get out of here and go home to my kids."

I wrote down the clinical information about the patient

without changing my expression or responding to Kelly's comment. We all knew the feeling of being forced to keep a patient alive long after it was determined the situation was hopeless. It was a futile battle that was more emotionally draining than almost any other nursing situation.

After arranging the facts by body systems, I looked them over once again and walked quietly into the glass-walled acute care room.

The rhythm of the respirator was in tune with the continuous hum of the building. The man's arms and legs were twitching, disturbing the plastic tubes that lay twisted across his naked chest and thighs.

I came close to the bed, which was cranked to the level of my waist, and looked at him carefully. With his slightly overweight, large-boned body, he filled the bed head to foot. A mist of sweat covered his balding head, and his skin was that particular gray color I knew well. The once-white adhesive tape, tightly wrapped in a thin strip around his mouth and cheeks, held a red-striped tube that invaded his airway and carried the warmed, moistened air from the respirator into his lungs.

I crossed the room again and pulled the solid blue curtain all the way around the glass, blocking the view of outsiders interested in watching.

Where to start? The mechanical assessment of the man's body was so like taking apart a dysfunctioning engine piece by piece. Neurological: focal seizures; all signs absent; no reflexes, no responses—no one home. Kelly had termed it "vegetable soufflé." Cardiovascular: heart rate, 150; blood pressure, 80 palpable. Skin: cool, wet, and mottled. Color: bluish gray, dusky. Drugs: procainamide, dopamine, and lidocaine. Pushed through his veins by more pieces of mechanical apparatus, they did their job to keep his heart pumping smoothly.

I replayed Kelly's report in my head. He had been alive and laughing yesterday. There had been a special gathering of the family to honor him: Grandpa, Dad. I could see images of the silly predinner joking and the fumbling backyard football, then the after-dinner Grandpa stories he told, keeping the younger children entranced. It all had taken place fewer than twenty-four hours ago.

I saw the small, dried crystals of blood clinging to his

nostril hairs and pictured the paramedics, their adrenaline running rampant, trying to push the tubes in without success. The man's broken ribs gave evidence of the prolonged cardiopulmonary resuscitation; so much effort without reward.

Spontaneously the seizures stopped, and I allowed the family in to be with him, one at a time.

His sister walked in first. Like him, she was large-boned. Seeing him, she made a half-waving sort of movement with her hand and laughed lightly while tears fell on her brother's arm. She stared at the place they had fallen but made no attempt to wipe them away. Without looking into his face, she shook her head and said in a very low voice, "Oh, Colonel, Colonel, good-bye now, dear, bye-bye."

She noticed me moving about on the other side of the bed and started to explain. "I called him Colonel all his life. He liked it. It was his nickname."

The woman stole a quick glance at her brother's face and walked away from the bed as if to leave. With a jerky motion she turned back and started to say something to him, but her mouth moved without the sounds. Putting her hand to her lips, she backed out of the room, still speaking silent words to her brother.

I stood motionless until I heard the waiting room door shut. Coming close to him again, I put my hand on his and held it. It was moist and warm. With the digital thermometer I quickly took his temperature; the bright red numbers stopped at 105.2. From my training I recalled having read somewhere: "Anything over 105 is incompatible with life." Incompatible with life. Simple. To the point.

Ten minutes later a grandchild, a thin boy in his late teens, walked stiffly into the room. He stared straight ahead as if prepared to fight the enemy which held his grandfather. The boy reached out to touch the older man's face and caught himself. He would not make this real. This was his grandfather, a man he had loved all his life. He would not give him up to the world of these ugly tubes and sterile smells. His grandpa was the smell of pipe tobacco and apples. He was the tall, balding man always telling stories. Gramps was the wisest man he'd ever known; he would not let him go.

Suddenly his shoulders began to shake, and his angular face distorted with the shape of his pain. He turned away quickly and left the room without saying a word or making any sound.

I went to the bed again and looked at the man's face. As I leaned close to him, my hand moved to his forehead and slowly wiped away the sweat. I pulled the bloody tape away from his upper lip and was surprised to see the full white mustache. For a time I looked carefully at his face and decided it was a kind one.

Pulling back the lids of his eyes, I found large and unresponsive pupils surrounded by a ring of light blue. I moved close to his ear and whispered. "Colonel, I'm here, do you know that? I am right here."

Down at the end of the bed I massaged his purple feet as they lay still and ice-cold. I thought about his life, his work, and wondered if he'd ever gone fishing. "What kind of man were you really?" I asked aloud. While listening to the answers of silence, I noticed the monitor: heart rate 70; blood pressure 74. He was slowing down despite the drugs.

Twenty minutes passed, and the soft, whooshing noise from the respirator lulled me into a kind of trance as I did my charting and prepared the paper work. A male voice startled me. Looking up, I saw a tall man with a middle-aged woman standing close to him. They looked worried and anxious.

"How's he doing?" the man asked, hope hanging on every word of the question.

"Not well," I answered. "He's very critical at this point."

The woman moved toward me slightly, wringing her hands. "Do you think he'll pull out of this? We've been his friends for so long. How long will he be in the hospital?"

I paused, staring directly at the woman. "He's not going to make it. His body is dying now . . . as we speak."

The man stepped toward me with a look that said he did not believe me; he wanted to bargain. "Look, if we go to San Francisco and hire the best specialists, that would help, wouldn't it?"

I stood up and approached them. "No. His brain is dead. He, the man, the person, really died last night; only his heart is beating and a machine is breathing for him. Not much else is functioning."

Both the man and the woman looked away from me, but not at each other. For a second I was afraid I'd said too much, too bluntly.

After a moment the man said, "Oh, dear God, I feel so bad." His eyes filled with tears, and the woman put her hand on his arm without looking at his face.

"He was very special, wasn't he?" I asked quietly.

There was a brief silence. Then the tall man answered me in a torrent of words that gained momentum as he spoke. "He was a wonderful man, the best of men. So intelligent, and boy, talk about a sense of humor!" The man threw his head back and laughed at the ceiling, though tears still dripped from his face. "He made everyone laugh. He tried to teach people how to feel good about their lives. He was a professor at Stanford, you know—very quick mind and yet always so gentle." He paused, then: "Special? Yes, he was definitely special."

The woman spoke up with a shaking voice. "Thank you, thank you so much for telling us the truth."

A lump came to my throat, and I could only respond with a smile. And with that they left me alone with my patient.

The thermometer now read less than 98.8 degrees. I felt the clamminess of his skin and had a half-formed thought of primitive things from the sea. I shuddered and walked to the outer door. Through the waiting room window I saw the white-haired woman still sitting on the couch. I opened the door and asked her to come in. It was her time with him.

She approached the bed very slowly, then touched his face and kissed him. "Papa? Papa, I love you so much. I always have, darling. Don't forget I love you so. I love you."

I pretended to rearrange the plastic tubes and gray monitor leads that were no longer of use. I was torn between curiosity and feeling intrusive, witnessing the years of love.

"During the night," the white-haired woman said, not taking her eyes off her husband, "he woke up several times, you know, the way we older people do, but the last time, when he walked back toward the bed, he called my name out. Just once. He looked so strange, lost really. Then he fell down, and I didn't know what to do. I was scared, and he wouldn't answer me, so I just kept talking to him, holding him, but he didn't say another word."

His wife opened her purse and took out an embroidered pink handkerchief and wet a tip of it with her saliva. With that she wiped away a smear of orange germicide from his chin. She picked up his cool, limp hand and put it softly to her cheek. "We were married forty-two years and loved each other every single day. He was my gift from God."

She stared down at him and kissed the palm of his hand. "I love you, my darling. Good-bye for now."

She put his hand down, closed her purse, and walked out of the room without saying another word. Forty-two years of loving, and in one instant it was history.

Thirty minutes later, as I was turning him onto his side, I felt another presence in the room. Looking up, I saw Dr. Skinner staring at us from the door.

"The head scan showed massive hemorrhage. The largest I've ever seen. Stop all the drugs. The family wants it that way."

"Okay," I said, but didn't move toward the intravenous lines. He felt like an intruder, and I wanted him to leave.

After a second he said, "He was dead before he even hit the floor." It was his explanation, his excuse. He shrugged and walked away.

Carefully letting down the side rails, I gently put my hands under the Colonel's shoulders and spoke to him in a slow, measured whisper.

"Did you feel all this love here today? You can leave this behind you now. It's all right, I promise."

My face touched his. "I'll stay with you. I'll be right here."

A soft buzzing drifted through the room, demanding attention, as a small red light flashed in harmony to the sound. Blood pressure 40, heart rate 32. I squeezed his hands and felt a pressure rise in my throat. The blurring image of his face was changed and molded through my tears.

I turned to the pole holding the blue intravenous fluid, the one that kept his blood pressure up, and turned the plastic stopcock to the "off" position; then the yellow fluid, the one that kept his heart beating smoothly . . . off.

"All the pain is over for you now. Let it go. Let go."

His skin was almost white, and the ring of blue surrounding his pupils had disappeared, leaving only the gray-black window open to finality.

Again the monitor flashed and buzzed as the agonal rhythm, the rhythm of death, slowly snaked its way across the screen . . . right to left. Blood pressure . . . zero.

The respirator seemed suddenly loud and obnoxious, diminishing the dignity of death. With one smooth, swift movement, I pulled the plug from the wall, creating silence.

For just a second his spirit and mine lived in that silence together. For just one moment I knew all the warmth and joy his spirit had ever given.

I removed all the tubes and tape from his body and washed him with the warm, soapy water reserved for the living. And as I bathed him, I softly hummed a lullaby, covered him with a clean, soft blanket, and said, "Good-bye, Colonel."

Just after midnight I walked through the empty waiting room, feeling drained. Yet, as I descended the eight flights of stairs and walked out of the hospital into the crisp night air, I carried something with me. He had never spoken to me, there had been no gestures, I'd won no visible battles; but I had touched him, and his spirit . . . lingered.

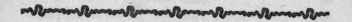

ONE

HALF-ASLEEP, MY CHEEKS still bearing patterns of pillow wrinkles, I walked behind my father and listened to the holes our footsteps made in the early-morning silence. Icy air bit the insides of our noses as we headed toward the forest which bordered our small provincial town. I could have traveled the route blind: two hundred steps down Wyman Street, turn right onto Riverside Avenue for a count of 231, blink twenty-six times after the big oak, and then to Schermerhorn Avenue, where the old railroad tracks showed through worn spots in the blacktop. On a count of three telephone poles after the tracks, we were almost there.

In the beginning it was only for the sheer joy of being with my father that I accompanied him to his target practice: the object of these rare predawn journeys. The first time I was allowed to hold the rifle, my father told me, tongue in cheek, to shoot in the general direction of the targets some sixty feet away. I mimicked everything I'd seen him do: feet wide apart, hold steady, squint one eye, concentrate on the tin cans with the bright red tomatoes painted on them, and slowly, carefully squeeze the trigger. As the can to the left flew wildly into the air, I made the can to the right disappear before the first one hit the ground. My father had me repeat the feat eight times in a row before he allowed himself to believe his eyes. From that day forward I was known in the family circle as "Tin Can Oakley," a name I grew to despise long before I was nine.

Hanging from my father's shoulder, the black rod of the

9

.22 swung slightly to the left, then back to the right with his every step. Trying to stay awake, I turned my gaze toward the sky. Birds perched on the telephone lines, looking for all the world like black notes in a bar of music. As they fluttered from one line to another, the tune constantly changed, like living sheets of music. Humming what I read, I distinctly heard the first few bars of "Mr. Sandman."

As we turned onto a dirt path, the clean, wet smell of the river came up strong. One hundred steps more, and the path first headed toward the water, then curved left into the woods.

When we entered the mass of white pines, I'd already set my mind on trying something difficult. The challenge of a live, moving target thrilled me. I had watched enough Saturday morning television to know how easy it was for the cowboys and Indians. Certainly there would be nothing to it.

And there wasn't.

The gray morning sky, the top of a white pine, and a small brown bird in flight were the only things I saw before I squeezed the trigger.

The bird cried out in surprise and fell, wings fluttering, toward the ground. Its body took forever to hit, as if it had sailed down rather than plummeted.

I ran to find my fallen target, glorious triumph pulsing through me until I reached the spot where the convulsing bird lay. Bewildered, I watched the trembling creature for a moment.

Sudden panic made my temples burn. Feeling a wild urge to do something, anything to make it stop shaking, I took the body in my hand, drew it close to my mouth, and blew puffs of air over its beak, while my fingers searched for the wound.

Warm, sticky blood oozed from a small spot under the right wing. I pressed my little finger over the hole and gently stroked the bird's head; it was like touching soft air.

In a second or two the fluttering lessened and finally stopped altogether. I felt for the vibrations of the tiny heart, but there was nothing. A strange, all-encompassing panic rose inside me and was more frightening than anything I'd ever experienced.

I had caused the death of a creature that coasted through clouds and sang exquisite songs on backyard fences. Surely I had done something which changed the world for the worse. From my guilt, the new importance I now gave to every living thing became a looming phantom shadow at my back. For this act of killing, I was certain I would die.

Whimpering, I grabbed for my father's waist and held on for dear life. "I hurt the bird, Dad. I killed it. Now he'll never fly again, and he can't go home. Oh, Daddy, help me."

As I pushed my face into the leather jacket that smelled of cedar, my head began to shake with the effort of holding back the sobs.

My father put his hands under my armpits and hoisted me up to his shoulder, where he stroked my hair, barely touching it, and whispered. "Ah, my, there's a girl, don't cry now, it's all right."

I took his giant hand in mine and studied it for the thousandth time; every one of his fingers had been broken at one point or another. Gnarled and bent, they reminded me of the witch's hands in my *Grimm's Fairy Tales.*

I shivered. The thought brought up the detailed drawings of the witch who killed and ate little children. Wasn't I just as ugly and bad as that very same witch?

My father spoke again, and the deep, raspy voice sent vibrations through my chest, calming me.

"Listen, Dolly," he said, using the nickname for the times I got a case of what he called the "sensitives." "I know how you feel. I felt that way once a long time ago, too. Remember I told you how I shot the poor rabbit? I—"

I interrupted, knowing by heart the story of his first hunting experience. But I also knew that as one of a family of ten he had been expected to put food on the table.

"But you were poor and had to eat the animals you killed. We aren't going to eat the birdie. I was just playing."

The thought of eating the small creature or any creature turned my stomach. I now pictured in cute, full-color Walt Disney animation every chicken, cow, deer, and fish ever killed for my stomach's benefit. A new wave of hard tears flooded out.

"It's all right, Dolly," my father said, stroking the back of my head. "It will pass."

After a few moments my after-a-hard-cry gasps subsided, and I remained in quiet, motionless limbo until the insistent chirping of a bird overhead cut through the void. "Look! Look!" I shouted, jumping out of my father's arms. "It's the mother bird looking for her little baby bird."

The added guilt and sorrow of the other bird's presence were more than I could stand. There was no question of what I had to do. Either I absolved myself of my crime right then, or I would surely die on the spot.

With my hands clenched and my feet spread apart in a stance that felt as if I were preparing to take on the world in some momentous fight, I lifted my face toward heaven and yelled into the sky, "I swear to God I will never, ever hurt or kill another living thing for the rest of my whole life."

The statement properly directed toward heaven, I felt I had righted myself with the living and the dead; I was absolved, and it was time to move on quickly before anyone changed his mind.

I turned to my father dry-eyed. "Let's bury him right here so his mom can come and visit him whenever she wants. Okay, Dad?"

My father's eyes filled with tears, and he pulled me close to him. Looking out from the nest his arms created, I stared at a single stream of sun that tinted the air with gold. Tiny rainbow circles swirled in the tears that still clung to my eyelashes. In place of the panic, a warm, peaceful feeling now lulled me.

Something important had happened. In the magic of a child's intuition, I was vaguely aware of a change.

The change was, I believe now, the beginning of a knowing of the heart. From that day of the bird, I began to watch carefully for the deep wounds that others hid but always carried with them. The more I saw, the faster came compassion, the tool of insight until my path was made perfectly clear. From the start there was no other choice; my purpose was to touch the wounds of others and then to heal.

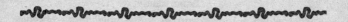

TWO

THE MAILMAN WAS MAKING his delivery just two houses away. When he got to my house, he would hand me an envelope which contained the blueprint for the rest of my life. I had been waiting for him since eight; the mail was always delivered at one.

Sitting on the front porch of my ninety-year-old wooden cottage, I played with my three-and-a-half-year-old son, Simon, teased our two altered cats, Emelio and Mooshie, swept the leaves from the steps, and contemplated the little house we'd been living in for three years.

Painted flamingo pink, a color Simon accurately described as "pukey," the inside of the cottage had a very different feeling from the 1936 Miami retirement center look of the outside. With its white wicker walls and brick fireplace complete with old-fashioned mantel, it was more New England than West Coast; that and the fact that the rent was insanely reasonable were the main reasons I had taken it at first sight, no questions asked.

It didn't matter that in the winter it was drafty and damp; that's what the fireplace was for. It didn't matter that the rats from the creek made their winter home in my kitchen cabinets; that's what the cats were for. As for the black widow spiders that hung around the woodpile in the backyard and the rumors that the front bedroom was haunted, I hadn't found good rationalizations yet, but I was working on them.

Built on a creek in the middle of town, the house was a fair distance back from the main street, but not so far away

13

that I couldn't see my neighbors and definitely not so far that I didn't know a block ahead of time when the mailman was coming.

I made note that the mailman had made it to the house next door and was now involved in a chatty conversation with my neighbor. They stood there discussing the town's sewer problems and the potholes which were slowly replacing the streets, while I sat on the porch, hyperventilating. Potholes and rainy-season flooding were a way of life in this little town; why did they have to pick today to research the complexities and possibilities of changing the situation? Obviously they had chosen today because they knew that for the first time in twenty-eight years I was desperate to get my mail. Why else?

Suddenly I was struck by the thought that the envelope I was obsessed with getting might not be in the day's mail. No, I knew that wasn't true because two days ago I personally had helped the Buchanan nursing department secretary put the 354 envelopes in the mailbag. Besides the small income, this was the main bonus in working as receptionist-typist in the student first-aid center; it was run by the nursing department. All the inside poop of the nursing program was bantered about right before my very ears.

Only three days ago the program secretary had asked if I wouldn't mind affixing 354 envelopes with 354 address labels that were hot off the computer printer. I affixed, perfectly aligning the little rectangular stick-on labels with the perimeters of the envelopes, knowing full well that only sixty of them would hold acceptance letters. The other 294 would hold letters that had words like "regretfully," "too bad," "tough luck," and "try again next year."

I recognized a few of the names on the labels, and my stomach ached for their owners. After three years in a row they might still be turned down. I didn't have three years to wait. My financial situation, which was on the extreme end of grim, dictated either I got in on my first application or I went back to being a legal secretary. The rather generous nursing student loan had only one string attached: You had to be a nursing student. That, plus help from the CETA program, would get me through with a little squeeze on an already tight budget. My ex-husband, Patrick, was struggling in the overflooded lawyer market, but he'd pledged to help out when he could.

The 107th label was mine. Letting it stick to the end of my index finger, I stared at it proudly until, one by one, all the horror stories I'd heard about first-time applicants crept in and bit my confidence causing it to wither up and die in front of me. "Only one-in-a-million chance," the rumor went, "of getting in on your first try, and, jeez, wasn't there one girl from Southern California who had applied seven times and was still waiting?"

I stuck the label on with two sets of crossed fingers, made the sign of the cross, sang a good-luck chant to Buddha, kissed all four corners of the envelope, and repeated the same prayer I had said over the mailbox when I sent off the application.

The crunching of dirt under leather soles brought me back to the painful realities of my present anxiety crisis. Jesus, Mary, 'n' Joseph, the mailman was walking down the driveway right toward me, smiling. How could the man be smiling? Did he know something I didn't?

He calmly handed me not one but two envelopes. My mouth was so dry I couldn't even say thank you, although I did manage to hyperventilate with a little more volume. He looked back over his shoulder only twice.

The envelopes both were from Buchanan College. My God, I thought, had they sent out an acceptance letter, then changed their minds? Did it have anything to do with the way I had put on the labels?

I sat down at my desk, twiddled with the letter opener, and found I just didn't have the guts to open the envelopes. I left them on my desk and put Simon down for his nap.

When I was finished, I sat down at my desk and stared at the envelopes carefully for a long time, as if I expected to receive the message through telepathy, then picked up the phone and dialed Janey's number.

"Hi. Did you open yours yet?" I asked before she even said hello.

She laughed one of her special laughs in reply. Janey was the owner of a laugh that made any problem seem ridiculous. The first time I heard it was the day we met, and despite the circumstances, it hooked me. I knew I had to get to know the person who could have a laughing fit while crunched under the chemistry lab counter waiting for someone's mistake to explode.

From the time the alarm sounded until the flying glass settled, I found out she was in my age bracket, was also raising a son the same age as Simon all by herself, and was waiting, too, to get into the nursing program, the only difference being this was her third try.

"I haven't checked my mail yet," she said calmly. "How about you?"

"For chrissake, Jane, how can you not be checking your mail? I've been waiting all morning."

"I'm used to this, remember? I take it you haven't opened your envelope yet." Janey clucked her tongue. "You're weird, Heron. You're probably sitting there staring at it unopened while we speak, Right?"

"Half-right. I'm staring at two envelopes, both from the college, and I haven't opened either one because I'm scared shitless. This is my life we're flippantly tossing around here, Jane."

"Look, I'll tell you what; why don't I go get my mail and we'll open them together over the phone? That way we can act as substitute suicide prevention volunteers for each other if we have to."

Janey, besides having a sense of humor, had the other essential ingredient for becoming a great nurse: basic common sense.

I waited until I heard the distant squeak of her mailbox to slit open the envelope with the crooked label. Peeking at the letterhead, I knew I was safe; it was only from the dean's office.

It was a mimeographed two-liner:

"Congratulations. Because of your academic achievement for this semester, you have been placed on the Honor Roll."

My heart jumped. Wow. The Honor Roll. I checked the name again. It was really mine. I was doing well; I was okay.

I wondered if my mother was turning in her grave; she so hated being wrong. After all, she had prophesied since I was born that I would never be capable of finding the intellectual or moral strength to go beyond the station of cleaning toilets.

For the years I endured her drunken abuse, I'd never been able to break through her icy righteousness, but following a natural course, the rejection turned to anger, and my rebellious side came forth with a strong sense of survival and perseverance. As soon as I was sure my younger siblings could defend themselves, I adopted a fearless wildness and escaped.

Trains running to unknown destinations always had an empty box-car in which to hide, and when my luck with abandoned farmhouses and boats ran out, I imposed on my wealthier friends' families for months before it was noticed I never went home.

Of course, I never really got away. Years later, long after my mother had been dead and buried, I carried on the battle with her loitering ghost. At the age of seventeen I had got as far as receiving a college catalog in the mail when my mother's prophecy loomed menacingly before me, ready to cut me down in a moment if I so much as tried to apply.

For the finishing touch, my high school counselor wisely predicted there would be no need for me ever to consider going to college because my most satisfying role in life (*he* said, patting my exposed knee) would be to put my future husband through school and be a devoted helpmate. It took brains and courage to go out there in the big, terrible world, he said; leave it to the men and stay home.

The confidence I needed to disagree had been shattered, and in the midst of feeling defeated, I was caught by the American June Bride Dream of love and security, manifesting itself in the form of a blue-eyed Irishman named Patrick. The result was to wake up in San Francisco as a full-fledged responsible married woman putting her husband through law school.

My need to learn was wrapped in tissue paper and put out of my reach while I rode the overcrowded number thirty bus posing as a legal secretary in the dry and humorless world of law and order.

Four years later I was still playing the role of a now frankly disillusioned, dissatisfied helpmate when a golden-haired son arrived and inadvertently jarred me into an acute awareness of my situation. The spirit which had been misplaced now clawed to get out. Weighing the pros and cons, I decided to crash the gates and run for the stars.

Patrick and I could no longer ignore the fact that it was time we retired from the stage of our failing marriage, and I packed my belongings in the back of my 1957 Chevy station wagon and moved, lock, stock, and baby, to the "country," just north of San Francisco. Surrounded by redwoods, mountains, and a slower, more peaceful way of life, I took steps to enter college and disprove my mother's toilet cleaner theory once and for all.

But Mother's ghost, still fighting, played back the old tapes about my deep-rooted selfishness and insisted my desire to learn about helping others was just another way to get attention.

That's untrue! I countered. *I'm willing to give up so much to try.*

Laughing, the ghost reminded me again I didn't have the intellectual strength to make it.

But why couldn't I try? I begged, hoping for something positive or even indifferent.

Try? the voice mocked. *How can a worthless idiot have such audacity? Stay in your place.*

Shaking my head, I backed away from the voice. After years of experience I should have known it was useless to argue with ghosts that would always have negative answers.

From the part of myself that reveled in being alive, a command stronger than any programmed shame took hold. I relaxed my white-knuckled grip, drew a deep breath, and jumped.

When I opened my eyes, I was in a world of new realities: enrolled as a student in Buchanan College, matriculated, if you please. True, at twenty-six I was a bit late out of the gate. To the young women I sat among, worries about crow's feet and sagging breasts were as foreign as diaper rash and colic. But conversely, microbiology, chemistry, and grade point averages were, to me, strange and wonderful things.

In just over two years I had taken every course even vaguely related to nursing. On a cold and rainy day, six months ago, I'd walked on legs of Jell-O to the campus mailbox, clutching my application for the college's nursing program. I remembered holding it over the slot and trying to swallow, though not one drop of saliva remained in the bed of cotton once known as my mouth.

Look, you guys up there, I prayed with a bargaining edge to my voice, *or whoever is in charge of this craziness down here, puleeezzzz, you've got to help me make it through. Let me learn how to help, and I won't let you down.*

I looked at the envelope lying in front of me. Inside was my answer.

"Hey! You there? Turkey head, I'm back." Janey's voice broke through. "Put aside the cyanide pills, and let's take a peek. Are you strong enough?"

"Ummm, yup," I answered, totally unsure.

"Ready?"

"Ready."

"Begin at the left corner and slit to the right corner at the count of three."

We both slit at the same time.

"Okay, crew, now pull out the letter and unfold it without looking at it," she continued, still calm.

My hands shook as I removed the paper and smoothed it out face down on the desk.

"Jane?" I said in a shaking voice.

"Yes?"

"Jane, are you ready to look?"

"Yes."

"On the count of three?"

"No!" Jane screamed.

"Why not?"

"Use four; it's my lucky number."

"Okay, Jane, four then."

Pause.

"One, two, three, four, LOOK!"

I think we both must have read the first six words at the same rate because we both screamed at exactly the same time.

"We are pleased to inform you . . ."—the most incredible, wonderful words in the entire language.

"Oh, my God, Janey, we did it!" I said, laughing and crying at the same time.

Janey screamed again. "We really did, didn't we? Does this mean a bottle of champagne?"

"This, my dear old girl, means two bottles of champagne, and I'm on my way to your house right now."

I hung up and danced until, on a particularly wild twirl, I landed in front of a wide-eyed, confused Simon.

"Is it time for French toast, Mama?"

I bent over and swept him off his feet. "Yes, sweetie, it's time for French toast and a new life for you and me."

"With honey on top?" he asked, his dimples getting deeper as he tried to match the width of his mother's smile.

"Yessiree . . . the sweetest honey in the world."

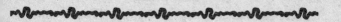

THREE

BY ANYONE'S STANDARDS first-year nursing school was a shock not only to the body but to the well-being of the mind.

Before two weeks had passed, I was convinced nursing school was a young woman's game; it wasn't meant for anyone over the age of twenty and certainly not for any person who enjoyed sleeping once in a while. How could there be time for sleep? Every week we were assigned several patient cases, each one requiring hours of research in order to come up with a flawless plan for nursing and medical care.

And then, if nursing care plans didn't occupy enough of our day and night, there was always studying to be done for the weekly test given every Friday afternoon, or we could always improve our charting skills by composing two to three pages of detailed descriptions of the bodily and mental functions of an imaginary patient.

There were major changes in life-styles, too. For example, the women who were divorced and had families to care for had daily nervous breakdowns in the closet. Our children rarely saw us (Mommy? Mommy who?), and friends and relatives eventually gave us up for missing in action or dead.

If we played with the idea of taking a day off for ourselves, there was always the cattle-prod thought that if we failed one test, or missed a clinical day at the hospital, or didn't hand in one care plan, we were out of the program with no chance

21

for readmission; there wasn't one of us who was willing to chance that.

Social life? Not that I personally had had any to begin with.

Since my divorce my time had been thinly spread among school, raising Simon, and a part-time job. Talking to myself and sleeping alone on the right side of my double bed had become a way of life. It wasn't too bad actually. There was always fascinating conversation and plenty of leg room.

Now even that part of my life was threatened; a growing stack of nursing textbooks began taking up more and more room on the left side of my bed, and I was being crowded out altogether. But it wasn't the crowding that was the main problem; the books, heavier than I, constantly caused me to roll toward the left. My nights were spent being poked in the eye by the corner of my nursing care plan book or being marked up by the assortment of pens I'd stuck between pages to keep my place. I'd wake up in the morning with major works of abstract art on my face.

At 5:00 A.M. poor Simon (most people thought Poor Simon was his real name because I was always referring to him by it, as in "Poor Simon did this" or "Poor Simon said . . .") was toted off to a baby-sitter who was kindhearted or crazy enough to take him in at that hour, then drive him to the campus nursery school when it opened at 7:00.

Dutifully carrying the little Spiderman duffel bag which contained a small bag of snacks and a change of clothes, he never complained. At times he actually seemed to like the idea of both of us going to "big people's school" at the same time.

When I picked him up from nursery school on clinical days, he'd throw open my cape so the kids could stare in amazed wonder and fear at my uniform and stethoscope. Beaming with pride, he'd climb up onto my hip and shout, "My mama's gonna be a nurse who doesn't give shots!"

This hazel-eyed midget was my first line of support. Not that Simon was always the perfectly behaved child, especially when he fell into one of his angry, stubborn moods, but somehow, he understood the enormousness of what I'd undertaken and pitched in whenever he could. If I'd dozed off over my books, he'd wake me with slobbery kisses on my nose, or if making dinner had slipped my mind, he'd bring me a carrot on a plate, complete with knife and fork.

Once a week his quiet home was invaded by the ten members of his mother's study group. Any other child might have been put off by the inconvenience of a gaggle of giggling, hysterical women all talking at once, passing him from one set of arms to another, fussing and cooing over his curls, but not Simon. Simon, I think, viewed those times as the "Anything Goes" years.

During the week, preparing and eating meals became such a major time problem that I finally settled for eating only self-packaged foods. Fast and simple, bananas, hard-boiled eggs, nuts, celery, and carrots could be stored in my purse or uniform pocket for a snack on the run. I'd always been thin; now I was trying for invisibility. Fortunately Simon was not a fussy eater since the baby-sitter provided breakfast, the nursery school, a hot lunch, and at dinner he was usually faced with a salad and soup made from last week's leftover vegetables.

Clothes? No problem there. Our uniforms were nondescript blue and white pin-striped sacks with large pockets to be worn with white stockings. All of us were convinced our school caps were someone's idea of a sick joke. They were cut to resemble the Golden Gate Bridge towers with the bay waters flowing underneath, and wearing one was like sporting a large but decorative white cardboard box. When the caps weren't getting caught in the IV tubing, they were being knocked off by bedside monitors or curtain rods, you name it. They were the bane of our clinical existence.

Dressing up in the few free hours we had outside the hospital or class was also easily accomplished; a simple bathrobe did nicely.

All in all, even with the hardships it imposed, the Buchanan nursing program had the reputation of being the best in Northern California. It'd come up with a way to jam four years' worth of information and experience into the space of two. The first year we learned the foundations of nursing and touched on all the body systems and their malfunctions and diseases, all the while getting a good dose of actual patient contact. In the second year our studies were to involve a more sophisticated level of medical knowledge and responsibility, but at this point in the first year, most of us couldn't allow ourselves even to have nightmares about that.

Buchanan's system of student rotation was extremely efficient. The class was first divided into four groups. Each group was assigned a different instructor with a different area of expertise. Each instructor was given privileges in a specific hospital where she could train us two days a week for two months. Then the groups rotated instructors, and we went into not only a new hospital but a new area of study as well.

As if we weren't scared enough, just before every rotation the groups tortured one another by spreading horror stories about the instructor they were currently studying under: "Have you had so-and-so yet? Next rotation? Well, if I were you, I'd worry. I have her now, and she is definitely the toughest. . . ."

Of the four first-year instructors, Karen, our neurology-physiology instructor, was, at thirty-five, the youngest. She held a master's in nursing education, was insanely witty, extremely bright, and, with an iron fist, demanded absolute perfection from her students. The best thing about going through her rotation was that somehow she managed to keep us laughing through our performance anxiety in the hospital and class—right up to the time we sat down to take our tests. The laughter would die immediately after we'd read the first essay question.

Victoria was our fifty-three-year-old Jill of All Trades instructor. Extremely adept in all fields of nursing but master of none, the tall, aloof brunette looked more like an older, sophisticated fashion model than a first-year instructor. She was meticulously groomed and expensively dressed, with every dyed hair always in place and every exquisite outfit tastefully complemented by matching accessories.

We found out through the greased grapevine of gossip that she was married to a millionaire, though none of us could ever figure out why she chose the stress of working in a nursing school, let alone work at all.

She never laughed and rarely smiled; Victoria was one of those people who seemed to exude unhappiness. But unlike most chronically unhappy people, she appeared to live in her melancholy state as comfortably as a blind man living in a house where he has memorized every inch.

Although she never crossed me personally, Victoria was responsible for the dismissal of eight students before the end of the year. It was with good reason we were terrified of her.

Burl, on the other hand, was so full of life and a sense of joy, anyone could have guessed her field was obstetrics and pediatrics just by looking at her. A solidly built white-haired grandmother, Burl was a retired army nurse who had single-handedly delivered enough babies from China to Kansas City to set a world record. The only thorn in Burl's side, other than a bad case of asthma, was a forced retirement staring at her from just around the corner. For Burl, that was like facing a firing squad. Her eyesight was going, it was true, and she was increasingly forgetful, but God, what a teacher!

Repeatedly she broke the rules for the sake of showing us a procedure or getting assignments for us she thought might be of value. She was frequently in trouble with the doctors for overstepping her bounds, but at the end of her rotation there were not many of us who couldn't have delivered a baby on the back of a galloping horse in a rainstorm.

Pearson, our general medical-surgical instructor, didn't appear, as far as we could tell, to have any personality at all. I couldn't say she was shy or aggressive, happy or unhappy. She had no opinions of her own, wasn't very animated, and was, well, like white bread pudding without the sugar. A dull woman at best.

Probably the most interesting thing about her was the fact that she was married to a man who could have passed for her twin brother. They had the same facial features, the same mousy brown hair, the same inane haircut, the same tall, macrobiotic-diet frame, and the same nonpersonality personality.

Janey and I guessed their home was done in dustless gray and hospital green. They probably had a coupon-organizing file and his and hers fruitwood clothes valets at the ends of their twin beds, which were pushed together. Since Pearson seemed totally devoid of any sexuality, we also came to the conclusion they both had been neutered.

Our laboratory workshops, study topics, and hospital assignments all were designed to complement one another. The first thing we learned, for instance, was how to reduce stress through therapeutic communication. That alone should have been a tip-off to what the rest of the year would be like.

On Friday we were given a study guide with the course objectives and a list of chapters and articles to read on the subject of how people, under the stress of injury or illness, react to the world and how the health professional can get them to communicate their feelings.

On Monday we met in the clinical laboratory, a converted classroom set up to look exactly like a hospital room, complete with a silicone dummy patient known as Catheter Cathy. Here, draped over chairs or lying about on the floor, we had a lecture and group discussion with our instructor. We reviewed the principles and reasons behind everything we did as nurses. For as long as I live, I will never forget principle one: "All communication begins with self."

Thus, after learning that knowing oneself takes a lifetime or two, we were free to move on to principle number two: "Injured or sick people have a greater need to communicate, for they fear they have lost control over their bodies and their surroundings." From this we were supposed to gather that the nurse is there to listen and guide these sick and injured back to their own power.

These first two principles were followed by hundreds more, each one forming the foundation of what we were all about. They were generally pretty interesting and, at times, right on the mark, but the rules we had to follow as nursing students sounded as if they were straight out of the book Florence Nightingale had written.

Designed to give the young student a strict, idealistic view of the way nurses *should* function, these antiquated rules were the cause of much wasted time and a lot of frustration. One rule that never made any sense to me stated we were not to write down any information in front of the patient. Supposedly it would diminish the patient's confidence in us. Therefore, we had to remember the entire physical assessment, including vital signs, lung sounds, heart sounds, etc., until we left the bedside.

I never did get the knack of remembering everything and would excuse myself every few minutes to go outside the room and write down notes on a scratch pad I'd hidden in my pocket. From some of the looks I got, I'm sure most of the patients must have thought I either was nuts or had a nasty case of the runs.

On Tuesday we returned to the lab to review problems we might run into and how to solve them: "Mr. Jones has had a heart attack and is afraid of becoming a cardiac invalid. When you enter the room to give him his bed bath, he picks up a vase of flowers and hurls it at you. What will you say?"

After discussion we broke up into pairs or small groups and practiced on each other what we'd learned about therapeutic communication. "So, ever since I got into this program, I've had nightmares that I've just been admitted to a padded cell in the psych unit and Pearson is my roommate. . . ."

On Wednesday and Thursday we went into the hospital and practiced on real, live sick people: "Yes, I know it's only seven A.M., Mrs. Celinski, but I thought you might like to tell me how you really feel about the recent loss of your gall bladder." Or: "Mr. Pappas, I see you've ripped out your IV and are packing your suitcase. Tell me, are you unhappy about being in the hospital?"

We sat next to the beds, wearing saintly expressions, and touched arms or gave bed baths while nodding our heads at the appropriate places and saying, "Yes, I understand, go on. . . ." This was in accordance with principle fourteen: "Physical touch communicates trust and an openness to listen."

Most of the things we learned usually worked; the patients responded to our gentle urgings by talking on about their secret fears, taking us into their lives like best friends, the way strangers stranded together in a bad situation often do. We weren't allowed to give advice or personal opinions, of course, for to say something like "I think your doctor is a jerk, Mrs. Way, and if I were you, I'd get rid of him before he kills you" erased all professionalism and the patients might withdraw their trust. But we did learn how to talk them through their various fears and help them make their own decisions.

At the end of the clinical day we met in an empty room to share and discuss our experiences. For every one experience

I shared, I heard fourteen in return. Sometimes funny, sometimes sad, the stories provided learning upon learning. There was rarely a dull moment, especially when our charting was critiqued by the group.

As students we wrote in three pages what it took the normal floor nurse one to three sentences to say. All of us wanted to be perfectly detailed, making sure we'd painted accurate clinical pictures of the patients. Descriptions of moles and corns and the size and placement of certain body parts were always overdone, but there was one from a piece of charting done by Nailbiting P.J. that took the prize.

Nailbiting P.J., the youngest and most anxious member of our group, had a driving desire to be the author of the best charting. In one herculean effort, her descriptive line in the gastrointestinal assessment of a patient read: "Patient passed flatus: two short, one long."

On Friday afternoons we were tested on what we had learned. That was fair, of course, but unbeknownst to us, our class had been chosen to be the guinea pigs for a brand-new format of testing which was, to put it mildly, at the extreme end of the difficult.

Not many weeks passed before the tests proved to be the weak link in the program. Like the other student rules, the one regarding tests was unrealistic and had failed to be updated when the new format was adopted. Once you had failed a test, you were on your way out the door; it didn't matter how good a student you were or how much time you had invested in the program.

The Friday afternoon post-test mass hysteria went on for months until the day when nine people from one group alone failed the same test. "One for all and all for one" was our battle cry as the entire class banded together and stormed into the director's office, demanding a new testing system.

It was hard to argue with an entire class, and the test format was changed to something more reasonable. Besides, the teaching staff could see that at the rate we were going, the graduating class of 1977 would have consisted of nothing more than a lot of bad memories drifting around an empty auditorium.

By the end of the first twelve weeks we'd covered most of the basics, like bed baths, vital signs, and sterile techniques, while becoming acclimated to the many mysterious and fascinating aspects of our new home, the hospital.

After I'd cared for fewer than fifty hospitalized patients, the institution I'd always called the cold white house of death began taking on a new face.

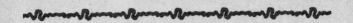

FOUR

I REALLY BEGAN TO GET an idea of what I was heading for during my obstetrics rotation with Burl.

Since Burl never knew whether or not there would be someone in labor when we showed up at the hospital in the morning, she had us write out a care plan based on the typical labor and delivery patient and told us to keep our fingers crossed in hope that someone's child would decide to be born on our obstetrics clinical day.

The night before my OB clinical I concluded that if I were lucky, I'd get a woman who had already vaginally delivered six children and would be doing her nails as she was rolled into the delivery room. If my luck held out, she would be attended by a seasoned OB doc and a labor and delivery nurse who wouldn't mind my breathing over their shoulders and mumbling questions through my mask.

When I arrived at the hospital, Burl's eyelids were twitching under her bifocals as she nervously played with her inhaler. These were bad signs.

"How do you feel today, Heron?" she asked with real purpose.

The twitching eyelids made me nervous. "Uh, fine. Why do you ask?"

She looked around as if she were going to rob a bank and pulled me over to the wall. "I've got a very exciting patient for you today, Heron. She's not really first-year material, but I couldn't pass up the opportunity. You'll learn a lot, and you might not see this again for a long time. Get into a scrub dress, and do a five-minute surgical scrub. I'll meet you outside L&D in ten minutes and tell you all about it.''

I did as I was told and within a few minutes was changed into surgical greens and standing at the scrub sink. Checking the clock, I attacked my right hand with the brush, scrubbing from fingertips to elbow until my skin was the appropriate shade of red.

I couldn't imagine what Burl had signed me up for. Twins or a breech delivery were common enough, and if it was something as strange as the world's first and only transsexual delivery, I doubt I would have been chosen to be in on it. Whatever it was, though, I knew I could throw away my normal labor and delivery care plan.

When I got to L&D, Burl was fairly twittering with excitement.

''I only have a minute to give you the basic scoop on your patient. Two more just went into labor, and another one is getting ready to deliver by C section. I don't know where I'm going to get the students to cover them unless I pull some of them from pediatrics.''

Her wheezing was so loud I could barely concentrate on what she was saying. She must have picked up on my distraction because she pulled the inhaler out of her lab coat, took a hit, and held her breath.

The edges of her lips were perceptibly blue when she exhaled with enough force to knock her off-balance.

''Your little lady is in big trouble,'' she gasped. ''Her name is Marie Hartley, she's twenty-six years old, this is her first baby, and she's severely preeclamptic.'' Burl lowered her voice and, with a furtive air, leaned close to me. I could smell the medication from the inhaler on her breath.

''Between you, me, and the IV pole, she's been badly mismanaged by some doctor I never heard of. He saw her in his office two days ago and told her to go easier on the salt, nothing else. Her body looks like a water balloon ready to burst, and her blood pressure was one-seventy over one-ten when she first came in.

''She told the nurse here that she's been eating only French bread, cold cuts, and canned soups for the last month because her headaches have been so severe; they were all she could keep down. She says she never received any kind of prenatal diet to follow, and her blood pressure, which has always run a little on the high side, wasn't checked at the last two office visits because the office nurse was too busy.''

Burl narrowed her eyes. "All the classic signs staring him in the face, and he never picked up on it. Can you believe that?''

My infatuation with the medical profession had not blinded me to some of the stupidity and sloppiness I'd already seen, and a flash of anger stung the pit of my stomach.

Preeclampsia wasn't a minor disorder; it was a killer disease. The preeclamptic woman was in danger of going into convulsions at any time. Once convulsions had started, there was a chance they couldn't be controlled and coma could follow. The mortality rate for both mother and child was high. Burl took off her glasses, rubbed her eyes, and continued.

"Yesterday the girl's mother flew out from the East Coast to help with the new baby, saw the condition her daughter was in, and brought her here, apparently just in the nick of time. She went into labor around two this morning.''

Burl pulled the inhaler out of her pocket again. "The prospective father was in Philadelphia on business but managed to catch a flight this morning. He's due to arrive in another couple of hours. Her mother has been asked to wait in the waiting room; she's too upset to be any use to Marie right now.''

Burl stopped twittering and looked grave. "Dr. Somers, the chief OB resident, and one of the senior OB nurses have been managing Marie's labor. This is serious business,'' she said, leaving no doubt in my mind it really was. "Do as much as you can to help. Remember it's important to keep her calm and comfortable, help monitor vital signs, and keep your eye peeled for everything that—''

The door to the room swung open, and a stocky middle-aged nurse hurried past us, never even noticing we were there. I zeroed in on her name tag. "Betty, RN—OB'' was the first line. The second read: "We Deliver.''

Burl stepped back to leave. "And, Heron, don't do anything that isn't within the scope of your skills, even if the nurse or doctor asks you to. Understand?''

I nodded, feeling my scared and insecure self gaining power.

Burl must have seen the crack in my calm façade because

she added, "You can do it, Heron. Just keep your thoughts straight."

She walked away in double time, took another hit off her inhaler, and held her breath all the way to the door.

Her confidence in me sat like a hundred-pound hump on my back. What if I screwed up and did something horribly wrong? What if I forgot what to do? What if . . .

The what-ifs went on for a few seconds until I caught myself playing my mother's role and stopped long enough to look at what I had to work with.

This was going to be my first cold-turkey experience. I didn't have a care plan all made out and memorized for pre-eclampsia, I hadn't studied the drugs the patient would be receiving, and I just barely knew what to expect. I was going to have to rely on intuition, common sense, and my existing knowledge of preeclampsia, which wasn't much.

Putting the facts in order dispelled most of my fears, and for a moment I felt a sense of adventure. Just like the first time I ever ran away from home, I was on my own, taking on the world.

I pushed open the door. The darkened labor room was half the size of a normal hospital room. To my left, in the middle of the wall, a monitor showed two heart patterns and several sets of numbers. The greenish light given off by the screen glowed brightly, giving the windowless room an eerie, futuristic look.

On the bed lay a pregnant woman drenched in sweat. Even though she looked exhausted, I would have guessed she was closer to eighteen than twenty-six. Her knees were bent, and under her buttocks was a blue plastic pad, heavily soiled with amniotic fluid, feces, and blood. Next to her was an IV pole on which hung a bottle labeled "Magnesium Sulfate."

I greeted the woman and pushed some of the dark, wet bangs out of her eyes. "My name's Echo, and I'm going to help take care of you today."

She raised a hand and weakly smiled in greeting. "Are you the student?" she asked hopefully.

I nodded. "I can stay with you until this afternoon. Did your nurse say where she was going? I need to talk to—"

Marie grabbed my hand and let out something between a grunt and a scream. Her face contorted, and I gaped as the large, shining dome of her belly rose and tightened into a peak. I couldn't remember my abdomen doing that during my contractions with Simon, but then again, I doubt I'd been watching very closely.

"Wait a minute! Hold on," I said, panicking. "It'll pass in a second. Breathe easy now. Hold on."

I looked out the small window of the door and started to sweat. Where the hell was everybody?

In answer to my silent question, Betty, the OB nurse who'd passed us in the hall, came charging in with an armful of clean pads and fresh sheets, focused immediately on Marie's face and belly, and shoved the pile into my arms. Sitting down, she lightly stroked Marie's abdomen in a circular motion.

"It's okay, Marie," she said soothingly. "Deep breath in, slowly . . . slowly . . . now, let it out slowly. Again. That's a girl. Good."

Marie's belly relaxed, and the nurse gave me a quick who-the-hell-are-you once-over. "You the student?" It was hard to tell whether she was an RN who liked students.

The RNs who liked us went out of their way to show us precious timesaving tricks they'd learned over the years and gave us reassurance and praise when we nervously did things right. I think they derived a great deal of satisfaction from teaching us, like the satisfaction a mother feels when passing on her special secrets to her daughter. The ones that had no use for us complained we only got in the way. I knew they must have been students at one time or another, and I couldn't imagine how anyone could forget what the ordeal was like.

Before I was through introducing myself, Betty interrupted hurriedly. "Marie is just a bit over nine centimeters dilated, so I'll be needing your help. I don't like the looks of the IV she has in now; I think it's infiltrated into the tissue, so I'd like you to start another one in her other arm. After you do that, grab a blood pressure. She'll need another dose of magnesium sulfate and a little morphine. When you—"

My tongue tripped over itself when I finally got it moving. "I, ah, can do only physical assessments, vitals, and comfort measures. I can also do some procedures like dressing changes, catheterizations, and vaginal exams, but they have to be supervised by my instructor or an RN."

The nurse's disappointment showed clearly. I decided to get in all the bad news on one dump. "I haven't studied intravenous administration of drugs yet. I haven't even given a shot intramuscularly yet."

I shut up. Apprehensively I waited for the huge sigh.

It came with an "Ahh, cripe!" attached to it. "Are you only a first-year student?" Betty, RN, asked in the darker shades of disgust. She spit out the word *first* as if it were unclean.

Behind us Marie's breath quickened, and another contraction turned her gently rolling belly into the Rock of Gibraltar. Betty looked at her watch, then at the monitor. I mimicked what I'd seen her do just a few minutes before and rubbed the taut abdomen, talking Marie through her breathing. "Big, slow breaths, sweetie." My voice was surprisingly calm. "It will pass soon, breathe the pain away, easy now."

When it was over, I took a quick blood pressure. "It's still high," I informed the room, "at one-sixty over a hundred."

"Okay," Betty said in a well-I-guess-we'll-have-to-make-do voice. "I'll start the IV and give the magnesium sulfate. You take the vital signs every fifteen minutes and keep the room quiet and dark. Time the contractions. If they start coming closer than two minutes apart, come and get me. Do her slow breathing with her during the contractions, and keep her clean. Try not to let her move around too much."

"Got it," I said, focusing in on the "come and get me" part. Oh, my God, I thought, did that mean she was going to leave me alone with the patient?

"Most important"—Betty stood and lowered her voice, hovering over me like the prophet of doom—"if you see her muscles twitching, or she goes into a full-blown seizure, stay with her, insure that her airway is open, and hit the red emergency bell behind you."

My external reaction to all this information was to sit rooted to the chair, nodding pleasantly; internally my sense of adventure had just dropped dead in its tracks.

Uncomfortable with talking about a patient in her presence (rule number 238), I looked over at Marie to see if she had heard Betty; her low, singsong moaning told me she hadn't.

With pure efficiency Betty quickly assembled the necessary equipment and started an IV line in Marie's right arm. Not one motion on her part was wasted or fumbled. I almost drooled. Someday I wanted to be just like that, the perfect nurse, keeping it all under control.

She injected the magnesium sulfate slowly into the new line while Marie watched, her golden brown eyes widening.

"Is that the stuff that burns me?" she asked apprehensively.

Betty answered apologetically that it was and then glanced my way. "Why don't you explain to Marie why we have to give her the magnesium sulfate?"

Before I could get a word out, Marie wrung her hands and started grimacing. "Oh, shit, I can feel the burning! God! I hate this almost more than the damned contractions! I feel like I'm on fire! Stop it, stop it! Goddammit, I said stop it!"

The pregnant woman raised herself off the bed to make a grab for the IV tubing. I caught her arm. "Marie, listen to me! That drug keeps you from having convulsions; that's what this preeclampsia is all about. We want you and the baby to be safe, and this medicine helps. Do you know that?"

She squeezed her eyes closed and nodded. Two tears rolled down her cheeks, melting me.

"I'm so afraid," she said so softly, I could barely hear her. "I'm so afraid that . . ."

I let her cry for a minute, then got a cold washcloth and wiped around her eyes and mouth. "When I had my baby," I said, remembering, "I was positive he was going to be born dead or have six heads and no eyes or nose. Every mother is fearful; it's natural."

Marie was not to be comforted by my simple explanation. "But see, I know there's something wrong. As soon as I walked in the door, the nurse got a worried look and put oxygen on me." Marie looked at me directly, searching my face for some understanding.

"There's so much more to this than just having a baby," she said. "I want this child more than anything else in my life. I already love it so much." Her voice broke. "Please help me. Don't let anything happen."

Awkwardly I put my arms around her and held her until I could get the knot out of my throat. "Okay, sweetie, I think I know how you feel, but don't forget that we're all going to work so nothing bad happens. So far everything is going really well, so let's concentrate on that."

Even though Betty had her back to us while she was fiddling with the monitor, I could tell from the way she held her head she was listening to every word. When I finished, she looked back over her shoulder and gave a short nod of approval.

Marie's face tightened as another contraction began, but this time her deep breathing was interrupted by sporadic grunting as she started bearing down with force. Betty noted the time and did another vaginal. "Take fast, shallow breaths. Pant like a dog, and try not to push."

"Okay!" she said when the contraction was over. "You and that baby of yours are going to meet very soon. With the next contraction, try not to push. Concentrate on your panting." Washing her hands at the sink, Betty spoke to me in a low voice. "I'm going to have Dr. Somers paged. I want you to watch this monitor very carefully." She pointed to the green, jiggly lines. "That's the mother's heartbeat, and this one is the baby's. If either one changes or looks different from the way they do now, come and get me right away.

"One of the interns should be watching out at the desk monitor, too, but we're really busy and understaffed, so I can't say for sure that someone will be watching every second. I'm relying on you to keep things running smoothly. I'll be gone for less than two minutes." Betty smiled while I quietly freaked out. I wondered if there were inhalers for anxiety attacks. "Don't panic" were her last words before the door closed.

I just hated the way people said things like "You can do it," "Don't panic," or "I have every faith in you" just before abandoning ship. It was probably the same for baby birds as they headed straight down after being pushed out of the nest.

I saw the renewed worry on Marie's face and felt embarrassed by my fear. She was the one who needed reassurance. Wiping the sweat off her face, I smiled and started to tell her how beautiful she looked, but she cut me off. "While Betty's gone, I want you to tell me the truth about what's wrong with my baby. I promise I won't get hysterical or anything."

It bothered me she thought that the doctors and nurses were keeping something from her or that they'd lied, but at the same time I knew why she felt that way. It was a daily occurrence in the hospital for doctors and nurses alike to lie to a patient because they thought it would upset him to know the truth. Even worse was the doctor who simply neglected to tell a patient he was having a heart attack or that the lab reports had come back positive for cancer. The nurse, bound by rules, had to hedge the patient's straightforward questions and create obviously flimsy excuses for answers.

Most people instinctively knew when they weren't being told what was wrong with them, and from what I could see, it only caused more suffering and anxiety than if they knew the truth of the matter. But even so, the rules being what they were, it was a rare nurse who went ahead and answered, "Yes, Mr. Jones, you *are* having a heart attack," before the doctor got around to delivering the news two days later.

"No one has lied to you, Marie. As far as we know right now, your baby is fine. Yes, everybody's acting concerned, but that's because of the preeclampsia, which is a potentially serious thing, but like I said, everything is going okay so far."

Marie relaxed. "Okay, I believe you, but you've got to tell me the minute something goes wrong. I want to know so I can help, too."

She'd made a good point, I thought. After all, there weren't many patients who wouldn't try all the harder to cooperate in fighting for their lives if they knew they were in danger.

Another contraction began, and I turned my attention to the monitor. Both heart rhythms jiggled around on the screen a bit, but nothing more. Marie tried to pant but gave up toward the end of the contraction and bore down.

"I can't help it," she grunted. "I've got to. The urge is too strong."

I moved to the end of the bed and took Betty's chair. "Next time I'll pant with you, and you concentrate on following my lead, okay?"

Marie nodded, and I saw the pad under her was soiled again. Pulling the pad out from under her, it slipped out of my hand and landed right side up on the floor. Peering over the side rails, Marie got a good look at the mess and made a face. "This isn't like all the movies with the men boiling hot water and everything clean and tidy, is it?"

"Nope," I answered, washing her off, "it sure isn't. It's more like rolling around in a freshly littered cow pasture."

Marie laughed and bit her lip. "Damn you, don't make me laugh!"

Without warning, the laugh turned to an uneven panting as another contraction started. I pivoted toward the monitor with the thought that the contraction had come too soon and saw the fetal heart rate drop from 130 to 50. The fetus was in distress. Either the baby was pressed against the cord, or something else was cutting off its oxygen supply.

"Stop pushing!" I yelled, but Marie was grunting and pushing with such force she didn't hear. Her legs and arms started twitching, as the dark, round top of the baby's head bulged from her vagina.

I had just touched the emergency bell when Betty and a man in surgical greens burst through the door and almost knocked me over. "The baby's heart slowed down to a rate of fifty, and she's twitching." I delivered my information to the backs of their heads; both of them were moving at greased-lightning speed. I guessed the "somebody" at the desk had been quick to send out the alarm about the baby's heart rate.

Betty handed me a filled syringe. "Here! give the magnesium sulfate quickly!"

I opened my mouth to protest, but she added, "Stat!" and spun around to turn up Marie's oxygen and unlock the wheels of the bed.

The man in greens was checking for the position of the baby's head and any problems with the fetal heart monitor wire. "Don't push! Pant, pant for all you're worth," he yelled. Nodding toward the IV tubing, he glanced over at me. "Hi. I'm Dr. Somers, glad to have you aboard, and don't let the grass grow while you give that magnesium. Thanks."

I found the rubber port in the tubing where Betty had given the drug before. Inserting the needle, I prayed Burl would understand. My hands were slippery with sweat and shaking so badly I could barely control the syringe.

Betty took the portable monitor from its home in the wall and placed it on a rolling stand. The baby's heart rate had picked up to a rate of 80, but that was still too slow.

Marie was making guttural sounds while panting like a crazy woman. "I've got to push!" She screamed and bore down.

"Don't!" Betty and I yelled simultaneously.

Preoccupied with the patterns on the monitor, Dr. Somers stood up quickly. "Okay, folks, we've got to get the baby out of there right now, so let's get this show on the road."

With Betty pushing the bed, Dr. Somers pulling and watching the monitor, and me guiding the IV poles and the monitor cart, it took exactly six seconds from the time we left the labor room to the time we flew through the doors of the large white delivery room.

Marie grabbed for my hand. "Tell me!" she demanded.

Bringing my lips close to her ear, I spoke rapidly. "Now is the time to really help us out. The baby needs more oxygen, and your muscles are getting hyper; but you are very close to delivering, and that's good. Just follow everything Dr. Somers says and you'll do fine." For a second I stared at the face blotched with blood vessels broken during her straining and prayed I was right.

"I'll do anything you say," she said calmly. "Just please make my baby okay."

With the pull sheet Dr. Somers and I eased her onto the delivery table and put her feet into the stirrups while Betty, now on automatic, grabbed a handful of masks and surgical gowns, prepared instruments, and opened sterile packets.

Dr. Somers pulled on his sterile gloves and sat down between Marie's feet.

The fetal heartbeat was still reading 80.

Trying to look reassuring, Dr. Somers picked up the pair of forceps and placed them under Marie's buttocks. His fingers felt the top of the baby's head. "Marie, I need you to push now!"

Not needing any encouragement, she pushed with her whole body, then stopped, breathing as if she'd just run a marathon.

A satisfied look crossed Dr. Somers's face. Pushing the forceps away, he made a small episiotomy incision. "Once more, Miss Marie!"

With the push the whole head of a tiny human being emerged, the face grimacing and squinting.

Dr. Somers slipped a bluish-looking umbilical cord from around the baby's neck and removed the monitor wire from the top of its head.

I took Marie's hand in mine. "Hey, you did it!"

Marie said nothing, mesmerized by what she saw in the mirror above the delivery table.

The doctor rotated the shoulders, then eased the rest of the small, perfectly formed body out of the birth canal. As soon as Betty suctioned out the mouth, his tiny squall reverberated through the room.

Dr. Somers's grave expression gave way to a wide, satisfied smile. "Whew!" he said, cutting the cord. "That baby is one smart little fella. He took one look at those forceps and knew it was time to get out of there on his own."

Betty checked the newborn over carefully, wrapped him in a warm blanket, and put the silver nitrate drops into his eyes, all the while humming a lively tune. Dr. Somers, waiting to deliver the placenta, whistled a harmonizing accompaniment.

When Betty laid the blue flannel package on Marie's slightly deflated belly, Marie touched the top of his head gently, as if she didn't believe he was real, then drew him up to her face with trembling hands. She kissed his red, wrinkled forehead.

"He's beautiful!" she said in a hoarse voice. "He's okay. I had a baby boy and I'm alive and he's alive. Oh, God, thank you. Thank you, everybody."

Thirty minutes later I walked into the sanctioned area known as the staff nurses' locker room.

Betty had given me her private key, explaining it was a present for not panicking. Who knows? Maybe she'd even decided first-year brats weren't so bad after all.

I filled the basin with soapy water and peeled off my stockings. Dampening a washcloth, I washed off the flakes of spattered blood and dried feces from my legs.

When I stood, I caught a glimpse of myself in the mirror over the sink and stared.

I still had on the green scrub dress, and the white surgical mask hung from my neck along with my stethoscope. The smile that formed came directly from my heart. It was so wide I could see the fillings in my back teeth.

I am going to be a nurse, I said to the image in the mirror, *and I love it. I love all of it.* I wept with the smile still on my face.

That was when Burl walked in.

I looked at her, helpless and a little embarrassed. "I'm so happy," I choked.

She sat me down on the bench behind us and patted my back for a long time. "It's an incredible profession, this job of nursing," she said finally when the tears had stopped.

"Do you ever get to know everything, Burl?"

"No, but you can spend a lifetime trying to learn it all."

I blew my nose, and Burl got up to leave. "You've got ten minutes to get to postclinical conference. Be on time."

The door hadn't closed all the way before Burl stuck her head back in. "By the way, Heron," she said, with a disapproving look over the top of her bifocals, "I hear you give a superb magnesium sulfate."

I laughed out loud, "Gulp!"

"I think we'd better get you through the first year before you start taking over." The door closed, but I heard her final remark: "Next thing you know, you'll be giving orders to the physicians."

I leaned back against the locker and hugged my knees to my chest. The memory of Marie's face when the baby was given to her danced before me, and my wide smile returned.

From one of my philosophy classes I remembered a small bit from a lecture on Eastern religions which stated that people who chose to devote their lives to helping others were spiritually tied to the world by golden chains. Their souls, being so confined, could never move any closer to the glory of Nirvana and would eventually stagnate and die.

Closing my eyes, I searched my supposedly stagnating soul and found nothing but clarity, strength, and joy.

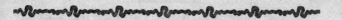

FIVE

ALTHOUGH THE BULK of us kept coming back every day, by the end of the first year many students had been dropped for failure to achieve the standards set by the program, or they had resigned because they couldn't stand the stress.

Despite my increasing number of gray hairs, I thought I was coping pretty well until a grinding ache in the pit of my stomach woke me up out of a sound sleep one morning at about four.

I drank a glass of milk and went back to bed never dreaming the ache would return every morning, each episode becoming more and more uncomfortable. Within a week the words *peptic ulcer* haunted me with every glass of half-and-half I drank.

Despite the ache, I said nothing. We had just finished studying the gastrointestinal system, and the chapter on peptic ulcers was still fresh in our minds. I didn't want to embarrass myself by letting everybody think I'd been fooled again by the old power-of-suggestion trick.

It's a well-known fact that every medical or nursing student will inevitably begin to imagine he has all the signs and symptoms of whatever malfunction he is currently learning about.

When we were studying basic cardiology, we all thought we were having angina and heart attacks. The same thing happened during our neuro section; there wasn't one student who didn't think she had a brain tumor. Our nursing class alone was keeping the local physicians in house payments.

I thought I'd learned my lesson when my doctor laughed me out of his office after I told him the brain tumor I thought I had two months earlier had turned into intermittent claudication of the wrists.

But this time was different, I was sure. The discomfort seemed so real, and taking antacids and eating ice cream soothed the weird, achy hunger feeling—just like in the books.

I thought of going to see my doctor, but the memory of his howling laughter temporarily numbed any pain I thought I was suffering.

And so I sat on the ache, thinking it was all in my mind right up until our group started studying drugs and their administration.

There were three main reasons for the drug section's being one of the most stressful of all our courses. One had to do with the immense volume of material to be learned, and another was that much of the administration of drugs involved mathematical skills. Few of us had advanced in mathematics beyond the mandatory, simpleton's college algebra designed for talented fifth graders.

The last reason was elementary: We actually had to administer drugs to patients, and that included giving shots.

The big day we all were dreading finally came toward the end of April. Each of our group was individually to demonstrate our first intramuscular injection on a conscious human who not only bled, but had active pain receptors.

On the appointed day Janey and I agreed to meet early in the clinical lab and practice on our oranges before the main event.

We all had our very own oranges with our names printed on them in Magic Marker. Each of us had spent endless hours hunched over a brightly colored sphere, holding it in one sweaty-palmed hand, while the other wiped it down with an alcohol pad. Concentrating with enough power to bend steel, we'd pierce our oranges, aspirate orange juice, and then inject sterile water. We all strove to perfect the wrist motion known as the "spearing quick flick."

Over and over again the spearing motion was repeated until the clinical lab smelled like the fruit section of a produce market. It wasn't at all unusual to walk into the lab and hear choruses of grunts and disappointed groans while orange practice was taking place. Sometimes even cries of pain could be heard as the acidic juice shot into the eye of a student holding her orange too close or as a needle missed the fruit altogether and instead found the palm of a hand.

Janey wasn't in the lab by the time I arrived, so I decided to get our oranges and prepare some syringes before she got there.

As I headed toward the cabinet with the fruit flies hanging around the outside, a noise from the laboratory kitchen caused me to stick my head around the corner and see who was there.

Janey stood against the sink, taking large gulps from a blue plastic bottle I recognized immediately as the same antacid I was taking for my hypochondriacal ulcer.

Seeing me, she stopped gulping and quickly hid the evidence in her purse.

"Oh, hi!" she said, smiling. "You're early!"

A white mustache left from the antacid hung on her upper lip.

I took the bottle out of her purse and held it up. It was almost empty. "You, too?" I asked.

Janey pointed to a small area of her upper abdomen. "A little pain right here that's worse in the morning and after pizza and salad?"

I sighed with relief and smiled. I wasn't the only one who still fell victim to the power of suggestion.

"Now what?" I asked. "Don't they have sanatoriums for people like us where we can go and rest for a year or so?"

Ignoring my question, I noticed Janey getting this dreamy, almost romantic look. "Ya know, Ec, it's really not that bad when you stop and think about it. I don't think I'd really mind so much going into my second year with a doctor-certified ulcer. It's kind of like being awarded a medal of courage. We earned this thing; we ought to be proud of it!"

"Oh, that's just great, Jane, great idea. I mean, sure, why not? Let's all go nuts. Hell, we'll just spear a little flesh and run right down to get our ulcer certificates." I gave Jane a long look. "You're getting weird on me, aren't you?"

Janey laughed, though not convincingly enough. "No, no, not at all. I just want to—"

"It's all right, Jane," I said, gently guiding her toward the lab. "A little fresh air, a little rest, and you'll be fine. It's the atmosphere here—all these hospitals and sick people. Believe me, I understand."

"I'm not crazy. I just think we deserve a little recognition for—"

I handed Jane her orange and gave her a warning look as we entered the lab. "Be quiet, Jane. No one else will understand."

"But—"

"Quiet. Look around you; then ask yourself honestly if this group wants to hear about ulcers and medals of courage."

In the lab a few of the students were nervously practicing their quick flicks; many were simply staring at the walls.

"Well, I guess . . ."

"Can it, Jane. Concentrate on your orange. The ulcers come later."

We'd just readied our oranges when Mrs. Zeitwitz, or Mrs. Z. as the students liked to call her, danced through the door, singing "God Bless America."

Mrs. Z. was somewhat off the beaten track for a clinical lab assistant, mostly because she was always so serene. Her patience with our fumblings was admirable, and I never once saw her lose her temper or raise her voice. She wore her long graying hair loose over her shoulders and usually dressed in a black turtleneck sweater, black tights, and lots of silver and turquoise jewelry. She reminded me of an old hippie or a born again beatnik. Understandably she was every student's favorite.

"Okay, girls, this is it," she said, rolling up her sleeves. "You're my last clinical group of the day, and I must say I can't really complain about the shots so far. I've only had two faints, three half sticks, and one crying jag."

A few scattered outbursts of nervous laughter rose from the students but died quickly.

Mrs. Z. scanned the group, and her smile faded a little.

"Oh, come on, girls, this isn't so hard. There's nothing to be nervous about. Now, I want you all to draw up a half a cc of saline with a five-eighth-inch, twenty-five-gauge needle on a three-cc syringe, and line up in front of me."

Mrs. Z. sat down, shuffled some alcohol pads, and waited. She looked a bit frayed around the edges, but after all, first intramuscular injections were always a hard day for the clinical lab assistant, especially when her muscles were being used as the target.

Janey and I stood in line together, discussing our twin ulcers and going over some of the finer points of pill pushing, when Mrs. Z. said the magic word to Janey. "Next?"

Timidly, Janey stepped forward, smiling. "I'm ready, Mrs. Z. Which arm would you like me to use?"

Mrs. Z. looked over her left arm, which was still bleeding from the last student's assault.

"Let's go for the right one this time, Jane. My left is needle fatigued."

Janey showed Mrs. Z. her syringe and waited for the nod of approval. Then, picking up an alcohol pad, she marked off the proper area for injection, removed the cap from the needle, raised her hand, and stopped.

Twenty or thirty seconds passed.

"Inject, dear," said Mrs. Z. quietly.

Nothing happened.

"Inject now, Jane, I'm ready." Mrs. Z. shifted her focus of attention from her arm to Janey and studied her face.

Janey did not move.

With controlled calmness, Mrs. Z. said the words again. "Inject, please, I'm waiting, Jane."

Jane remained frozen in position.

Standing directly behind her, I stared with some interest at the back of Janey's head. I was impressed by the way the ends of her hair rhythmically jumped with the pounding of her heart.

I looked over her shoulder.

In a white-knuckled grip Janey's left hand held Mrs. Z.'s upper arm. Under her blanched fingers, I could see little bruises forming on Mrs. Z.'s skin. Poised above Mrs. Z.'s well-punctured, skinny deltoid muscle was Janey's quivering right hand. Like a vise grip, her small fingers held on to the syringe.

"Inject, Jane. It won't hurt me. Just go ahead and do it. Now, dear."

I thought I heard an edge to Mrs. Z.'s voice I'd never heard before: understandable considering the circumstances. Her forearm was now turning a mottled blue just below where Janey was cutting off the circulation.

Janey finally stirred. "Can't. Can't do this. Oh! No. Can't . . ." She was whispering so softly I had to lean over her shoulder to hear her. She managed to speak without moving her mouth, but it had been well over five minutes since she'd moved anything at all. I noticed her eyes glazing over from not blinking.

Mrs. Z., recognizing terror, said in the same evenly modulated voice, "Well, dear, why don't you just go back over to your orange and practice a few more times, then give it another try after the other girls have had their turns?"

The room was instantly silent. Disgrace had fallen on one of us; being sent back to your orange was like a prize fighter's being sent out of the ring back to a sawdust punching bag.

Janey still did not move, and I watched her freckles fade and blend into the gray color of the rest of her skin.

"I'm going to be sick," she whispered, again without moving her mouth. I knew if she ever flunked nursing, she had a great future in ventriloquism.

With a surprising amount of agility for a woman her age, Mrs. Z. pried her arm out of Janey's grasp and jumped back in one faster-than-the-eye-can-see move.

All eyes were now on Janey.

She stood like a mannequin whose props had been taken away; same position except now, instead of Mrs. Z.'s arm, her left hand held a death grip on thin air.

"Can't do it. Can't do it. Sick, oh, no . . ."

Janey stared straight ahead.

We'd all heard of nursing students cracking and going over the edge, but most of us had already placed bets on Penny Mummy with her fear of hospitals and her contact dermatitis allergy to alcohol swabs. I'd never dreamed Janey would be the one to go as a victim of simple performance anxiety.

Gently I put my arm around her waist and tried to pull her into a chair. No luck. She was rooted.

"Janey!" I shouted into her ear. "Janey, do you hear me?"

I thought I saw a nostril quiver, but it was only the reflection off a drop of sweat at the end of her nose.

I pulled her left arm out of position, and while another student massaged her fingers, I put steady pressure on Janey's raised arm until it rested stiffly at her side.

Next, the legs. Jamming a chair into the back of her knees worked quite well in overcoming Janey's strictly vertical position.

No one needed a mind reader to know the question everyone was asking but was afraid to voice aloud: Who was going to disengage the syringe from Janey's hand?

The small needle tip, sparkling with sharpness, looked like a deadly weapon.

I could feel the attention of the room shift. When I looked up, all eyes were trained on me. The message was clear: I was her best friend; the job was mine.

Gently, ever so gently, I grabbed Janey's right wrist and twisted it until she let out a little scream. Something in Janey snapped, but it wasn't her wrist.

She smiled faintly, said my name once, and, with a swiftness I have never seen in any human being, lifted my arm and executed the most professional intramuscular injection anyone had done that day. Her spearing quick flick was outstanding.

I didn't feel a thing.

Everyone was stunned into silence, except Janey. Suddenly she came to life and began to chatter a mile a minute.

"Well, now, how about that? Not bad, huh? I guess I can just throw this old orange right into the old compost heap, huh? Yep, nothing to it, just spear and flick. Not a speck of blood, not an ounce of pain. Anyone want to lend me an arm? Say, how about you, Mrs. Z.? Want to see that again?"

Mrs. Z. was quick to answer. "Ah, no, dear, that was just fine. Why don't you go to the library and study up on next week's topic of intravenous techniques?"

The spell broken, some of the students went back to their oranges, while others re-formed a line in front of Mrs. Z.

I sidled up to Janey.

"Say there, Jane, how're you doing?" I asked nonchalantly. I was afraid anything might push her over the edge again.

"Fine, Ec, why do you ask?"

Was she blocking, or had I imagined the whole thing?

"You, ah, seemed to have a bit of trouble there for a minute. You had me worried. I thought maybe you were going to chicken out, you know?"

Janey reacted rather strongly, I thought.

"Chicken out?" she screamed. "Precision injection, and you call it 'Chicken out'?"

"Now, Jane, I didn't say—"

"Oh, yes, you did. I heard you! Let's see how well you do, shall we? Let's just test you out, hotshot. Here's my arm; go ahead!"

Janey got me where I lived; I could not pass up a good challenge.

Since she had given me her first injection, it would be proper clinical etiquette to reciprocate. I could pump an orange full of water as well as the best of them; an arm certainly wouldn't be any different.

It was settled. I readied my syringe and prepped her upper arm with an alcohol swab. Janey's eyes were squeezed shut, and her head was turned as far away from her arm as was muscularly possible. I could feel her pulse through her fleshy upper arm; it was bounding and fast.

I made the mistake of hesitating. Here I was, ready to stab this perfectly normal arm with a piece of sharpened steel. Horrible visions of sticking the needle all the way through her bone and not being able to get it out wreaked havoc with my nerves.

The smell of the alcohol drying turned my ulcerous stomach upside down.

I shook off the negative thoughts, prepared my wrist with a few practice flicks, and removed the cap.

The needle looked dangerous, and my instincts told me to stop fooling around and put the cap back on before somebody got hurt.

"Inject! Come on, Ec, I'm waiting. Let's get this over with!"

For some strange reason, Janey's voice sounded as if it were coming from the inside of a tube very far away.

I picked out a freckle on Janey's arm to be the bull's-eye and raised my hand.

The freckle got smaller and fuzzier, and I felt as if a thousand tiny needles were injecting Novocaine into my body.

Just before everything went black, I thought I heard someone say ever so sweetly, "Inject, dear, inject."

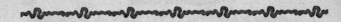

SIX

MAY CAME INTO TOWN masquerading as July, and the promise of a long, hot summer got under every schoolkid's skin. Sneakers squeaked with impatience on classroom floors while their wearers waited for the sound of the last bell to free them once and for all to the world of skateboards, bicycles, and yet-to-be-built secret forts.

Not that we were any different. With only two more weeks of school it was difficult going home each day to labor over care plans in the winter setting of our desks while the sun beckoned us to warm afternoon walks along the ocean.

Somehow I had managed to stay on the bucking bronco of nursing school for the entire year, but after the fainting fiasco and the debut of my duodenal ulcer, I knew my body was trying to tell me it was time for a break. Besides, Simon's Spiderman duffel bag was so badly tattered and torn it couldn't have lasted much longer.

We'd started the year as an enthusiastic, hefty class of sixty and were exiting for summer vacation as an exhausted, anorexic group of thirty-four. But just because we all were tired didn't mean the pace was going to slow down. On the contrary, the last couple of weeks were the busiest.

While we crammed for finals, our instructors made lists of clinical skills and experiences we each had to complete before the end of the year. My list consisted of clinical time in the operating and emergency rooms; it would have included intramuscular injections if it hadn't been for Mrs. Z.

One morning, as I was on my way into a patient's room,

Mrs. Z. approached and asked me to follow her to pediatrics. She told me there was an eight-year-old boy scheduled for a tonsillectomy who needed his preop injection; I was her first choice of students to do the job.

After an uncontrolled outburst of laughter I reminded her I was the very same person she'd revived a few weeks earlier on the laboratory floor. Not only that, I said, but whoever heard of giving a first injection to a child?

Mrs. Z. smiled slyly and pooh-poohed my arguments while she dragged me through a teddy bear-decaled door.

Brooks Crabtree III, a pampered and precocious little darling, sat like a docile lamb while I explained how the magic medicine would take him to dreamland. To make the whole procedure even more appetizing, I threw in that when he woke up, he'd have all the ice cream and soda he wanted.

His response? "Screw off, bitch," to be exact. Genuinely surprised, I told him he sounded angry and suggested his angry feelings probably came from being scared. I said that as soon as he got the medicine part over with, he'd feel much better.

Darling Brooks bit my hand, then executed a follow-up kick to my right rib cage. He gave the scene added color by screaming obscenities one should be over forty to use. By the time the techs pulled him down off the water pipes, I *wanted* to inject him.

Mrs. Z. watched the whole circus, wearing a smug expression, and when I finally injected the little rump without so much as turning a hair, she clapped.

From then on it was easy giving injections; all I had to do was imagine Brooks Crabtree III under the needle.

I was finishing the year with Pearson. That really wasn't so bad; it was like finishing the year by myself. Actually Pearson was a welcome break. I was tired of having my life dominated by a different strong personality every two and a half months. Pearson was the only instructor I could go home and forget about.

In the first week of the final two weeks Pearson assigned me to the operating room. It was reminiscent of my days in Anatomy and Physiology class, the exception being that these bodies weren't covered with fur and they bled blood rather than formaldehyde.

In two days I witnessed three orthopedic surgeries, one

nose job, one hysterectomy, and the removal of a shattered plastic dildo from someone's lower bowel.

It didn't take a sharp observer to realize the OR staff was not like any other group or unit in the hospital. It doesn't really deal with the patient as a whole; it deals only with an anesthetized person who needs some body work. Unless the surgery involves the head, the surgeon rarely sees the patient's face.

By the end of my first surgery I'd come to two firm conclusions: One, I would never have surgery done unless absolutely necessary, and two, the responsibility of the anesthesiologist and surgeon was staggering. These were the jobs someone who knew what they really entailed might go into thinking, *Well*, somebody *has to do it*.

A surgeon's mistake has to be one of the deadliest. It isn't like prescribing the wrong medication or putting someone on the wrong diet; a surgeon's mistake is instantaneous. An accidental nick here, a wrong cut there—by the time it's made, it's either almost too late or just too late, period.

The anesthesiologist's job isn't much better, although it includes a lot of the basics, like keeping the patient alive. He breathes for the patient, watches the monitor and vital signs, and keeps the person floating at the perfect level of deep sleep.

Thus, considering the nature of their work, it didn't surprise me that the surgical staff was a pretty funny bunch. I think it's safe to say that most operating rooms are the birthplaces of hospital jokes.

As soon as the patient stops counting backwards, and the draping and initial cutting are done, the anesthesiologist usually starts the ball rolling with something like "Hey, have you guys heard the one about the doctor and the rabbi?" From there the surgeon does a few takeoff jokes, and then circulating and scrub nurses add their two cents, and so on and so forth, right until the last stitch or staple is inserted.

Surgeons came in all shapes and flavors. Most of them were good, one or two were excellent, and a rare one was dangerous.

Dr. Bell was the best general surgeon I ever saw. Physically he resembled Abraham Lincoln, and his temperament was what I imagined a combination of Lincoln and Mrs. Z. might have been: kind, eager to teach, and never a raised voice to anyone.

The moment Dr. Bell saw a student in the OR, he ordered her to move from the outskirts and get as close to the operating table as possible. If the student was short, he requested the circulating nurse to find a stepstool. He explained everything he did, going into detail about what organ attached to what or what nerve or vessel had to be carefully avoided and why. He was a rare doctor if only because after twenty years of performing surgery, he was still fascinated by the inner workings of the human body.

On the farthest end of the stick from Dr. Bell was an orthopedic surgeon by the name of Dr. Drigely. In contrast with Dr. Bell's calm perfection, Drigely was a five foot ten inch, 240 pound disaster. Nervous and slightly shifty, he projected more the image of a fat used-car salesman than that of a surgeon.

As soon as he opened his mouth, one's attention was drawn to the extensive gold fillings in his front teeth. The next thing one noticed was that he had a tendency to cover anyone he talked to with a fine mist of saliva.

The first time I had a chance to watch Dr. Drigely at work was a hip pinning on an eighty-year-old woman who had fallen at home and broken the head of her femur. Drigely examined her on the ward and filled out the surgical consent form for the placement of a pin in the right hip.

The surgical nurse had finished gathering the supplies needed to position the hip for surgery, when Drigely waddled into the room, making jokes and bragging about his new sailboat. It was easy to see he was uncomfortable trying to be one of the boys; his jokes fell flat, the anesthesiologist was clearly uninterested in carrying on a conversation with him, and the nurses were on the thin side of civil.

As they began to position the patient onto her left side, the circulating nurse and the anesthesiologist suddenly shot looks of concern at each other. Clenching his jaw, the anesthesiologist loudly cleared his throat.

"Seems to be quite a bit of bruising on the opposite side, Drigely. I thought the consent stated the *right* hip?"

Freezing, Drigely seemed puzzled for a moment, then giggled like a nervous teenager and flushed a deep red color.

The anesthesiologist stepped back, slipped his surgical cap

off his head, then back on, like a baseball pitcher on the mound. "How 'bout we take a look at the road maps, eh, Drigely?"

"Aye, right you are, matey!" he said, looking toward the empty x-ray screen. "Nurse! Put up the x-rays."

The circulating nurse inserted the films of the woman's hip on the lighted opaque box.

Now, I have always had more than my share of trouble remembering my right from my left, but it was immediately obvious which hip needed pinning.

Drigely's wrinkled forehead was pouring sweat like a faucet. He took the films down, turned them around, and stood back. He stepped forward, turned them back again, and looked. It was when he turned one upside down and started wringing his pudgy hands that the anesthesiologist, now standing with his hand over his face, angrily screamed out the obvious news.

My second experience with Drigely occurred later the same day. The case didn't actually begin as a scheduled surgery; it started in the cast room as a simple procedure of cutting a window in the body cast of a teen-age boy. One week before, the boy had crushed his pelvis and broken every bone in his legs in a motorcycle versus tree accident.

After six days of hospitalization, the nurses noted that the boy's white count was elevated, and he'd started to run a low-grade fever. He complained of a burning sensation in his left leg but couldn't pinpoint exactly where it originated.

By feeling the outside of the cast, one nurse found a "hot spot" and immediately informed Drigely of the problem, suggesting at the same time that cutting a window out of the cast might be a good idea.

I guess Drigely didn't recognize me without my surgical mask because as soon as I wheeled the patient into the cast room, he proceeded to describe his new boat all over again and tell the same jokes. I noticed the boat had grown a few feet, and the jokes fell a little flatter, but what got to me the most was that nothing in the man's presence indicated he'd been at all humbled by the morning's episode in OR.

After the preliminary explanation of what he planned to do, Drigely emphatically informed both me and the patient that the procedure had to be quick; his sailing lesson was scheduled to begin in forty-five minutes.

I wiped a few of the larger droplets of spittle from my cheek and stepped out of range.

With the cast cutter he sawed a five-by-five square over the spot the nurse had designated and lifted out the window. An oblong pool of brown pus covered the middle of the exposed leg. Around the spot, rings of necrosis and spreading infection faded from black to deep purple to bright red.

Obviously, when Drigely applied the cast, he had failed to notice a small, open wound, which was more than likely the parent of what we were looking at now.

Drigely's eyes bugged, and he quickly set the window back into the cast. It was the action of a man who, opening a door upon some horrifying scene, closed it, hoping it would disappear.

The young man lifted up on his elbows and started to yell. "What the fuck was *that*, man?"

Drigely's face turned red, right down to the last of his four chins. If I thought the sweat had poured from him earlier in the day, it was gushing now.

"Ah, it's nothing, son, just a little dead skin that needs some cleaning up."

"A little dead skin? Man, that shit looked infected as hell. Christ, that's probably why I've been sick. Oh, man, I'm gonna lose my damned leg!"

Drigely turned defensive, more than likely wondering if his sailboat could be taken away in a malpractice suit.

"Don't use that language!" Drigely spit like an out-of-control child. "I told you I'd clean it up, so pipe down!"

Intimidated, the boy lay back down to stare helplessly at the ceiling. I wanted to say something like "Your leg will be fine" or "Don't worry" but couldn't. Drigely's nervousness made me uneasy.

He wiped his forehead with a damp-looking handkerchief. "Get me a basin of hydrogen peroxide and a bottle of Betadine solution." He took off his black-and-white checkered jacket, which resembled a horse blanket, and rolled up the sleeves of his perspiration-stained shirt. As an afterthought he added, "And while you're at it, grab one of those disposable instrument sets. I'll get this young man cleaned up in a jiffy and still be on time for that lesson." He stood there smiling and sweating.

I left the cast room to gather the things Drigely had ordered while my intuition nagged, telling me something was not right. Hydrogen peroxide, Betadine, and a three-piece instrument set were not going to take care of that degree of infection.

On what would have been considered an insane urge by most students and staff, I made a spontaneous detour into the surgeons' lounge.

Dr. Bell was stretched out on the couch, reading a newspaper. He turned a page and noticed me.

Terrified, I couldn't believe I was actually doing this. I thought of forgetting the whole thing and asking him some ridiculous question, like could I take a look at the sports section, when I remembered principle number sixteen: "A nurse acts first and foremost in the patient's best interest."

It was enough to hold on to.

"Ah, Dr. Bell, may I speak with you for just a second?"

He put down his paper and regarded me as I twisted my fingers around one another. I was trying to control my hyperventilation long enough to get out the problem.

"Certainly. What's going on?"

"You see, sir, I'm helping Dr. Drigely in the cast room with a patient who has a badly infected leg, and I thought you could just, you know, sort of pass by and take a look and maybe give some suggestions?"

Dr. Bell stared for a moment, and I got the sinking feeling I'd made a grave error.

"I'm not quite sure what you're asking me to do. You should know I can't interfere with another physician's treatment of a patient without being consulted."

I got desperate. Saving the teen-ager's leg suddenly became the most important thing in the world. I didn't give a damn about the etiquette and ethics of the physicians' brotherly code; it wasn't worth a future amputation.

"Please, Dr. Bell. The patient is only nineteen years old, and I thought maybe you could say you were looking for something in the cast room and take a quick look over his shoulder. All Drigely—I mean, all Dr. Drigely plans to do is to clean it out and put a bandage over it. He says he has to be somewhere in about thirty minutes." I relaxed my shoulders. "Look, Dr. Bell, I'm no surgeon, but I think the leg needs more than a little swab job."

That was my last appeal. I saw it had had no effect when

Dr. Bell shook his head. "No, I'm sorry, I can't do that. It isn't ethical, and I'm sure Dr. Drigely knows what he's doing."

I started to argue that Drigely never seemed to know what he was doing, but I was already way beyond the bounds of what might be considered standard operating procedure for a student nurse.

My Abraham Lincoln image of Dr. Bell disintegrated, and I returned to the cast room depressed.

Arranging the supplies on a sterile tray, I tried to think of a way to rectify the situation and came up with zero. Of course, my store of rationalizations opened and spilled forth, but I couldn't buy any of them.

Drigely took me aside and insisted I put up a drape sheet to block the patient's view of the infected leg. He told me it would be psychologically damaging to the boy to watch the procedure. I wanted to tell him about the psychological damage going on in my own mind.

I put the drape sheet over a foot cradle at the level of the boy's waist and stood next to his head. I tried engaging the boy in conversation by telling him about my father's 1927 Indian Chief motorcycle.

Drigely removed the window and carelessly scooped out the pus with a couple of gauze pads.

I started pausing between words.

Drigely poured in the hydrogen peroxide, and the liquid fizzed up into a mass of white foam which spilled over and onto the floor. Added to my worries was the fact the boy felt nothing but a little pressure.

By the time Drigely started poking blindly around the hole, I'd out and out lost my train of thought and was stuttering.

Satisfied with his work, Drigely wiped out the remaining foam and poured in some Betadine solution.

"There! All done. We can go ahead and pack this little scrape and get our young man back to his room and start some IV antibiotics on him."

Drigely's enthusiasm failed to affect me. I was facing a sleepless night, knowing the wound would keep infecting. My only recourse was to tell the head nurse. Not that that would change much; right or wrong, physicians had a great deal of power over what would be done and when.

I was opening the first packet of bandaging gauze when

Dr. Bell stepped into the room. "Afternoon, Drigely. Just looking for a plastic long arm splint. Don't let me interrupt what you're doing."

I had to hide my grin. Bell deserved an Academy Award.

Drigely's forehead poured forth another waterfall of sweat. I saw him grope blindly for the cast window and pushed it out of his reach.

Dr. Bell, under pretense of searching for the splint, walked past the gurney and did a vaudevillianlike double take of the infected leg. He made a long, low whistle.

"I see you've got a nasty hour's worth of debridement to do there, Drigely." He gazed thoughtfully at the Betadine-stained rot. "You know, if I remember rightly, operating room D is free for the afternoon. If you'd like, I'll tell them to get it ready for you."

An irritated sigh escaped from Drigely's tense, mountainous body and made his jowls jiggle.

"Yeah, sure. I was just going to send the girl over there myself to see if anything was open."

I caught my tongue between my teeth and forced a colorful comment down for my ulcer to snack on.

Dr. Bell winked at me. "The debridement process is tedious, but you might find it interesting." He glanced over at Drigely. "You wouldn't mind having the student observe, would you, Drigely?"

The glint in Drigely's eyes looked like that of a trapped rat.

I did find the process tedious, though not very interesting. Dr. Drigely didn't talk much, but that was okay with me. I had the satisfaction of knowing a young man would walk out of the hospital and through the rest of his life on two legs instead of one.

I never did mention it to Pearson, of course, but Janey heard the story in detail. The next morning she presented me with a jockstrap bearing the note "For the nurse who's got a lot of . . . moxie."

My last assignment of the year was in the emergency room. With no care plans or charting, I figured it would be an absolute breeze: a day of watching a few bread knife lacerations being sutured, perhaps wrapping sprained ankles, and maybe culturing a sore throat or two.

I followed the red neon signs to the double blue doors marked "Emergency." In the waiting room the patients, mostly poor, mostly angry, sat staring at each other. The pneumatic doors swung open and hissed, urging me to move forward, into the world of on-the-spot medicine.

Just at the end of the black runner I stopped, overwhelmed by the turmoil and noise.

Separated by only a few feet of space and flimsy curtains, five gurneys plus one institutional crib were lined up side by side against the wall. Every available space was occupied. My eyes drawn to the color red, I saw a young woman on the farthest gurney from me lying with both her legs in cardboard splints and her face and arms crusted with blood. She was crying for someone named David and begging God to make everything go away. A paramedic was holding her hand, speaking to her, trying to get some kind of history.

The child in the crib was on its knees, hind end stuck in the air. Instead of crying, he was whining in a thin, continuous wail. A laboratory technician prepared the tubes to draw blood, while the mother stood next to the crib, arms crossed over her chest. "This is fucking ridiculous!" she yelled when she caught my eye. "Where the hell is the goddamned doctor? I need to get to work!"

The curtains were pulled around the gurney in the middle, labeled "Bed Three," but I could hear moaning. A tiny old woman, who muttered to herself as she worked, mopped the smears and specks of blood from the floor in front of the gurneys. A middle-aged man in a three-piece suit sat on the end of one of the gurneys watching her while he held an ice pack to his foot. He was smiling and shaking his head. Just why wasn't clear.

Bed three moaned again, retched, and cried in harmony with the baby's wail. An old man, lying on the gurney next to the crib, started from an apparent deep sleep and yelled out several times for a nurse. One of the float nurses tried to calm him, but he went on yelling despite her. The clerk, with her hand over one ear, answered the constantly ringing phones while two paramedics joked loudly over the noise. The sounds all blended into a song of human frailty.

Off to the sides of the main room flanking the clerk's desk, were two smaller rooms. The room, to the right, marked "Trauma," was closed, and the one to the left, marked "Minor Surgery—Suture,'' held two more gurneys, one of which was occupied. In the back, on the small table used by the staff to chart, two policemen were engrossed in filling out report forms.

Before I had a chance to move my feet, the trauma room door opened and a blond nurse appeared, looking as if she needed some assistance. When she saw me, she smiled and yelled to no one in particular, "The student is here. I'll have her help with the stab wound."

Hurrying over, she introduced herself as Katy Rankin and led me toward the suture room, speaking rapidly.

"Oh, boy, am I glad to see you! We are desperate for the extra help this morning. I've got the two floats, and it's still nuts down here. I don't know what the heck is going on around this county, but we've been going like crazy for the last two days. I think everybody and his brother have decided to hurt themselves.

"I'm sorry I don't have the time now, but if we slow down later, I'll show you where everything is. For right now you'll just have to search around until you find what the doc needs."

From the suture room doorway I saw an obese man lying face down on the gurney, muttering obscenities with a slurred Spanish accent. Using a pair of long surgical tweezers, a woman about my age sat on a rollaway stool, intently searching through the five-inch gash decorating the roll of extra flesh near the lower part of his back.

Katy gently shoved me into the room. "Here's someone to assist you if you need it, Doc. I've given ipecac to the overdose, and I'm still waiting for her to vomit." With that, she disappeared back into the trauma room.

The woman didn't look up from what she was doing, and for a moment I wondered if she was aware of my presence. I moved closer to the gurney. From the depths of the gash the woman extracted a jagged piece of green glass and held it up to the surgical lamp.

"Aha! Emerald treasures from the Isle of Fat," she said, smiling. The glare of the light whited out the lenses of her glasses so I could not see her eyes.

Dropping the piece of glass onto the white sterile sheet, she examined it carefully, turning it over a few times with the tweezers. "A gem of the cheap port variety, I believe."

It wasn't until I leaned closer for a better look that the woman noticed me.

"Oh, hello. I see by your uniform that you have chosen to pursue a career in the depressing and generally unrewarding profession of medicine. Since that qualifies you as being as maladjusted as the rest of us who work here, would you kindly, as your first task of the day, bring me another bottle of sterile saline so I might wash out the rest of the wine bottle from this distinguished guest of ours?"

Luckily the cabinet which held the saline stood right in front of me. I was reaching up for a bottle when the man, motivated by some internal unrest, turned over and rolled off the gurney. The tray of surgical instruments crashed to the floor.

The six-foot, 225-pound monster lumbered unsteadily toward the door, swearing in the guttural voice common to long time drunks. "Son of a bitch! I ain't takin' this bullshit from nobody no more. I'm gettin' out of here!"

The doctor, still holding the sterile tweezers, calmly rolled over to the door and placed herself in front of the man. "Come on, get back onto the gurney, big fella," she said wearily. "I'm not done with you yet."

The man took two more steps toward the door. "Git out of my way, bitch!"

She stood up and barred the door with her reedy five-foot-two-inch frame. "Back on the gurney, buster. I've got to fix you up before they'll take you in down at the jail. They'd prefer you didn't bleed all over their new sheets."

The man lunged at her and missed by two feet, hitting the wall headfirst.

Still maintaining the sterility of her gloves and tweezers, she glanced down at him while he scrambled, trying unsuccessfully to get on his feet.

"Are you absolutely sure you want to go into this field?" she asked me.

Before I could think of a good answer, she said, "Don't ever accuse me of not trying to discourage you," and walked out to the wall where the officers were still filling in their reports. She tapped one on the shoulder. "Excuse me, but our friend in there has become a bit animated. He needs to be handcuffed to the gurney before I can continue practicing the art of medicine on him. Would you be so kind?"

Discarding the no longer sterile gloves, she turned to me.
"Well, if we really sprang from apes, this guy's family were
lousy leapers." She took my hand and shook it vigorously.
"And now for formal introductions. I'm Dr. Mahoney, also
known as Susan or you might also hear me sometimes referred to as 'hey, shithead' or simply 'bitch.' I work in this
nut house. Who are you?"

When I told her my name, the standard look of disbelief
crossed her face. This was followed by the standard question:
"That's not really your name, is it?"

I gave the standard answer. "Yes, it is, and no, I did not
change it during the sixties."

Dr. Mahoney gave me the standard look of suspicion and
let it go. I was glad; it was too busy for me to go into the
rest of the standard answer, which involved the story about
my sister, Storm.

"Okay, Reverberation, as soon as this charming fellow is
securely handcuffed, I'll irrigate him, and then I'd like you
to bring him over to x-ray to check for any more surprise
packages his drinking buddy may have left inside him. He's
lucky he's fat and the other guy was too drunk to find another
empty bottle."

Dr. Mahoney sighed. "Not that he's long for this world
anyway. He has the body of a seventy-five-year-old who's
acutely ill. He is, in fact, only thirty-five, been doing drugs
and booze since he was nine.

"They drag him in off the streets once every few weeks.
His liver is shot, and the rest of him is so screwed up I don't
know why we bother. I wish he'd just do it up big and get it
over with someday. I'm tired of dealing with him."

My face had a habit of betraying everything I felt, and Dr.
Mahoney read the shock clearly.

"Oh, don't listen to me," she said. "I've been up all night,
and I have to come back tomorrow. I'm exhausted and on the
edge of a nervous breakdown, that's all; it's nothing unusual."

I watched her move away from the counter, talking to herself. "Okay, first I'll irrigate this guy, then get to the crib.
After that it's the motorcycle accident, then the OD in the
trauma room. Menowitz can take care of the minor stuff when
he gets here." Turning, she yelled out to the clerk, "Irene,
see if you can find out what's taking Menowitz so long to get

here. If you find him, tell him to hurry up. I'm swamped. I need relief before I go out of my—''

Red-faced with anger, the mother of the child in the crib approached Dr. Mahoney. The noise suddenly abated. All eyes were on the two women in the middle of the room, and there was a clear sense of impending trouble. "I've been waiting two hours and forty minutes for someone to tell me what's wrong with my child," the woman yelled. "What kind of place is this? I'll tell you right now, I'll never come here again. This is absurd. Why can't you hurry? I'm going to be late for work and I can't—''

Dr. Mahoney took the woman's hand and spoke kindly. "I don't blame you, but I'm going as fast as I can. Try to be patient for a little while longer. Another doctor will be here soon to help out.''

There was a pause before the woman exhaled and let her body relax out of the defensive stance. "Look, I don't want to cause trouble, I just want to get out of here. It's driving me crazy, all this noise.''

"I know, and I'm sorry, but that's the way it is here. If you want to take a break and go for a walk around the lobby, that's fine.'' Dr. Mahoney held up her hands and made an announcement to the room. "I'll get to every one of you. Poor babies, I know you're sick or hurt, but it's been a long haul this morning. Forgive me.''

Turning, Dr. Mahoney indicated she needed me to help her in the suture room again. I noticed much of the tension had disappeared; even the moaning had stopped from bed three.

Almost an hour had passed when I returned from x-ray with the glass-free but still unsewn man. The main room had now taken on another, completely different face; all but two of the gurneys were empty, and the room was almost silent.

The overdose had been moved from the trauma room to bed two, had vomited up most of her pills, and replaced them with a glass of our liquid charcoal. Tearfully she told her tale to the worker from the crisis unit: She was so alone, and the attempt was, she sobbed, a cry for help, a need for attention, a plea for someone to notice. The message through her words said, "Please, somebody, love me. Love me, because it's too hard to love myself.''

I watched Katy and another nurse help the woman dress.

There was little compassion and a great deal of impatience. They treated her as if she had done something wrong and shameful. I wondered, were our lives so charmed on this other side of the stage that we could afford to be so callous? If the woman had had a sprained ankle, I was sure she would have been treated differently, with more respect. But she'd done something socially unacceptable and was being treated accordingly.

My illusion that all people were created equal in the eyes of the medical world shattered, and the broken pieces were added to my pile of other defunct fantasies.

Bed five was taken by a nose versus baseball bat victim. I observed that the short, red-haired man prodding the painful proboscis was definitely not Dr. Mahoney. He could, however, very easily have been Harpo Marx.

Katy finished discharging her overdose to the care of the crisis people and led me into the trauma room. "This is where we see our critical patients. Codes or anybody who looks like they might start going down the tubes are automatically brought in here.

"You have to develop an eye for the people who need to be in this room. I've seen people walk in off the street, looking maybe just a little off, complaining of some minor problem, and before I even had them undressed, they've gone out on me."

There was only one gurney in the room. "What happens if there are two codes at the same time?" I asked.

"Good question. Two days ago we had an eight-year-old boy and his mother in the main room side by side. They had been in a one-car accident, and on cursory exam we thought they were okay.

"Meanwhile, in here we were working on a twenty-six-year-old woman contractor who fell from the roof of a house and landed on her head. She came in from the field in full arrest." Katy backed into the gurney and sat down. "So anyway, Susan was running the code in here when all of a sudden the mother of this eight-year-old starts screaming that her son is sick. When I went out to check, the boy was in full arrest. I think we pulled every available doc that was in the house at the time."

Goose bumps covered my arms just imagining the chaos. "And?"

"The lady who fell off the roof didn't make it, but the young boy did. He's still in ICU, hanging in there like an old trooper."

The red-haired man walked into the trauma room and threw a patient chart onto the gurney. It landed a couple of inches away from Katy.

"This isn't the place for personal conversations," he said dispassionately. "I want bed five taken over to x-ray for facial bones, and I'll need some assistance with the stab wound in the suture room when you come back."

Katy flared. "It isn't a personal conversation, Dr. Menowitz," she said to his back. "And have you ever heard the word *please*?"

He ignored her and sat down at the small bit of walled-off counter space which served as the doctors' desk.

Katy gritted her teeth. "Oooooh! I hate it when he treats us like that! It's hard enough working here without that attitude."

"Who is that, and where's Dr. Mahoney?"

"That friendly guy is Dr. Morton Menowitz. He came on duty just after you went to x-ray. He's Dr. Mahoney's relief."

I was disappointed. Not only was Dr. Mahoney friendlier, but she provided some comic relief. Dr. Menowitz looked as if he needed a good laxative.

Katy looked at the expression on my face and laughed. "Not that I should talk, but don't let him get to you. He definitely has his quirks, but they all do, you know," Katy whispered to me. "You just have to work with them long enough to know what they like or don't like."

"What's this guy's problem area?" I asked. "I definitely don't want to tread on his quirk."

"Dr. Menowitz has a need to feel like he's the one in charge. He has a bad case of what we refer to as the 'hey, boy' attitude."

"The 'hey, boy' attitude?"

"Oh, you know that syndrome by now, don't you?" Katy walked toward bed five. "Like when a doctor starts with the do-this-do-that-chop-chop-bend-over-and-give-my-ass-a-kiss-don't-forget-I'm-the-doctor-and-you're-the-handmaiden kind of attitude."

"Oh, yeah, *that* attitude," I said, rubbing my chin, "the one involving the fragile ego."

"*Very* fragile, but under it all, especially when he's in a good mood, he's okay. Just let him know when he's over-stepped his bounds, and he usually backs off."

"No, that's okay, Katy, I'd prefer not to, thanks. Remember, I'm just a student, and he's God. He probably takes nursing students home, varnishes them in his garage, and uses them for coffee tables."

Until Katy returned from x-ray, I successfully avoided Dr. Menowitz by looking through all the cabinets, trying to memorize where everything was kept. Speed was the essential ingredient to working in ER, and the most speed came from knowing exactly where to find everything from a sterile specimen cup to the pacemaker cabinet.

After the drunken stab wound had been signed out to the police, and the broken nose sent home, Katy took me into another side room used for the gynecology-obstetrics cases. She was demonstrating some of the unusual contortions the pelvic exam table was capable of when the county radio suddenly came to life with a squawk of static and several different-pitched tones.

Katy picked up the receiver. "This is Redwood Base, MICN Rankin, go ahead."

A small masculine voice came from the radio. "Redwood Base, this is ambulance twenty-five. We are en route to your facility code two. On board we have a fourteen-year-old male in moderate distress. How do you copy?"

Katy pressed the transmitter button on the mike. "Copy ten-two. Go ahead, ambulance twenty-five."

"Patient's mother states he had a syncopal episode about thirty minutes ago. At this time patient is pale and tremulous. His skin is dry and warm. No lumps, bumps, cuts, or bruises found. BP is eighty over sixty; pulse is one-ten. Respirations are twenty-four with normal effort. Patient has no other history of syncope, takes no meds, and has no allergies. He's alert and oriented. Do you request any further information, Redwoods?"

The voice was replaced by static until Katy pressed the transmitter button. "What is your ETA, twenty-five?"

Static waved again. "We're at your back door now."

"Ten-four, twenty-five, see you in a second. This is KMMS six forty-seven clear."

Dr. Menowitz rolled his chair around to the radio. "Probably just another overhysterical mother making her contribution to the ambulance company fund," he said dryly.

Ignoring him, Katy directed me over to bed one. "Let's put this kid here. I'm going to have you be the nurse on this case. Do you feel comfortable with that?"

"Sure," I said, "if Dr. Menowitz tries to bite me, I'll let you know."

The hissing sound of the automatic doors heralded the arrival of two uniformed ambulance drivers pushing a stretcher.

The boy was lying flat, trembling. As soon as he slid off the stretcher onto the bed, I rumpled up his short black hair and touched the white skin of his cheek, gathering data as I went along. So far, he'd transferred himself with no motor weakness or balance malfunction; his grips on the side rails were equal and strong. His skin was pale, cool, and moist.

"Hi, what's your name?" I asked.

The boy's teeth were chattering, and his eyes were closed. "Tony Hamilton," he answered in a cracking halfway-to-manhood voice.

"How're you feeling, Tony?"

"Okay, 'cept a headache."

"Headache, huh? Show me where it hurts on your head."

He locked his fingers and, starting at his forehead, slid his hands over the top of his head and stopped at the nape of his neck. He covered his closed eyes with his hands. "All over. It hurts all over."

"Why are you shaking?"

"I dunno. I'm cold, I think. I don't know for sure. My head hurts real bad."

"Do you know where you are?"

He still wouldn't open his eyes. "Yeah, the hospital."

"Okay, we're coming in for the finish now, Tony. Can you tell me the time, and do you know what day of the week this is?"

"I guess it's Tuesday, about nine-thirty. I've got to be at a math final in a half an hour."

"Right again, but forget about your final for now. You can make it up later. Now, if you answer this next one right, you get the prize."

I reached into my pocket and pulled out Simon's pocket present of the day.

His habit of sneaking little surprises into the deep hidden

pocket of my uniform had started a few weeks after school began. Every morning, just before we left for the sitter's he'd make me close my eyes while he wiggled his hand all the way to the bottom of the pocket and deposited his goody. His variety of gifts ranged from pieces of gum or candy to not so little toy trucks. He promised me they all were guaranteed to bring good luck. Today he'd left me a plastic replica of Bullwinkle the Moose.

"Now, Tony, for one thousand dollars in Monopoly money, who's this?"

The curtains of thick black lashes slowly parted, and a pair of dark brown eyes stared first at the little plastic toy and then up at me as if I were crazy.

The pupils were equal and reactive to light.

"Huh?"

"I said, who is this?" I held the toy closer to him. "It's very important that you answer me correctly." I didn't smile.

"It's a plastic Bullwinkle."

Oriented to person, place, time, and thing.

I got a warm blanket from the warmer and covered him, then took his blood pressure: 90 over 50. Heart rate 100. Respirations 20. Temperature 98.1. Nothing remarkable.

When Tony's mother arrived, I brought her back to sit with him. She was concerned, but down-to-earth and reasonable; not the type to overreact.

"Tony got up at his usual time this morning and took his shower," she began. "When he got downstairs, I had his breakfast ready for him, but he said he had a headache and felt sick to his stomach."

She sat down on the gurney, and the boy curled his hand next to her thigh. He was just close enough to her to have comfort from her presence without betraying his oncoming manhood.

"I suggested he stay home, but he refused. He said he had two finals today and couldn't miss them. He's been studying so hard I didn't insist."

She looked over her son's face with concern.

"He'd gone upstairs to take some aspirin for his headache when I heard a crash. I found him passed out cold on the bathroom floor. He was white as a sheet.

"He came to right away and said his head hurt. He looked so pale I called the ambulance. I feel silly now."

"You shouldn't feel that way. I think most mothers would have done exactly what you did. I'll ask Dr. Menowitz to take a look at him. Hold on."

Dr. Menowitz was sitting behind the small room divider at his counter space, writing instructions on the chart of a patient with a badly sprained wrist.

Smiling, I had started to put the chart down on the counter when the man shot me a hostile look that would have frozen flames. I forgot about any introductions and shrank back from the hard face, totally intimidated.

"The fourteen-year-old boy who fainted is on bed one. His mom is with him. He's pretty pale and complaining of a severe headache."

Dr. Menowitz sighed impatiently before I could continue. "Is this an emergency?"

I wasn't sure how to answer the question. "Well, no, I mean, he's having pain, he's—I don't know, his mother is—"

"If he isn't in need of my immediate attention, tag the chart and put it in bed one's slot. I'll get to him when it's his turn."

He waved the chart away with a flick of his wrist.

At the clerk's desk a container of three different-colored plastic strips sat next to the chart rack.

The clerk, a matronly-looking woman named Irene, patted my arm and whispered, "Don't let the jerk get to you. He isn't worth it." She picked out a red strip and explained how to tag the charts.

A red strip indicated the nurses had evaluated the patient, taken his vital signs, and set up any equipment that might be necessary.

The chart was blue-tagged by the doctor when the patient was ready for discharge or needed something like a medication or a dressing. A yellow tag alerted the clerk to orders for lab work or x-rays.

Uncomfortably aware of the boy's pain left unattended, I put a red tag on the chart and put it in the slot. It was the only one in the rack.

Katy called me into the suture room to help her apply a plaster splint to the sprained wrist. I was holding the setting splint when Dr. Menowitz stormed in and threw the red-tagged chart onto the plaster cart. "I'd like to know how the hell I'm supposed to examine the patient while he's still in his clothes!'' he yelled at Katy.

"Dr. Menowitz, I'm the one who signed him in," I said sheepishly.

Ignoring my admission of guilt, Menowitz continued to address Katy. "Why is it we can't have qualified help in this department? Why do I have to put up with incompetents like this?" He jerked his thumb in my direction.

The elderly patient whose splint was rapidly drying under my hand, stared at the floor, embarrassed by the doctor's display of anger.

"Get this patient properly readied for me," he ordered.

My anger, like a tidal wave, choked me. The thought that the boy would have to wait another ten minutes for the pompous Dr. Menowitz drove me to the point of wanting to scream.

"Ooops." Katy put her hand over her mouth. "I forgot to tell you to fully undress the boy." She started out of the room. "You stay here and I'll help the kid get into an exam gown."

I handed her the splinted wrist. "No, Katy, let me do it. I want to finish taking care of Tony, and I don't want to back down from this Dr. Menowitz asshole."

"Okay." Katy shrugged. "Have it your way." She made it sound like a warning.

Tony was still holding his head. His mother pointed to an emesis basin half-filled with greenish bile.

Not wanting to disturb him, I touched his shoulder lightly. "Tony, I've got to get you into a gown before the doctor can examine you."

Stoically, Tony sat up, and his mother helped him undress. When I slipped the gown over his thin shoulders, he threw up over the front of my uniform. Ashamed, he hid his face and cried. I tried to reassure him, but he was too sick to care.

I cleaned myself off and took the chart to Dr. Menowitz. "Bed one is in a gown."

He sighed. "Are you hard-of-hearing, or do you just have a poor memory?" Condescension iced his voice. "I told you to put the chart in the slot."

"But you wanted the patient in a gown," I protested. "I thought you were ready to see him."

Morton Menowitz swiveled in his chair and picked up the phone.

I stared at the red, curly hairs on the back of his neck and tried to imagine how anyone could love such a man. At some time he must have had a mother and a father who loved him . . . maybe.

His level of arrogance made me want to hurl obscenities. Instead, I went to the bathroom and pounded the sink with my fist.

When I returned, Dr. Menowitz had examined Tony and ordered a number of basic blood tests. I found Menowitz in the suture room, removing a crimson handkerchief from the hand of a twenty-nine-year-old carpenter who'd partially severed the tips of two fingers with a Skil Saw.

The patient and I smiled at each other.

"I see you did a great job on those fingers," I said.

"Yeah." The man laughed. "I've heard this emergency room is famous for its embroidery. I thought I'd give it a try."

Dr. Menowitz turned around and fixed me with one of his Antarctic specials. "Do you mind? I don't think we need an audience for this."

The man, not noticing the tension, interrupted. "Oh, I don't mind if she's here. She can distract me while you're sewing me up, Doc."

Menowitz made a face as if he were sucking on lemons. "I *do* mind, however." He looked over my head, his eyes searching the main room.

"Miss Rankin! Come in here. I need some help with this thumb."

Katy stuck her head around the corner. "Sorry, Dr. Menowitz, but I'm helping hold the boy for his blood work, and the float is at lunch. The student is right there. She can help you."

Menowitz sighed. It was the kind of stage sigh drama students often overdo. "Bring me some seven and a half gloves, and one percent Xylocaine plain, and I'll want some five-O prolene with the small needle."

I remembered where the gloves were; the Xylocaine I had to search for but, after four wrong drawers, found it on top of the syringe cabinet; as for the 5-0 prolene, I had no idea what it was, let alone where to find it.

Too intimidated to ask for directions, I searched for anything that said "5-0 prolene," going from cabinet to shelf to boxes on the floor.

Menowitz sat back and dramatically drummed his fingers on the aluminum suture tray. He let me go on for a few minutes while he milked the scene for everything it was worth.

"What *are* you doing?" he asked finally.

"I'm looking for the five-O prolene. I can't find it."

Menowitz took off his exam gloves and threw them on the floor. The guy was a regular Camille.

He pushed me out of his way and stalked to the far wall cabinet where the suture material was held. There, in the center of the cabinet, was a small drawer marked "5-0 prolene" in tiny silver letters you needed good eyes or a magnifying glass to read.

Pulling out a couple of packets, he started a mumbled monologue it didn't take any straining of the ears to hear. "Goddamned incompetent moron . . ."

With that not only had Dr. Menowitz found the 5-0 prolene, but he'd found the end of my rope. My head cocked to one side, I walked stiffly out of the room.

On the other side of the door, I started counting to ten.

Katy walked by and stopped in her tracks. "Jeez, what's the matter with you? You look totally—"

Menowitz charged out of the door at my count of five. Working the muscles of his jaw, he looked like Mickey Rooney in a fit of rage. "How dare you walk out in the middle of a surgical procedure? I ought to report you to your instructor. I won't tolerate—"

I cut him off at the pass. Dr. Menowitz didn't know it, but he was about to get a firsthand look at a newly developed part of my psyche. Under my mother's harsh rule, expressing anger and defending myself were among the top-ranked offenses. Brutally punished for any infraction of those laws, I'd spent years beating therapists' couch pillows and reading self-help books on repressed anger.

Although I regressed occasionally, I was making headway by at least being able to recognize my anger . . . and my fear of it. Little by little I'd started setting limits and tried to assert myself as constructively as possible. I'd let Dr. Menowitz tread too long.

"Don't talk to me in that tone of voice, Dr. Menowitz, and don't use that language in front of me or a patient again. Who do you think you are? I'm a human being, and I expect to be treated like one. This is a teaching hospital for student nurses, and I am trying to learn; but you've insulted me in front of not only Katy but several patients as well, and I don't have to take that."

I lowered my voice, trying to reach the balance between assertiveness and aggression. "I've done nothing wrong, and the only person who needs to be written up is you. You're a physician, someone who is supposed to act with dignity."

I stepped back.

Dr. Menowitz opened and closed his mouth, but nothing came out. I focused on two moles at the corner of his left eye and held my ground, waiting for a reply. Nothing came, but he did find his legs and stomped back into the suture room.

Feeling as if I were getting back on a horse after it had bucked me off, I followed him and handed him another package of sterile gloves.

He hesitated before taking them, but when he did, he said "thank you" for the first time since I'd laid eyes on him.

I was puzzled when the results of Tony's lab tests were all within normal ranges, but Dr. Menowitz seemed unimpressed. Tony's mother stood up expectantly when Dr. Menowitz stepped over to the gurney.

"Well, your son's blood work is normal, and with the exception of his headache, Tony appears to be in good shape. Neurologically I can't see any deficits. He may have picked up a virus, or he may be nervous about finals; all those things could bring on the headache and nausea. I don't think it's anything to worry about."

Mrs. Hamilton's eyes lit up with relief. "Oh, thank God! Isn't that great, Tony?"

Tony kept his hands over his eyes and didn't respond.

"Should I keep him home from school for a few days?"

"He can go back to school whenever he feels better," Dr. Menowitz said. As he passed me, he added under his breath, "Or as soon as finals are over."

Dr. Menowitz made a hasty note on the chart and handed it to me. "You can have him get dressed to go now." He smirked. "Please?"

Under the "patient instructions," I read: "Rest. Diet as

...rated. Return to normal activity as tolerated. Aspirin or analgesic of choice for headache.''

Under "diagnosis" he'd written: "Acute adolescent anxiety reaction to academic stress."

I carried the chart over to bed one and quietly drew back a corner of the curtain. Tony had not moved, and Mrs. Hamilton was tenderly urging him to sit up.

I stood back and regarded the boy. Somewhere along the course of the year, while the foundation was being set, each one of the students was unknowingly involved in the process of finding her own special talent. For some it was having the knack to deal with children; some took to surgery; others did well as leaders. Janey, with her quick and highly organized thought process, was a great diagnostician. She could look at a patient's laboratory values, fit it all together like a jigsaw puzzle, and come up with the right diagnosis and treatment without ever seeing the patient in the flesh.

For me, numbers and data on report slips were useful guides, but they didn't keep up with the inconsistencies of the human body. My special knack came in the form of a sixth sense for recognizing trouble before it showed itself.

I turned on my heel and went to Dr. Menowitz's desk. He did not look at me but stopped writing. "Don't tell me you have more to add to your flowing description of my faults?"

I laughed, although Katy, who was eating her lunch, put down her fork, ready for another confrontation.

"No, but I don't feel comfortable with your diagnosis of the Hamilton boy."

Dr. Menowitz sat back in his chair and crossed his arms over his chest regarding me with what I thought looked like mild amusement. "Really? What is it that you find 'discomforting,' Miss . . . ?"

"Heron."

"Miss Heron?"

"Well, this boy just doesn't seem like a kid who would get that upset over finals. His mom says he's an A student."

Dr. Menowitz smiled wisely. "All the more reason for him to be stressed. He's a budding type A personality, Miss Heron. This type usually experiences migraines, ulcers, and other problems associated with highly strung individuals."

If my ulcer could have laughed, it would have.

"I still don't agree. The boy doesn't have the obsessive

rigidity of the type A. I'm only guessing, but I think there's something wrong, and don't forget, he did have a syncopal episode."

"And what would you like me to do, Miss Heron?"

The cold, sarcastic edge was creeping back into his voice, and I looked furtively over at Katy, who now sat with her head in her hands, staring at her tray.

"Well, how about calling in a neurologist?" I suggested, not sure how I felt about another confrontation so soon after the last one.

Dr. Menowitz took the suggestion better than I thought he would.

"He's not going to find anything more than I did, which is nothing. The family history is negative for syncope, migraines, or any other neurological problems. Vital signs are good; blood work is normal; there's no evidence of trauma; all his neurological reflexes are intact. What do you think I missed?"

"I don't know enough about neurology to answer that, but my intuition is telling me something's wrong."

I saw the you-must-be-kidding look start in one eye and spread across his face. "I know that sounds like a soothsayer speaking, but I listen to my intuition when it sounds off. It's pretty accurate."

Menowitz placed his elbows on top of his counter space and covered his face with his hands, the same way Katy had. I looked at both of them. So much for first impressions, I thought.

"Clerk! Get Dr. Schupbach on the phone," he yelled through his hands. "Dr. Schupbach is one of our better neurologists." He peeked through his fingers. "Is your intuition happy now, Miss Heron?"

"Well, it's very much relieved. Thanks a lot, Dr. Menowitz."

"Don't thank me, Miss Heron. Just tell me how much longer I have to be subjected to your intuition?"

Katy hastily answered for me. "She's here until three P.M. today and tomorrow."

Menowitz picked up his pen and resumed writing. "Whew! I'm off tomorrow! Thank God for small favors."

Dr. Schupbach showed up thirty minutes later to examine Tony. While I eagerly awaited the outcome, we treated an embedded tick's head, a grease burn, a minor motorcycle accident with a fractured collarbone, and a second overdose.

Dr. Schupbach came out from behind the curtain and approached the desk. "I'm going to order a CAT scan for this kid," he said writing the order on the chart. "I've got a feeling something isn't right somewhere."

Dr. Menowitz whipped around and stared at me. "Tell the truth, Miss Heron. Did you bribe this man?"

I held my hand over my heart. "I swear I did not."

Menowitz shook his head and almost laughed. "Jesus! I'm working with a bunch of crackpot psychics. I can't even trust my own colleagues."

Dr. Schupbach looked at me for an explanation.

I shrugged. "Private joke."

At 2:50, I wheeled Tony over to the scanner on my way to postconference and wished him luck. Into his hand I pressed the plastic Bullwinkle. "It's an incredible good-luck charm," I said seriously, "personally blessed and given to me by St. Simon." Tony again looked at me as if I'd lost my mind. "Never mind. Just hold on to it."

In conference, Pearson completely ignored my experience with Tony and Dr. Menowitz and wanted to concentrate on how we had treated the embedded tick's head. For Pearson, that was par for the course.

That evening I made a real dinner for Simon: green salad, roast chicken, mashed potatoes with the skins left on, fresh vegetables, and, for dessert, his favorite, French toast smothered in real Vermont maple syrup.

While we ate, I told him all the stories about the patients we'd seen and was glad to see he was fascinated. He wanted to know how we sewed the man's fingers back on, and did it hurt, and just exactly what was the magic medicine made out of. We got into deeper discussions about the lady who took too many pills and the safety of motorcycles, but what made me laugh was having to tell Simon the tick story six times before he'd go to sleep.

In contrast with the previous morning, the ER was almost deserted. Dr. Bell was removing a mole from a young woman's leg as an outpatient procedure, and Dr. Mahoney was just examining an early-morning commuter whiplash.

Katy welcomed me warmly. "You should have been here yesterday when the Hamilton boy came back from the scanner."

"Oh?" I said. My stomach tightened.

"The scan showed a small bleed into the ventricles. He'd blown one of the vessels in the back of his brain. Dr. Schupbach had him in surgery before five P.M. He came in this morning to tell us Tony's upstairs in ICU, doing great. I don't know what tipped you off, but you hit it right.

"I couldn't believe Menowitz went along with you. He was flabbergasted. You're in with him now; he even asked me what your first name was, and as far as I know, Menowitz hasn't called anybody by a first name in years."

Dr. Mahoney came around to the back and collapsed into a chair. "Oh, shades of silence and peace. The crazed mobs of injured are at bay." She pushed her straight ash brown hair from her face with a blue plastic headband.

"Good morning, Echo-in-the-Mountains." Behind her hand she spoke to Katy in a stage whisper. "The fledgling masochist is back for more."

I sat down and shook my head. "Listen, you guys, I like ER, I really do. The nurses here move a little closer to the physician's role and out of the second-class-citizen mode. You get results right away and get to see the patients walk out. On the floors you can wait six months, and sometimes you never get results. It's fast; you have to know a little bit about everything." I looked inquiringly at Dr. Mahoney. "Why don't you like it?"

"Not so fast, Sound Wave. Your assumption is erroneous. I *do* like it. I'd even go so far as to say I love it, I wouldn't do any other kind of work, but when you do it every day, and over and over again you see the same crocks who take time away from the people who really need it, you have a tendency to become bitter." She stopped just long enough to take a breath.

"And don't forget the overabundance of enchanted wealthy in this county who demand you drop everything to cater to them.

"Two days ago a woman whose husband makes a seven-figure salary came in here while we were in the middle of a code and demanded I leave the code and tend to her cut finger so she could make it on time to her tennis date."

She shook her head, "Do you know what that does to your belief in humanity? Or if that doesn't do it for you, try dealing with the same junkies ODing every other day. We try to keep them alive, and when we do save them, all they do is curse you out because you've ruined their highs. I even had one come in in full arrest, and after we brought him back, he signed out against medical advice, waited for me in the parking lot and then robbed me when I got off duty."

She paused. "And that's not all. Two weeks later the same guy came in in full arrest, and I had to save him all over again."

Dr. Mahoney laughed and wagged her finger at me. "Honey, let me tell you, it ain't easy. Keeping a sense of humor is the one thing that keeps me going. Everybody in this business has to have some way to release, or you'll go crazy . . . or, even worse, end up like Menowitz."

"Ah, don't let her scare you, Ec," said Katy stepping in. "Don't overlook what keeps us here."

I waited for the secret words to be dropped.

"It's the excitement, you know. Everybody ends up getting addicted to the constant state of crisis. It's a rush never knowing what's coming through the doors next. I've been working ER for eight years, and I could never go back to working on the floors. That would be like moving from New York City to Silent Springs, Utah, population twenty-four."

Irene walked back and honored me by placing a new chart in my hands. I read the complaint aloud: "Patient states stomach refuses to communicate with him."

"Now that's what I call real rush material, Katy," I said.

Dr. Mahoney took the chart and reread the complaint.

"You know," she said, "just this morning I found myself half-asleep, staring at the cereal, waiting for it to give me the promised get-up-and-go. I woke up fifteen minutes later with my head in the bowl, breathing milk. If this is an omen of what the rest of the day is going to be like, I think I should have stayed in the bowl."

The old black man, wearing one shoe for comfort, and one for a rainy day, shuffled at his own pace into the space of bed four.

Orville Robinson was eighty-four years old, though he looked at least twenty years younger.

"Sit right up here on this gurney, Mr. Robinson, and let me take your blood pressure and pulse."

Mr. Robinson hoisted his skinny body onto the gurney. " 'Taint got no bad heart, missy. It's my stomach dat's ailin' me."

Instantly I liked the man. The sound of his southern, bumpy voice and the smell of strong coffee on his breath brought me back to my brief searching time of riding the rails. He was so like the hobos who'd kept me from harm and entertained me with achingly good stories Edgar Allan Poe and Erma Bombeck might have envied.

"Mr. Robinson, this is what we do to everybody that comes in here."

With raised eyebrows I told him his blood pressure was 200 over 110.

"Dat's 'cause my stomach quit talkin' to me. I told you dat, missy."

"Exactly what do you mean, 'quit talkin',' Mr. Robinson?"

"Well, it jest stopped callin' up for somethin' couple of days ago."

"Callin' up?"

"Yep. Like, say, if my stomach called up for greens, I et greens. If it called up for ribs, I et ribs. See, dat way me and my stomach, we stayed friends. It never gave me no trouble till now."

"Okay, Orville, I got it now. Maybe I can get Dr. Mahoney to see if she can talk to your stomach. How's that?"

"My stomach says dat sound fine, missy."

Mr. Robinson was a character I would have liked to sit down with for a long conversation, but when I red-tagged his chart, I found three more charts of patients waiting to be brought back.

That, I discovered, was the weak link in working ER. There was no time to spend with the people you treated. The contact we had was intimate but brief. We never saw them again unless they were repeaters.

Katy brought back a swollen bee sting, while I escorted in an acute asthma attack and a dog bite to the face. Katy topped those with bringing in a human bite to the buttocks, and Dr. Mahoney's picks included a thirty-eight-year-old bag lady who hadn't taken her rubber rain boots off in four months and a hallucinating twenty-two-year-old PCP overdose who broke three of his teeth biting the brass buckles on the four-point leather restraints that just barely held him down on the gurney.

Between the choking stench of moldy feet and the terrified ravings about stalking giants that looked like Nixon, it was hard to choose which one should win the grand prize.

By noon the main room was quiet again. I never did get to talk to Mr. Robinson again but saw that he'd been admitted with a diagnosis of "stomach mass; rule out malignant tumor." The dog bite and the human bite were referred to a plastic surgeon, and both of Dr. Mahoney's prizes were admitted to Unit D, the psycho ward.

"We've been awarded a break for lunch by the controller of emergency traffic in the sky," said Dr. Mahoney while all three of us crowded around the sink, scrubbing our hands.

"I am so tired I think I'm going to spend my lunch break on bed one taking a nap," said Katy.

Dr. Mahoney interrupted. "Listen, girls, by the time three o'clock rolls around we're going to—"

We all stopped and listened. In the distance beyond the doors we heard a screeching wail. No one moved until a shrill buzz caused all of us to jump as if we'd hit a bump.

The room surged with the electricity of our adrenaline.

Katy and Dr. Mahoney flew in different directions. Katy went for the doors; Dr. Mahoney to the trauma room. Only Irene sat, unmoving, her hand on the phone.

"What's going on?" I asked, totally bewildered.

Irene answered me without turning around. Her eyes were riveted on the automatic doors. "A single buzz means a nurse is needed in the lobby to triage simple problems like lacerations or sprains. A double buzz means all hell has broken loose and is headed this way."

I started for the double doors. Passing the main door to the trauma room, I saw Dr. Mahoney in a plastic apron, switching on all the lights.

Just as the toe of my nursing shoe hit the black runner of the doors, Katy charged in, holding a bundle wrapped in a red-checked tablecloth.

A disheveled-looking woman clawed at Katy's back, screaming. As soon as she saw me, she let go of Katy's uniform and fell to her knees, bawling helplessly. I bent down next to her, held her hands, and told her not to worry, it would be okay.

From the trauma room Katy yelled to Irene. "Call a house code! Stat! And get a pediatrician down here!"

Irene picked up the phone, and the overhead house speakers belched out the page: "Attention, all personnel. Code blue, emergency room. Any pediatrician to the emergency room, stat!"

No sooner had she replaced the phone than the pneumatic doors hissed and a herd of lab and respiratory techs rushed in past us. A second later a pediatrician, his tie flying behind him like a wind-direction ribbon, ran in the side door and slid on smooth-soled shoes the last five feet into the trauma room. The heavy door shut with a final bang.

Pregnant and out of breath, the supervisor nurse was the last one to arrive. She helped the whimpering, crying woman out the side door toward the quiet room.

I opened the trauma room door a crack and slipped in.

Concentrated around the gurney, there existed a state of well-ordered pandemonium. All I could see of the patient was a small hand with water-wrinkled fingers and a bit of wet, matted blond hair around a child's shoulder. My heart sank; the hand was almost the same size as Simon's.

Dr. Mahoney was tense but in control. As she tried to intubate the child with the smallest endotracheal tube I had ever seen, there was absolutely no sign of the wise-cracking comedienne who had been so entertaining only a few moments ago. The respiratory tech stood by, holding a breathing bag no bigger than his fist. The pediatrician was inserting an IV, while Katy did CPR, her eyes glued to the monitor.

"Stop CPR!" Dr. Mahoney commanded. All eyes went to the monitor. There was absolute silence as the straight line continued to cut the screen in half.

She placed her stethoscope on the child's chest and listened for equal lung sounds as the respiratory tech pushed puffs of air into the child's lungs through the endotracheal tube.

"Okay. Resume CPR, Katy. Lab, get a blood gas if you can." Dr. Mahoney checked the child's pupils and addressed the room in general: "Fixed and dilated. This isn't looking like a happy ending, folks."

She noticed the number of extra people in the room and

sternly ordered anybody who didn't have a specific job to do to leave the room.

I had turned to go when she called to me. "Echo, Katy got a little information from the neighbor boy, but try to find out the details of what happened from the mother, specifically how long the child was under."

Irene provided me with a last name for the child's mother, and I headed toward the quiet room.

The quiet room was the hospital's answer to a chapel. I figured it must have been one of the administration's afterthoughts because it looked as if it might once have been a storage closet. It was just big enough to hold a love seat and a chair. The side table was the resting place for a Gideons Bible and a depressing white lamp designed to look like a large pineapple. The giant photographlike wallpaper depicted a sunny forest setting with a dirt path running through the middle.

I think the idea was if you wanted to forget your troubles, all you had to do was mentally step into the picture and run away.

This idea was lost on Mrs. Hughes. The distraught woman stared wide-eyed at the orange-carpeted floor. The supervisor sat with her, trying to talk her into taking a cup of tea. The child's mother wasn't listening.

As soon as I walked into the room, Mrs. Hughes stood. "What's wrong with my baby? I want to know what you're doing to her." Her voice rose to a hoarse scream. "I want to see Amy. Is she crying for me? Tell me! Tell me! I've got to see her. I'm going in to see her."

In her hysteria she pushed past me, toward the door. I grabbed her shoulders, and the supervisor took her by the waist. Together we guided her back to the couch. I put an arm around her shoulder. She was trembling.

I thought that if for just a split second I changed places with the woman, it would help me say just the right words, the ones I'd want to hear.

I closed my eyes and saw Simon's hand instead of Amy's. My guts turned inside out.

The only "right" words were "Your daughter is fine"; anything else was torture.

"You can't see Amy yet, Mrs. Hughes. The doctors and nurses are still"—I almost said "working on her" and cen-

sored the harshness of the phrase—"are still trying very hard
to help her." The woman twisted the hem of her skirt and
rocked back and forth whispering in anxious repetition, "Oh,
God, oh, God, oh, God, oh—"

"Mrs. Hughes, I know this is very hard, but you have to
tell me what happened. The doctors need to know so they
can help Amy better."

The supervisor noiselessly left the room.

Mrs. Hughes continued to hug herself and rock. About five
or six minutes passed. Suddenly she straightened her back
and spoke in a clear, calm voice.

"I put Amy down for a nap about ten this morning and
went into the living room to take a nap myself. We'd been up
since six-thirty, so we both were tired. I woke up at eleven
and made some soup and sandwiches for Amy's lunch. When
Amy still hadn't gotten up by eleven-thirty, I went in to check
on her. That's when I saw she wasn't in her bed.

"I started looking through the house, calling her. Sometimes she likes to play hide-and-seek with me; but the house
seemed too quiet, and she didn't answer. I think that's when
I started to panic. The next door neighbor's boy heard me
yelling and came over to help search for her.

"I was going through the closet in our bedroom when I
thought about the pool. She has no fear of water, you know,
so we built a fence around it with a double lock on the gate.
I'm sure I locked it after our swim this morning. . . ."

Mrs. Hughes dug her fingernails into her scalp and whined.

I flashed on the little wrinkled fingers and the damp strands
of hair. I pieced together the rest of the story and felt suddenly ill. Among the fears in my own secret vault was my
fear of drowning. In my mind no death was worse, not even
burning.

I rubbed the woman's back gently, until she stopped the
awful sound.

"It's all right," I said, swallowing hard, "you don't need
to tell me any more."

Mrs. Hughes wiped some tears away with a shredded
Kleenex. "No. I want to tell you. It helps me get it all
straight. I ran out to the yard and saw the pool gate was open.
The boy was standing at the deep end of the pool, looking
down. I had asked him what he was looking at when he yelled
at me to stay where I was and jumped in.

"I made it as far as the gate and saw Amy's blue overalls next to the diving board. I couldn't look into the pool. I thought I was going to go crazy waiting for the boy to come up. I was so scared I didn't know what to do. I had all these terrible thoughts.

"I don't remember much else except seeing Amy's red shirt and some of her hair. Her eyes were half-open, but she wasn't crying. The boy took the tablecloth off the patio table and wrapped her up so I couldn't see her.

"I knew the boy was scared, too, but he kept telling me Amy was okay and we had to get to the hospital right away. In the car I remember asking him, 'Are you sure she's okay? Are you sure?' and he kept saying, 'I'm sure. Just go to the hospital.' I must have driven like a maniac. I don't remember anything until the nurse took her from the boy. I was afraid I wouldn't see her again."

The woman stopped rocking.

"She hasn't had lunch. Would you tell the nurses to make sure she gets some food and find out when I can see her? Please. I want to see her."

I had to clear my throat before speaking. "I'll tell the doctor what you told me, and I'll see when you can go in."

I called the supervisor back and went to the trauma room.

The ambience of the room was changed. Only Katy, Dr. Mahoney, and the pediatrician were still there. The pediatrician talked quietly to Dr. Mahoney by the door. He had his hand on her arm, and her head was bowed. Katy was cleaning the debris from around the child's body.

The monitor had been turned off, and the leads hung uselessly off the side rails, the pediatric electrodes still attached. The endotracheal tube remained in place along with the IVs, everything in miniature, waiting for the coroner.

I forced myself to look at the child. I was stunned by how unnatural it seemed for a child to be so still; even a sleeping child was a study of constant, subtle movement. She was about the same age as Simon. Her eyes were half-open, but without life. Two pink plastic elephant barrettes were askew, still clipped in her damp hair. I unclipped one and straightened it.

Dr. Mahoney came over. "What did the mother tell you?"

"They both took a nap, and she thought the child was

asleep. She even made her lunch before she went to check on her.''

Dr. Mahoney sucked in a breath. "Goddammit to hell." The comment was laced with anger and sadness. I wondered how much of the anger had to do with being beaten by death.

"This child had to have been underwater for at least forty minutes before she was found."

My imagination played a grim scene of the child struggling furiously to reach the top of the pool, while her mother serenely slept only a few yards away. I shuddered and covered my face.

Dr. Mahoney sucked in her breath through clenched teeth. "Jesus! Can you imagine living with that for the rest of your life?"

A minute went by before either of us spoke again.

"Echo, I'd like you to break the news to the mother." I opened my mouth to protest, but Dr. Mahoney held up her hand. "I *know* it's highly unusual for you to be the one to break the news, but the supervisor said you've established some rapport with her. I'll be over in a few minutes to help. I've already told the father over the phone. Someone he works with is driving him over to pick up his wife."

She walked a few feet away and remembered something. "Another thing you should know: This was their only child."

Katy was roughly wiping off the intubation instruments. She looked worn-out.

"How do I do that, Katy?" I pleaded. "How do I tell a woman her child is dead?"

Katy answered in a short-tempered way without looking up. "You just do, that's all. You'd better get used to it if you're going into this business. They should teach you about the realities of this job; people, including babies and kids, die, you know?"

I felt the lump rising in my throat just at the thought of facing Mrs. Hughes with the news. "Katy, what if I cry?"

"So? You cry. Where's the law that says you can't cry? Jesus, Echo, face it, you're human; you can cry with a patient or the people who care about that person. Nursing isn't always the happiest profession in the world. The instructors make you think it's a crime to show any emotion in front of a patient. They give you that crap about maintaining strict professionalism and all, and it's not true."

She picked up the tray and headed toward the supply room. "Look, just do it and get it over with. Don't make a federal case out of it. You'll just make it harder on yourself."

As soon as I opened the door to the quiet room, I lost my nerve and started tearing. The supervisor saw me first and immediately knew. She came to the door and gave my arm a tight squeeze, then slipped out behind me.

Mrs. Hughes stood up from the couch and grabbed for my hands again. "How's my baby? Can I see her yet?"

I could not stand to see the pleading face and looked away. I felt her eyes searching my profile. When I finally looked at her, she read the news in my eyes.

She dropped my hands as if they were poisonous snakes. "What is it? What's wrong with Amy? Oh, my God, please, no!"

I cried openly, trying to tell her. "Amy isn't—Amy isn't okay. They did everything they could. Everybody tried so hard to make her live, but it was too late. Amy—"

Mrs. Hughes shrieked, holding her head. "No! No! No! You liar! You liar! What are you saying? Give me my baby! I want to see Amy right now!" She made a move for the door.

I turned her around and held her. "Amy is dead."

She went stiff the way I'd seen people do just before they have seizures. "Mrs. Hughes, listen to me. Your husband's on his way, and Dr. Mahoney will be here in a minute."

The woman cried out, then sank down to the floor, holding her stomach. "No, please tell me it's not true. Please say it's not true."

I knelt next to her and started to put my arms around her when she slapped me away.

"This isn't happening. Tell me this isn't really happening. Please."

I shook my head. "I can't. I have a boy her age. I know . . ." Crying, I took her head in my hands and put it on my shoulder.

"My baby," she cried, lost in her pain. "Oh, my God, please, not my baby."

Nothing I thought of saying would come close to touching the woman's anguish. In the end I said nothing at all and rocked her in my arms until Dr. Mahoney arrived.

For the rest of the afternoon everyone was quiet. There

was no more laughing or light conversation. No one wanted lunch.

Mr. and Mrs. Hughes came in to see their child before she was taken away by the coroner. Mr. Hughes looked in from the doorway and covered his eyes with his hand. He said only, "Oh, dear God, no," and sobbed openly, leaning against the doorjamb.

Mrs. Hughes inched toward her daughter, holding both hands tightly over her mouth. She got right up next to her, touched the little face, then slid her hand under the child's back and lifted her effortlessly into the cradle of her arms.

Slowly, methodically, she peeled the tape off Amy's arm and removed the IV. Next, she eased the endotracheal tube out of Amy's throat and flung it violently away from her and her child. It was her way of spitting in the face of death.

Dr. Mahoney started to protest but changed her mind and left the family alone.

Between patients, Dr. Mahoney went to the doctors' sleep room and locked the door.

The docs who usually came into ER for a cup of coffee and small talk heard the news and stayed away. Only two came in to ask for details. Katy told me they both were the parents of young children.

Simon danced through my thoughts constantly for the remaining hours in ER. I couldn't wait to see him. I wanted to reacquaint myself with every inch of skin and every hair on his body. I wanted to feel his platinum curls under my fingers and memorize how the wrinkles appeared around his eyes when he laughed his hard laughter over himself passing wind or the funny songs he created to entertain himself. I wanted to breathe in the baby sweat smell from the top of his head when I kissed him. I would record and learn the way his child's logic cut through all the unnecessary fluff and got to the heart of a matter.

And if I ever had to give him up to death, I thought, I would have those small things forever.

Driving to the campus, I cried, thinking of Mrs. Hughes. Would she and Amy's father share the grief, or would there be accusations to pull them apart? How would they get through the hours and days of empty time?

And what about the future when the sting of agony wasn't so sharp? Would a long-buried toy found between the cushions of a chair or in the back of a closet reopen their hearts to the memory of today?

I spotted Simon across the nursery school's large playroom, absent-mindedly picking his nose while listening to a story about a friendly bear. I sent him a secret message of love and waited for him to turn around.

He ran to me, and I enveloped him in my cape, holding the top of his curly head in the crook of my neck for just a moment longer than usual.

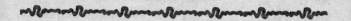

SEVEN

ON THE FIRST MORNING of freedom I awoke in my book-free bed to find Simon crawling up next to me with his determined I-want-something look.

"Mama?"

Yawning: "What?"

"Mama, I want something."

"What?" One eye opens.

Fidgeting closer to my head, he said, "You know."

"Do you want French toast?" I asked, wiping away the winkies from the one opened eye.

He gave a crooked sideward shake of the head that meant no.

"Do you want to fill your pool in the backyard and ask Clark to come and play?"

He placed a hand on his hip, denoting exasperation. "Pssssssh, nooooooo!"

"I know. You want to go for a bicycle ride."

Negative nod to the tenth power.

"Okay, Simon, I give up. My mind-reading days are over. What *do* you want?"

Crawling to the edge of the bed, he pointed out the window to the smoky blue-gray mountain that separates our village from the ocean.

"I want to go up there to find the bears and the magic places."

I couldn't have come up with a better idea myself.

* * *

Simon and I milked the summer days for all they were worth. Although the bears eluded us, we found everything we wished for in magic places not far from our cottage on an old cowpath that led up to the mountain.

Breathing in the sunny air, we were free for an hour or a whole day to wander unhurriedly over the seldom-traveled trail. We walked through the golden, rolling hills until cars and houses were gone from our sight and patches of tall grass gave out the sweet, dry odor that Simon said was nature's candy smell. After we had pushed and pulled each other up slopes, the patch of redwoods appeared just in time to give us a cool and fragrant canopy under which we devoured a lunch of thermos-cold milk and peanut butter sandwiches.

Lying head to head, we traced shapes around the soapsuds clouds through the maze of redwood branches.

"See the witch with the big nose over there? . . . Look, see her eye? She's got only one funny-looking eye . . . see her now?"

Rested, we'd move on into the wind, then bear off to the right where the redwoods abruptly ended at the foot of one last steep hill. Raising our eyebrows (or "blathums," as Simon was wont to call them) at each other was our cue to take off running.

Simon always reached the top first. Pointing vigorously, he'd send the piercing treble voice he used for dire emergencies down the hill to where my running had slowed to spurts of crawling.

"It's *still* there, Mama! It hasn't gone away!" His amazement would be as genuine as on the first day he had seen the other side of the ridge.

Below us the expanse of silver-blue ocean went on forever, filling up the whole of our sight and what looked like the entire rest of the world. Whooping, we'd take off running over the field, across the road to the shore, to touch the waves, just to make sure it was not some grandiose optical illusion.

Sand castles and shell knights came to life under Simon's small hands while I indulged in the art of watching the ocean's endless dance, both of us unaware of our being restored.

When the wind raised goose bumps, we headed back home, taking the time for learning. Using the words my father had taught me, I passed on bits of knowledge about the trees, plants, and the ways of the earth. I answered thousands of Simon's questions, then watched the formation of his universe, listening to his complex interpretations of what was taken in as useful information and what was discarded.

More times than not, we trudged home to find Janey and her son waiting on the front porch, their grocery bags sitting in the shade of the trumpet tree.

These spontaneous combined dinner efforts always provided perfect conclusions to perfect days. While our look-alike tow-headed sons played in any one of their imaginary worlds, Janey and I, like two old-fashioned country women, cooked and talked, filling in the blanks in our lives, quietly enjoying the slow process of friends growing closer. Together we'd put the trials and tribulations of the year into perspective and within minutes be weak from roaring laughter, dropping food and breaking dishes that our hands had become too "silly" to hold. We made solemn vows that nothing would make us lose our objectivity during the next year; our senses of humor would *not* fail us.

Toward the middle of August I stood in the center of my garden and studied the way the morning sun lit the feathery leaves of the tomato plants. Everything had changed overnight. The light was pale and not quite as warm as before. The air held a hint of dry leaves and pumpkins. It was almost autumn, time to begin again.

I introduced the idea of a second year of nursery school to Simon by letting him choose his new duffel bag. He decided on one with Kermit the Frog's perpetually smiling, perpetually green face displayed on all four sides.

The night before classes began, I read him the fairy tale about the grasshopper and the ant. At the end, after explaining the moral, I said it was time for us to work again like the ant.

Simon told me he supposed he could stand one more year, but that was his absolute limit. Sighing off into sleep, he added, "After this year, Mama, you have to be a nurse by yourself. I'll be too busy in kindergarten to help you anymore."

Our class met as a whole in the old tower building auditorium. We had filled out; the vacancies provided by the poor unfortunates of the first year were taken by women, mostly licensed vocational nurses who had challenged the entrance exam and passed. We were back up to a fat and sassy forty-eight students, and glad for the new blood. Everyone wore the golden, relaxed glow California summers tend to leave on people. I decided to keep track of how many days passed before it disappeared; I was banking on six—or seven max.

The second-year instructors introduced themselves and mingled among us. With the exception of Miss Telmack, who after every one of her moist Jell-O handshakes, surreptitiously wiped her hand off on the side of her dress, the women seemed to be a comfortable, easygoing group.

Once the meeting had been called to order, all of them, even Miss Telmack, gave us the impression they were on our side. "If you've gotten this far," Miss Telmack said, turning her palms upward and shrugging one shoulder, "you'll more than likely make it the rest of the way."

That broke the tension. It was a statement which would be referred to by every one of us at least a million times before the end of the year. Sighs of relief and a swell of happy chatter flooded over the room. A few of us applauded.

Tessie, the perky middle-aged woman who was to be our group's first rotation instructor, increased the feelings of good will by asking what *we* wanted changed within the structure of the program. The first request was unanimous: We called out for the abolition of the caps.

The four women bent their heads together in a two-second deliberation and gave us the thumbs-up sign.

Tessie held up her hand to abort the wild cheers. "*And* we've decided to allow you to wear pants suit uniforms this year so you all can run even faster than you did last year."

Laughter blended with the applause.

Forty-eight caps, like so many mutant Frisbees, were unpinned and flung into the air.

We were off and running down the home stretch.

Our group's training commenced in a large county hospital situated in the predominantly black community of Oakland. A more valuable setting for the observation of such an enormous variety of complex medical problems would have been hard to find. It was an institution where every bed was always filled and the nurses were grossly understaffed. We enjoyed the luxury of being considered a valuable, necessary part of the staff and were assigned sicker, more complicated patients.

For the purpose of polishing and perfecting our clinical skills and exercising our stores of knowledge, we now were given license to make decisions on our own, no longer under the constant supervision of the instructors. The resultant feeling that each patient was our sole responsibility gave each of us incentive to strive for our best.

Truly a teaching institution, the hospital played host to three different nursing schools and a myriad of interns and residents who loved to instruct. Whether it was to show off or just strong physical interest in some of the attractive students, they were cornucopias of information about anything we needed to know. All we had to do was ask one simple question, and we got full lectures, reading lists, and papers on the subject. The instructors thought the camaraderie between the docs and the students was wonderful. They encouraged us to pick their brains but sternly reminded us to steer wide and clear of the linen closets.

Tessie, in her down-to-earth way, believed in teaching on-the-job reality. She looked at nursing from an extremely practical viewpoint. To increase the overall quality of our care, for instance, she'd add up what every hour of hospitalization cost a patient, then multiply that number by how many hours we were assigned to care for him.

"This patient," she'd say, showing us the back of an old envelope on which she'd set her calculation, "is paying about thirty dollars an hour just for your skills alone. That's a lot of money; give them care that feels expensive."

Tessie knew the monetary value of every pill, procedure, and supply ever used. Once, while I awkwardly struggled to apply a dressing to a patient's oddly-shaped abdomen, Tessie came over and pulled out her pocket calculator. "That dressing," she said, pressing the little buttons faster than I could see her fingers move, "is costing this patient twelve dollars. I want you to redo it and give her something that *looks* like a twelve-dollar dressing. The way it is now, it looks more like you got it at a rummage sale for two bucks."

I had to pinch my nose to keep the snorting laugh back, but after that I never did a dressing that didn't look as if it had come straight from Neiman-Marcus.

Tessie's new home for us was the intensive care unit. Here, we were to be broken into medical life in the fast lane, or as Tessie put it, "In this place, just when you think you know it all, you'll turn around and meet a brand-new set of problems and catastrophes guaranteed to keep you on your toes and thinking."

On the morning of our first ICU clinical, Tessie gathered Nailbiting P.J., Janey, and me together in the conference room. After rolling out the respirator she'd been training us on for a week, she lifted off its dust cover.

"Before I turn you loose on the patients, I want to stress once more a few of the main things you must be mindful of when taking care of someone on a respirator."

Without even glancing in P.J.'s direction, she reached over to pull P.J.'s fingers away from her mouth and continued speaking.

"This machine is usually the patient's only air supply. Make sure it's delivering the right concentration of oxygen at the right rate through a patent, leak-free tubing system.

"Next, don't forget that endotracheal tube is shoved down into the patient's trachea. This means irritation to the lining of the respiratory tract, and more often than not, there will be a lot of secretions building up on the inside of the tube. Even if the patient seems to be coughing up a lot of mucus on his own, you've got to suction frequently to get everything out of there. If it's left in, it gets thick and sticky and forms plugs that will eventually occlude the tube. The next thing you know, your patient will be hypoxic; *don't* let it get that far."

She walked around to the side of the machine, ignoring P.J., who was back to biting her nails.

"Now this part is very important, so listen up. Pay attention to your alarms. Don't ever get lax about them. These alarms are on this machine for a reason. Listen to them when they talk to you."

Tessie pointed to a small black button in the upper right portion of the control panel. It was barely noticeable, crammed in between the numerous other knobs and buttons.

"I haven't shown you this little device because I never want to see any of you using it . . . ever. It is the one feature of the machine I'd like to see done away with forever; its function is to silence the alarms.

"A lot of nurses flip it on when they disconnect the tubing from the endotracheal tube so they can suction without all the alarms going off and waking up the people in the morgue."

P.J. burst into a wild giggle until she noticed the rest of us weren't even smiling. She coughed a little, then quieted.

"As I was saying," said Tessie, "it's all right to do that, except that once in a while, people forget to switch it off. It's an easy mistake to make."

Tessie had not removed her eyes from the button since she started talking about it.

"That means if the patient somehow disconnects from the respirator while you're away from the bedside, or if your attention is elsewhere, your patient can go without being oxygenated and you won't know about it, especially if he's heavily sedated and receiving curare.

"It sounds like such a dumb mistake to make, and right now you're saying to yourself, 'That'll never happen to *me*" but it does happen to nurses just like you."

Tessie didn't say anything more for a long time. The silence was just on the edge of being uncomfortable when she started again. She didn't look at us, and the statement was made slowly, quietly. "When we were rookies, one of my closest friends was responsible for the death of a young woman because of that little button. That, ladies, was the end of her promising career as a critical care nurse."

There was another long pause while she put the cover back on the machine.

"The moral of this story is, Don't learn the hard way; unless you want to court disaster and a lifetime of self-recrimination, hands off this button. You can put up with the noise for the few seconds it takes to suction or retape the tube."

After Tessie had put away the machine, she came back to us smiling.

"Last but not least, it's a good policy to keep the respirator patient's hands restrained, no matter how 'with it' he or she appears to be. In this hospital it's left to your discretion; in others it's standard policy. Don't be fooled by the alert patient. That tube is extremely uncomfortable, and most of them want to get it out any way they can.

Tessie clapped her hands. "Okay, girls, go out there and do your stuff!"

Eager and scared, the three of us headed off for our assigned respirator patients.

The ICU was one huge, open room done entirely in spring green. With green curtains between the eight beds, green walls, green floors, and green scrub dresses, the windowless, softly lit unit would have been hypnotically relaxing if it weren't for the constant noise of the respirators, the alarms, and the nauseating sound of suctioning.

P.J. was responsible for B bed, the twenty-seven-year-old Japanese motorcyclist who had encountered an automobile while traveling up the wrong side of the highway. Helmetless, his head and face had paved a goodly portion of roadway before he finally came to a halt a hundred feet from the initial crash.

The surgeons who had wired his skull together were waiting to see if the brain inside would function before attempting to reconstruct some kind of face. For the time being, the concave bowl of red pulp with the two lidless dark eyes staring from its middle would be protected with sterile saline-soaked pads.

Next bed over from him was one of Janey's patients, a petite sixteen-year-old girl who, on a popular, crowded beach, put a creative touch to her attempted suicide. Witnesses said she spread out her towel, carefully applied tanning lotion, then, within a few minutes, chugged down the better portion of a fifth of hundred-proof whiskey. She buried the bottle upright in the sand next to her, then lay down on her stomach to worship the last of the late-season sun.

A passing off-duty paramedic's suspicion was aroused when he saw her in the same relaxed tanning position long after the sun had ceased to shine. She arrived in emergency with a core body temperature of 94 and was barely breathing.

At 0.6 she took first prize for having the highest blood alcohol level for a surviving nonalcoholic in the history of the hospital. While jokes and reminiscences about hangovers floated freely among the interns and residents making rounds on her, there was, as in the case of her Japanese neighbor, some question about how much of her brain had been permanently "pickled."

Janey was also given a spur-of-the-moment assignment to

recover a fresh post-operative patient. The surgery schedule told us the patient was in for the removal of a bezoar.

We hurried to the ICU book cabinet where we found *bezoar* defined as "a mass formed in the stomach by the compaction of repeatedly ingested materials such as hair, bones, and fingernails."

According to our conclusions, the patient was someone who ate parts of cars or licked his dog clean.

The surgical resident accompanied the man back to the unit. For our amusement, he presented the three of us with the bezoar tightly wrapped in a blue sterile towel.

Expecting something spectacular like parts of door handles and headlights, mixed together with fragments of a miniature fox terrier, we were almost disappointed. The fist-size conglomeration consisted of what could only be described as a hairy steak studded with fingernails.

Obviously undaunted, P.J. regarded the mess from a distance and continued to bite her fingernails, while Janey and I kissed the idea of lunch good-bye. It was a vision not easily forgotten, not to mention the fact that it smelled like something left to die and gone to hell and back.

I was in charge of G bed, a burly, baldheaded man who looked like the character from the Mr. Clean advertisements.

For a man who suffered from serious cardiovascular disease, Rexford Moore appeared to be in remarkably good health. Ever since his lungs had filled with the fluid his heart was too weak to keep circulating, he'd been on a respirator. After several days Mr. Moore's fluid load had been reduced with medications, and he was being weaned off the machine. Instead of breathing for him completely, the respirator was now set to deliver only a few extra breaths per minute to supplement his few shallow ones.

The nurses left his hands untied most of the time so that he might write notes for things he needed. Next to his bed I found a stack of one-sided bits of conversation written in a bold, though shaky hand.

When I introduced myself, Mr. Moore nodded toward the pad of paper and pencil on the shelf next to his bed. I untied the long cotton straps and gave him the writing materials. Standing there, I felt ridiculous holding the man's hands on leashes.

His first note read like a long Burma Shave jingle:

Howdy Miss Heron: I'm Rex Moore/that's for sure/ but my friends don't botch/they call me Scotch./So don't be shy/give it a try/and we'll be friends/until the end./I see by your eyes/you don't trust my ties/but trust me so/you can let go/and have no fear/I'll stay right here/and I won't rave/if you let me shave./I won't knick the tube/'cause I'm no boob.

Added at the bottom of the page was "P.S. Are you married?"

Though his poetry left something to be desired, I laughed and let go of the straps. "No, I'm not married, and yes, I'll get a shave kit for you."

I was pleased the man was so alert and oriented. Because I was thinking more with my heart than my head, the desire to extend a friendly gesture won out over Tessie's warning; I kept a close eye on him but left his hands unrestrained.

Scotch shaved and bathed himself, did his own oral care, careful not to disturb the tube, and, despite a brief feeling of air hunger, insisted he felt strong enough to dangle his legs over the side of the bed.

About ten-thirty I sat down to chart, feeling satisfied with the way the morning had gone. Scotch's heart rate and BP were up slightly, and he seemed a little restless but was content to work on a crossword puzzle. To me it was logical he might be overtired from the morning's activities, and I hoped he might doze off for a nap.

Fifteen minutes later a pencil whizzed past the end of my nose just as the respirator's alarms sounded off. Looking agitated and dusky around the gills, Scotch swung his legs over the side of the bed and roughly pulled out his IV before I could get past my stunned panic and onto my feet.

The monitor showed a drastic increase in his rate, and he was having a few dangerous, irregular beats called premature ventricular contractions, also known as PVCs.

When his hand went for the tube, I dived across the bed. "Stop!" I screamed into his ear, trying to pry his fingers away from the tube. The man looked at me as if he'd never seen me before and ended my futile struggle by giving the tube one strong yank.

Strips of adhesive tape, rendered useless by his sweat, hung like white streamers from the tube's end.

He retched once and, staring abstractedly ahead of himself, started in the direction of the exit doors across the room. His monitor leads, like rubber bands stretched to their limit, ripped off his chest and snapped back, hitting the wall.

Taking hold of his waist with both arms, I yelled for help over the noise of the respirators. By the time Janey responded, Scotch had dragged me ten feet into the main room. "Stop him!" I yelled.

Janey tried pushing him back, but he knocked her down with one swing of his arm. Full of spirit, she rolled once and grappled for his left leg. Just then P.J., like Wonder Woman, came flying out of nowhere and jumped onto Scotch's back.

I recognized the scene from an early Frankenstein movie as the hulk of a man, now gray in color, stiff-leggedly dragged the three of us across the room as if we were no more than mosquitoes. Inside my head the weird place of humor opened, and I laughed hysterically until I cracked my head on P.J.'s chin.

Two of the ICU nurses working on the far side of the room took note of the strange grouping of bodies moving toward the doors and sounded the general alarm for help. They joined the menagerie and grabbed for Scotch's other leg. All of us were screaming different, conflicting commands at each other. Scotch was the only one who stayed silent, his purpose clear.

Suddenly Tessie was there, pulling one of the overstuffed lounge chairs out from the corner. She pushed it in front of him.

Blinded by P.J.'s red, nail-bitten fingers draped over his eyes, Scotch walked right into it. With one hand Tessie pivoted him around and into the chair.

Brought in by the alarm, a group of doctors and nurses carried the kicking and biting man back to his bed and reintubated him. Tessie established another IV line and drew a blood sample to determine Scotch's oxygen level. I kept taking his blood pressure, trying to keep busy so I could put off looking at Tessie for as long as possible.

Thirty minutes later Scotch lay quiet, restored to a healthy pink color, his BP and heart rate running normally. Tessie watched me clean up the mess around the bed. I moved fast, trying to make myself appear too harried for a talk.

With a sigh Tessie pressed the heels of her hands over her eyes, then slid them down her face before starting in.

"You know, I *knew* it was going to be one of you three when I heard the alarm."

I kept my eyes focused on my hands.

"Would you like to tell me what happened?"

I couldn't really tell if Tessie meant the question to sound so captious, but that's the way I took it.

"I don't know." I shrugged. "One minute he was fine, and the next he was hypoxic and crazy."

I broke off and redirected my interest to clearing away wrappers and rolls of tape. Tessie waited patiently for the rest of the explanation.

I resigned myself to telling her everything. "I left his hands untied, he seemed so alert. Besides one episode of air hunger, he never got short of breath. I mean, really, Tessie, this man was writing *jingles*, for Christ's sake! I never thought he'd pull the tube out, but he did—just like you said."

Tessie took the information calmly.

"Okay, so how do you feel?" she asked.

My voice croaked from all the yelling I'd done. "Shitty. I'm glad he's okay, but I still feel lousy."

Tessie smiled. "That's about right. If you felt like dancing, I'd be worried. At least that's one mistake you'll never repeat."

She leaned over and pulled something off the bedside monitor. "Now, let me show you what happened."

To the light, Tessie held up the old endotracheal tube.

"Take a look for yourself."

The end of the tube was almost occluded with a mucus plug as solid as concrete.

"Did you suction Mr. Moore?"

"Yes, twice."

"And what did you get when you suctioned him?"

"Nothing. He didn't have any secretions at all."

Tessie threw the culprit tube into the garbage.

"Aha! That's what you thought. Herein lies another lesson for you never to forget. Mr. Moore has pulmonary edema; he should have had *some* secretions, even if they were minimal. When you aren't getting anything out when you suction, use a few cc's of sterile saline to irrigate the tube and soften any plugs that might be forming. Mr. Moore was slowly suffocating because of that plug.''

I rolled my eyes with exasperation. ''I can't believe he waited until my shift to go crazy. He's probably been growing that plug for the last three days just waiting for me to take care of him.''

I stared into a fold of green curtain and remembered the vows of objectivity and humor Janey and I made in my kitchen. The thought of all of us piling onto a hulking blue patient who walked like Frankenstein *was* kind of funny, I supposed, but I couldn't get past my momentary depression to laugh again.

''Hypoxia can make people very weird, very fast, Echo. As a general rule of thumb, I allow for the possibility of anything's happening right up until a patient gets in his car to go home.''

She scrubbed her hands over the sink and dried them, then came over and gave me a quick hug. ''Don't look so sad. The patient is okay, and two lessons have been etched forever on your brain.''

''Yeah, but what a way to learn!'' I still felt stubbornly miserable.

Tessie laughed at me. ''Sometimes it's the only way to learn.''

I opened my mouth to drive the incident into the ground, but she walked away and left me talking to myself. From the end of the hall she called back, ''Stop dwelling on it, and proceed with laughter. Class dismissed!''

Besides respirators and the monetary value of health care, Tessie taught us how to sidestep burnout.

''Start early,'' she said in our first impromptu health worker's support session. ''Avoid the rush of burnout victims, and start talking. The amount of death and other sad things we see is enough to make anybody crazy. Share all that garbage with somebody. Tell one of your group about how bad you felt when that patient of yours died; tell anybody who's going to give you support about the medication error you made and how scared you were. You're asking for trouble when you hold things in, or as my instructor used to tell me, 'Talk it out before you walk it home.' ''

Tessie was right, of course, though some of the girls thought the idea of burnout at a student level was ridiculous. Too many of the group still held in the things which bothered them, insisting they could work out their difficulties on their own. As one who spilled her guts at the first chance, I tried to tell them not to be embarrassed, that we were all in the same sinking boat, but the effort was to no avail.

It was Robert who sent the message home and made believers out of all of us.

Robert was a brilliant and devoted resident who thought, like most young doctors, he could cure the world. The many bitter disappointments which most times outweighed the rewards of healing hadn't changed his mind as it had the others; Robert never stopped believing that if he tried hard enough, the crippled would stand up and run.

He was always there when his patients needed him, always on top of the problem. He took a maximum caseload and extended himself way beyond the limits. When his patients felt pain, he felt responsible; when they died, he cried and tortured himself with the idea there was something he could have done differently in order to save them.

Robert was the all-around giver. He lent what little money he had, did favors, covered shifts for any of his colleagues who had good sob stories, and listened to everybody else's problems. Robert had the unusual capacity to be completely tolerant of other people's pain.

From what I could tell, he never asked for anything for himself, though I doubt if anyone ever took the time to listen to him. Everyone was so busy taking that no one noticed Robert was being used up.

Halloween day the staff broke rules and dressed up. Nurses painted glittery stars or hearts on each other's faces, while the interns and residents donned fake glasses and noses and attached urinary catheters to the seats of their pants for tails.

I'd seen Robert that morning while I researched my assignment. He wore a pair of wide bright red suspenders and a white, painted-on smile. I didn't notice anything else about him that seemed unusual; he was Robert being good old Robert. Like everybody else, I never thought to look past the painted smile.

Just after lunch I was sedating an agitated DTs patient when out of the corner of my eye a brief dark shadow passed the windows. Thinking it might be a large sea bird come inland too far, I looked over the sill and saw a body, like a crumpled puppet without strings, sprawled in the parking lot below. A gust of wind rearranged the back of the white lab coat; one side of the wide, red suspenders had come unsnapped from the impact.

Robert's suicide note included an outline of care for a few of his sicker patients and begged forgiveness from the people who might be put out by his death.

The hospital held an informal memorial service during which the director of the psychiatric unit gave a short speech about suicide's being one of the unresolvable deaths for those left behind. In an attempt not to have the tragedy repeated, she and the chaplain offered their services to hospital personnel.

So, even in death, Robert gave more than he knew. Among the students, as well as the staff, there was a noticeable increase in friendly touches, concerned looks, and inquiries of "You okay?" or "Want to talk about it?" In November we changed instructors. Though none of us wanted to cut ties with Tessie (she explained it was just our abandonment fears resurfacing from childhood), we were happy to be moving on to the various general medical wards.

We were informed we'd be staying at the Oakland hospital, but under the supervision of Miss Geraldine Telmack.

My rotation with Miss Telmack did not go quickly. She didn't like me very much, and told me so in a special one-to-one conference three weeks into my rotation with her.

Picking nervously at the corner of her desk pad, she said she'd heard about my reputation for being one of the better students, but as far as she could see, I didn't amount to a hill of common beans. She said I was too "cocky" for a student and summed up the rest of her complaints by informing me I had an attitude problem just like her sister, Mavis. Other than reminding her of Mavis, I never knew what she really had against me, but she was on my back from the first day right up until the last.

Nothing I did was right. No matter how well I'd done something, Miss Telmack would find the flaw. My care plans weren't *focused* enough, my charting was too brief, I "dawdled'' over my patients, my hair was touching my collar, my fancy twelve-dollar dressings took too long, *and*, she added, my sense of humor was too "odd" for the patients; she swore they were laughing *at* me, not *with* me. The list of my short-comings was endless, according to Miss Telmack.

Miss Telmack drove me up the walls, and I talked to any-body who would listen about my ordeals with her. Janey, of course, got the brunt of most of it. The first thing she'd ask when seeing me was not "How are you?" but "How's Miss Telmack treating you?" As light and happy as I tried to be around him, Simon, the perceptive child, sensed my tension and started including little notes with his pocket presents. With a few exceptions, they always read the same: "Simon luvz mama." He signed them off with a happy face done in yellow crayon.

It was a well-known fact that I was a holiday hater, but this year I could not wait for Christmas. This year the closer the day came, the happier I felt; I knew when I left for holiday break, I would be leaving Miss Telmack forever.

It was 6:00 A.M. and still dark outside when I picked up my last assignment of what I would always refer to as the "Terrormack Rotation." I was so happy, I forgot myself and hummed "Jingle Bells," a song that hadn't passed my Scroogeian lips for years.

The three-by-five card bore two lines of Miss Telmack's impeccable printing in black ink.

Second Year—Heron:
Ward Six Bed Five—Patient: Wilson, Richard

My initial surprise changed into suspicion. *One* patient? Why only one when, in the past, each of us had always been assigned three or more?

Janey came up behind me and peered over my shoulder. "Wow! Lucky girl! How do you rate anyway? And here I thought Miss Telmack didn't like you very much."

I turned to look at Janey and laughed. I recognized the look common to us all—exhaustion.

"The important question here, Janey, is not whether Ger-aldine Telmack really likes me or not; the suitcases under your eyes tell me the important question is, How much sleep did you get last night?"

Janey stifled a yawn, which made us both laugh.

"It's the drugs," she said, making her hands tremble like someone having "withdrawal willies." "I was up until two A.M. beefing up my drug box."

"Well, from the looks of those bags, I'd say you'd been researching the drugs on a personal level rather than a cerebral one."

From her 1942 leather book bag, Janey pulled a clear plastic recipe box two-thirds full with three-by-five cards. She handled it as if it contained all the answers to the unsolvable mysteries of life.

She held the box out to me. "Look," she said in a whispery voice, "look into my fake crystal ball and see your future."

What she was holding under my nose represented the nursing student's most valued possession. We all started our own drug boxes the day we started worrying about pharmacology. Laboriously we researched every drug we'd ever heard of, given, or hoped to give, wrote every bit of information down, and then filed it in an old recipe box or, in my case, a shoebox. We equated the number of cards we accumulated with our level of pharmacological expertise.

At five every clinical morning, to help pass the forty-minute drive to Oakland, our car pool played Name That Drug. As we clutched our file boxes on our laps (rarely did we let them out of our sight), somebody would give out several pieces of information about a drug, and each of us got a chance at naming it correctly.

The drug hysteria was all due to the fact that the art of pill pushing had changed over the years. It wasn't like in the old movies anymore where the nurse walked into the patient's room and gently, but with determination, insisted the patient take the little white tablet, explaining only, "It's good for you," and walked out.

Now, when a nurse approached the meds cabinet, she was facing a major job. Not only did we have to know the drug thoroughly, including things like how it acted chemically, what it did in the body, side effects, contraindications, and proper dosages, but we practically had to stand on our heads before we could give it. We had to make sure the patient had no allergies to it, then check to see if it would react with any of the other medications he was taking. The last thing done before it was actually swallowed or injected was to triple check the drug with the patient nursing information card, known as the Kardex, the doctor's order, the medication chart, the patient's armband, and, finally, the patient himself.

We were told that if it ever came down to going to court on a medication error, it would not carry any weight that we'd cared for Mr. Smith for three days in a row and knew him better than we knew our own father. We *still* had to ask him what his name was and check that armband.

I looked away from Janey's file box and turned my attention back to my assignment card. "I don't need to see the future to know that Miss Telmack has something very special lined up just for me with this Richard Wilson."

Janey started to say something but swiftly pulled herself away from the wall she'd been leaning against and hurried toward the nursing station. As she passed me, she whispered out of the corner of her mouth, "Cheez it, sister, it's de cops!"

The crisp squeak of nursing shoes hitting the polished hospital floor and the smell of fresh starch told me Miss Telmack was approaching.

"Heron?" she shrieked into the back of my head. Geraldine Telmack had a voice exactly like that of an army sergeant.

I pretended to study my assignment card with profound interest. "Yes, Miss Telmack."

"Why aren't you going over the nursing Kardex and the patient's chart?"

"I haven't gotten to it yet, Miss Telmack. I just arrived approximately three and one half minutes ago."

"That's three wasted minutes as far as I'm concerned. If I were you, I'd put the snotty attitude aside and study this patient's chart with the utmost care. You'll be running into some special problems with this young man, and I'll be curious to see how you'll do as the 'top student' around here." Sarcasm coated the military voice.

While my stomach was busy burning new corners into its ulcer, Miss Telmack turned and left. I watched her nursing cap bounce up and down in time with the squeak of her step and, after the fashion of P.J., bit my left index fingernail until it bled.

"Sure, Miss Telmack," I called after her just softly enough so I knew she would not hear me. "Anything you say."

Then, putting my snotty attitude aside, I almost ran to the chart to find out why my task for the day was so "difficult."

Wilson, Richard. Age, twenty-five. Diagnosis, chronic myelocytic leukemia, terminal stage.

So? I'd taken care of young people before, and I'd cared for quite a few terminal cancer patients, so what?

Reading over the Kardex, I learned the young man had played professional baseball for a year before his illness, and his closest relatives included his mother and one sister. After many hospitalizations in which his condition had slowly deteriorated, this was considered his last admission. He'd been in a semicoma for twenty-four hours, and both his liver and kidneys were shutting down. In the box at the right-hand lower corner of the Kardex, written in red ink was a notation which designated the patient as a "no code."

"No codes" were the medical world's way of saying a patient was not to be resuscitated if he had either a cardiac or a respiratory arrest. It meant we were to let him die in peace.

Mr. Wilson had only two medications ordered: morphine and Valium, both to be given prn, or as needed. The main emphasis seemed to be on his need for personal care measures: turning; bathing; anything that made his death as smooth and comfortable as possible.

I flipped through the chart and read the intern's and resident's progress notes. All of them were pretty much the same: The man roused only to painful stimuli. His prognosis was nil, and most of the docs were confident Richard Wilson would not live out the day.

At 7:00 A.M. sharp all of us assembled in the nurses' lounge for our preclinical conference. Miss Telmack presided at the head of the table, looking particularly pleased with herself.

Janey reviewed her three patients and explained how she planned to care for each one. Her elderly male patient with congestive heart failure needed careful respiratory assessments and instruction on taking his medications and the importance of a low-salt diet. The thirty-two-year-old drug abuser with bacterial endocarditis needed close monitoring not only of her vital signs but also of any visitor possibly bringing in heroin to her. Last but not least was the sixty-one-year-old alcohol withdrawal syndrome who needed to be sedated for impending DTs and seizures.

The rest of the girls were assigned the regular garden variety of patients: strokes, overdoses, renal disease, cancer, heart attacks, gastrointestinal bleeders, post trauma, and so on and so forth. By the time it was my turn to give report, I was embarrassed to admit I had only one patient in the terminal stage of leukemia, only two medications to give, and some simple comfort measures to perform.

I'm sure everybody wondered, but nobody asked what was going on, especially since Miss Telmack wore a smug, almost spiteful grin throughout my report and concentrated on tapping her pencil eraser on the table.

Usually ready with criticism at the drop of a hat, willing to suggest and point out faulty reasoning on a moment's notice, Miss Telmack uttered not one word while I explained what my plans were. I almost begged her to spill forth even one or two caustic remarks just so I'd feel comfortable.

My pitifully simple report took all of two minutes, and that was with padding.

Several of the girls looked at each other and raised their eyebrows.

Finally, Miss Telmack stood up, and although she appeared to be addressing the entire table of students, my paranoia was functioning at top level: I just knew she was speaking only to me.

"I'll meet you back here in four hours. You may not see me, but just keep in mind I'll be watching every move you make."

Big Brother Telmack smiled maliciously.

Janey squeezed my hand under the table and looked at me as if I'd just received my termination notice.

Richard Wilson was beautiful. The young man, a mulatto, had smooth golden brown satin for skin. Unblemished, it was stretched thinly over wide, high cheekbones.

He lay bathed in sweat, and his bed was soiled with small smears of feces and blood. I reached over to touch his forehead and pulled my hand away as if I'd touched fire. The whites of his eyes were all I could see from the half-closed lids.

"Richard?" One. "Richard?" Two. "Richard!" Three. No response.

I'd never gotten used to the practice of pricking someone with a needle to test pain response, so I pinched his upper arm instead. He groaned and seemed to struggle to open his eyes. Briefly I saw the dark brown irises rolled side to side, then back up into his head.

I took his blood pressure. It was alarmingly low: 68 over 40. Adrenaline rushed through me but was tempered by the red-inked "no code." Sliding the bedside chart from its slot, I checked to see when he'd got his last dose of morphine. Less than forty minutes before, he'd been given ten milligrams all in one shot. Over the last few hours I saw that he'd been receiving as much every hour and a half.

I checked the medication order, reading it over several times: "Morphine sulfate, five to ten milligrams, IV, every one hour, prn pain."

According to my morphine card, this was a substantial dose for most normal people, let alone someone whose drug-clearing functions were as compromised as Richard's. If he were to continue receiving the morphine as frequently as was ordered, it would build up in his system and eventually suppress his respirations enough for him to arrest.

I put away the chart. I realized it was standard practice to heavily sedate patients in situations like this, but I'd blocked out the possibility that I, personally, would ever be faced with having to do it.

Placing a large bath towel in a plastic bag, I poured liquid soap and tepid water over it, then laid the bag against Richard. The minute it touched his arm, he made a low guttural sound and gritted his teeth. His body stiffened.

I felt for his pulse; it was thready and weak. His blood pressure read 70 over 38; it was too low, especially for someone in pain.

Fully panicked, I ran into the next room, where I knew Janey would be giving her congestive heart failure patient a bath.

I stopped short in the doorway. Janey was sitting on the bed leaning over an old man, his white head resting on her shoulder. They both were crying. Patting her back, he spoke in broken English.

"I was only four years old when the soldiers come and kill

my mother and father. I watch everything very scared until they put the potato sack on me and throw me over the wall to the convent. The nuns, they took care of me, but I never saw no one in my family again. I was lucky, the soldiers did not kill the children then. . . .''

I turned away, unwilling to dispel the intimacy of the moment. It was almost frightening when I thought of how close people allowed themselves to be with us; we were given such easy access to their souls. We were like housekeepers given the keys to every room and finding the skeletons and long-hidden cobwebs no one else ever saw.

I dashed back to the room to check Mr. Wilson once more before I stat-paged Miss Telmack, but she was already there, standing by the bedside, taking his blood pressure. As soon as I walked in the door, she turned around, her face twisted with anger.

"Where have you been? What gives you license to leave this patient and gallivant around?"

From her tone I knew better than to give anything but a straight answer. "I went for help," I said, feeling renewed panic. "I couldn't find anybody, so I was going to stat-page you, I swear it!" The impulse to cross my heart and hope to die came very close to being played out.

The glare from Miss Telmack's eyes softened to a suspicious stare. She opened her mouth to say something, but I cut her off before she could get the lead.

"I don't know what to do. His pressure is only seventy systolic, but he's in agony. If I give him any morphine, I'm afraid it'll drop his pressure all the way out. I was going to bathe him and try to change the bed, but he's in so much pain. He's burning up, too. I haven't taken his temp yet, but I know it's—"

I was astounded to see Miss Telmack break into the smug little smile again. For a moment I hated her with frightening intensity.

"Uh-huh," she said, folding her arms over her chest, "and now what will you do? This is the big time, little girl. Let's say you're all alone on the floor with six difficult patients and no backup to help. What are you going to do with Mr. Wilson?"

"I'm going to call the doctor and ask him if—"

She snapped at me, still snickering, "You don't have time

to call the doctor, and he's not going to help you anyway. He wrote the order just this morning. He knows the situation as well as you do! Besides, he's too busy to listen to you snivel."

"But, Miss Telmack," I whispered, "that's asking the nurses to kill the patient!"

Miss Telmack looked shocked, then angry. "How dare you call what we're doing for this man killing!" she shouted. "You are helping him be pain-free during his last, agonizing hours. And welcome to the real world of nursing, Heron."

I was horrified. This was something new to me, and I was not prepared in any way to deal with it. I closed my eyes to shut out the image of Miss Telmack for a moment, just to clear my mind.

Instead of a calming picture of the ocean, my mind fogged up with mental images of myself wiping off the rubber medication port and injecting the morphine, watching it swirl toward his vein, closer until . . . internal hysteria.

"I can't do that!" I said in a terrified whisper. I opened my eyes and looked at Miss Telmack. "I won't do that! I won't sedate this man and have his death on my conscience for the rest of my life! I couldn't live with myself. You can flunk me, you can do whatever you want, but I won't do that!"

I searched Miss Telmack's face. The smug smile was still there, but I saw something else now, too. It looked, and for a second felt, like compassion, sadness, and wisdom all mixed together.

"Okay, Heron, let's get his bath done, and get something in him to bring down that fever. You can deal with the medication when we finish."

She'd let the matter drop too quickly, and my internal antenna went to full power. A sense of foreboding hung over my heart like a hundred millstones.

Miss Telmack removed Mr. Wilson's gown as I spread the large soapy towel over his naked body. Working from the shoulders down, we rubbed his skin so gently we seemed not to be touching him at all. But by the time we washed his feet, his low moaning had changed to weak, high-pitched yelping.

Dripping with sweat, I clenched my teeth. I could feel Miss Telmack glancing up at me every once in a while, waiting for me to say something. The bed bath and changing of soiled linen were basic nursing care for every patient, but I was not following the common practice of medicating a patient in pain before the bath was started.

Turning him onto his side and gently inching him to the far side of the bed, I washed his back and buttocks, then spread out the fresh linen on my side of the bed. After rolling him back over the bump of old linen and wet towels, Miss Telmack finished by making up the other half of the bed and taking a rectal temperature: 102.8. Quickly she inserted an aspirin suppository.

Pumping up the cuff, I prayed his pressure would be up so I could medicate him.

"Eighty over forty-two," I said, burning with anxiety. Richard Wilson was still screaming weakly. I wished I could stop the screams without silencing the man forever.

"Yes? So now what? What are you going to do, Heron?"

"I don't know. I want to wait a little. When his pressure hits eighty-five, I'll give him three milligrams of MS to start."

Miss Telmack looked at me in rage. "Listen to this man. He is suffering! *What* is your problem with letting this man die a peaceful death? Explain it to me, Heron, because I don't think anyone else is going to understand why you're putting him through this either."

I looked at Richard Wilson, the young man, the baseball player, and I remembered a seven-year-old me standing over a dead sparrow and throwing vows to the sky never to kill any living thing.

"Miss Telmack, please listen. I don't want to cause this man's death. I'm scared. I want . . ." My voice broke.

Miss Telmack pulled me into the hallway, and we both leaned against the wall. Nurses were hurrying in and out of rooms all around us, while a small group of interns were doing rounds with the chief resident in the next ward.

"Helping people get well is the easy side of nursing." Miss Telmack's voice turned soft. "The other side isn't as pleasant, but it's a fact. We're here to help people die, too. When death is inevitable, you need to be there to make that event as smooth as possible for the patient. You can't let this young man down. He needs your help."

What she said sounded right, but I knew it still boiled down to my going in there and giving Richard Wilson one or two more doses of morphine.

"Have you ever done this?" I asked.

Miss Telmack nodded without hesitation. "Lots of times, and I only hope that if I ever end up in the same way, someone will do it for me."

There was such finality to her tone I believed her.

"Heron, haven't you ever been in so much physical pain that you wanted someone just to put you out of your misery?"

I thought back to the time I severed my Achilles tendon with a rusty garden hoe, and even to Simon's birth, but for the life of me, I couldn't remember the pain's being *that* bad.

"No. Not anything bad enough for that."

Miss Telmack let out a resigned sigh. "Okay, Heron, it's up to you, but I want you to stay in there with him and watch him carefully. I'll give you a few minutes to rethink this. If you change your mind, page me. Otherwise, I'll be back to check on you."

She made a notation on a small pad of paper that she'd pulled from her pocket and stuck the pencil back into the high mound of teased hair under her cap. She went a few steps away. "Just think on this, Heron: This young man has no chance for life. He will never wake up and go play baseball again."

I stayed still for a moment after Miss Telmack left, unconsciously running my fingers over the face of my man-size silver watch. I flipped it over to read the inscription: "To Nurse Wretched—We Love You." I thought fondly of the friends and neighbors who had presented it to me soon after I was accepted into the program. I wondered what they would think if they saw me now trying to decide if I was going to deliberately medicate a twenty-five-year-old dying man possibly out of existence. I looked at Mr. Wilson. He was still moaning.

I tried to brush his teeth, but his gums bled so badly I stopped. Instead, I squirted mouthwash in between his teeth with an irrigation syringe, suctioning at the same time so he wouldn't aspirate.

Five minutes later his blood pressure hit 82, and I paged Miss Telmack to supervise me while I gave the morphine.

While I waited for her, I tried to keep myself from feeling scared. I stared at the handsome young man and then into the hallway. Closing my eyes against the hospital greenness, I tried to be Richard Wilson.

I feel the sheets and the hard mattress under my thin body and take in a breath. I am suffocating; my lungs feel like lead. Intense pain is present in every part of my body, and I want to yell or howl, but I can't; my tongue is too cracked and swollen, and I'm too weak to make the effort.

I smell disinfectant, urine, and the stench of my own breath tinged with old blood. My stomach revolts, and the spinning nausea swirls in my throat. I am burning from some internal fire raging out of control, and even the thin cotton sheet covering me feels like coarse sandpaper. The overhead paging system constantly belches messages in a nasal, twanging voice that stabs at my throbbing head.

In the next bed over, the confused old man with the broken hip passes wind with astounding volume, then rattles his side rail and curses.

Oh, God, I think, *please, somebody, please make all this stop!*

I opened my eyes. Miss Telmack stood in front of me wearing a look of distrust. "You okay, Heron? You look pale."

"I'm okay. I was trying to feel what it's like to be him." I looked over at Richard.

Miss Telmack rolled her eyes. She'd never given much merit to my practice of trying to experience the essence of another person.

In spite of herself, she asked, "Oh, yeah? Well, how does it feel?"

"Not so good. I want to give him some morphine, but not his maximum dose. His BP is up a little, so I thought I could take the edge off with five milligrams."

"Five milligrams won't even begin to touch him," Miss Telmack snapped. "You'll be wasting your time and mine. You give what you have to give to take the patient out of pain. This man's drug tolerance is high, but I'll be conservative. Give him eight milligrams now and another five after lunch."

"I can't do that," I mumbled, looking away from her.

Miss Telmack took in a deep breath and let it out slowly. "Okay, Heron, you just wrote your own ticket. After lunch I want you to go to the conference room and stay there. Study, think, do anything, but just don't let me see you back on the floors. I'm taking over the care of this patient now. You're relieved for midday conference."

She turned away and pulled the narcotics cabinet key from

her pocket, heading for the nursing station. I didn't know what to do. Never before had any student from our class been ordered off the floor.

Taking the long way around, I walked toward the conference room, feeling guilty, scared, and embarrassed. I was hoping I'd run into Tessie. I even toyed with the idea of paging her, but I knew there wouldn't be enough time.

I sat through midday conference in a cold sweat. Janey, in a real talking streak, took up most of the thirty minutes discussing her patients. Miss Telmack didn't say a word about what had just taken place between us.

"You all are dismissed for lunch; thirty minutes, then straight back to your assignments."

She didn't even give a side glance in my direction.

In the cafeteria I saw Miss Telmack and the head nurse of ward six having what appeared to be a serious discussion by the coffee machine. They stopped as soon as they saw me and walked away.

I was sitting with a cup of broth, my stomach tied in knots, by the time Janey sat down next to me with her plate. I looked up just in time to see her stethoscope slide from around her neck and land squarely in the middle of her mashed potatoes.

With a napkin she nonchalantly wiped it off and checked my face to see why I wasn't laughing.

"Say, girl, you look like you just got a positive rabbit test and an eviction notice at the same time. What's up?"

"I've been pulled from the floor, Janey. Miss Telmack has assumed care of my patient."

Janey choked. "What?"

"I was afraid to give him his morphine because his BP was too low, and he's already having problems breathing. I didn't want to be the one to push him over the edge."

The knot moved from my stomach to my throat.

"Oh, shit! What are you going to do, or maybe I should ask, What is Geraldine going to do to you?"

I pushed away the broth, still untouched. "I don't know. I've been thinking maybe nursing isn't for me after all, you know? Maybe I should go back to being a legal secretary or something benign where I don't have to make decisions about ending someone's life for him. I don't want anybody to suffer, Janey, but I don't want to be the one who does him in either."

Janey held my hand while I babbled out the whole story.

"In some ways, I know Miss Telmack is right," I said in conclusion, "but I just wish I'd had more time to think about this."

Janey spoke up in a low, serious voice. "What would you have thought, Echo? Miss Telmack gave you this assignment because she knows how sensitive you are; she knew this would be a really tough problem for you. We're all going to have to face this sooner or later; maybe she wanted you to set the example for the rest of us, you know, like If-she-can-do-it-it'll-be-easy-for-the-rest-of-you type of thing."

I realized part of what Janey said was true. No matter what her motives were, Miss Telmack had given me the chance to deal with the problem with her rather than on my own.

"I guess it's one of those things that are left out of the nursing textbooks, isn't it?" Janey asked, looking at me as if I were a lost child. She calmed me, and I loved her for it.

I shook my head and played with the now-congealed broth, making it stick to the sides of the cup. Janey got up to leave, gathering my purse as well as her own. She helped me out of my chair the same way she might have a ninety-year-old arthritic.

"Come on, Ec, look at it this way: The next time you have to face this, you'll be one ahead of the game."

The next time. I guessed there would be a lot of next times. Nurses heavily sedated Richard Wilsons every day in hospitals all over the world. Did it *ever* get easy? I wondered.

Alone in the conference room, I put my head down on the table and closed my eyes. On the back sides of my eyelids I saw Richard Wilson lying in his bed and wondered how he was. I knew he wasn't going to live no matter what any of us did.

I got up and paced back and forth in the small room, feeling closed in. Peeking from a crack in the door, I waited until the hall was empty and made a break for the elevator. It was one twenty-five. I had an hour and thirty-five minutes to myself.

Having hit a button, I slid down through space toward the second floor and the hospital chapel.

My simple spiritual beliefs did not belong to any one

church, nor did I follow any particular teachings, but I was drawn to the hollow silence common in most holy places.

I remembered one wintry night back in the days when churches were left unlocked and I was in search of a warm place in which to hide, I sneaked into a local church not far from my home. Feeling safe and protected, I stood by the confessional boxes and wrapped myself in the thick wine-colored velvet curtains. The pervading wax smell of the devotional candles inspired me to dream of miracles. I eventually fell asleep at the feet of the beautiful lady statue, hoping she would shed her stone shell and take me away to a house that smelled like fresh-baked pies. She would love me forever, of course, and the gentle person I'd imagined her to be would never get drunk and yell awful things or threaten to kill me in my sleep.

When I woke up, I found out miracles never happen when you want them to, but I'd discovered another place where I could be left alone to think.

Rumor had it that the elaborate hospital chapel was almost always empty, with the exception of the times it was supposedly used as a trysting place for hasty and subdued romantic interludes. I was relieved to find only half the rumor was true: The place was deserted. I sat down in the farthest corner of the room where the soft lights did not reach. When my eyes accommodated themselves to the darkness, I saw the pews were padded with teal blue velvet, and the altar was carved from a block of white marble.

Mostly because of exhaustion, I gazed, transfixed, at the dark fruitwood crucifix suspended from the ceiling. A white porcelain Jesus, looking quite comfortable, stared down at his wounded feet.

Would *He* have objected to a shot of morphine while dying on the cross? Probably. I dimly remembered from the catechism classes I was forced to attend, the nuns trying so hard to teach us, the sinful children that "His" (bow your head, irreverent girl) suffering was for a grand purpose; somehow it proved a point.

Richard Wilson didn't have a point to prove. His was needless suffering; he was going to die of his disease no matter what we did.

If I hastened the process of his death, didn't that make me a murderer? In my mind I heard the nuns repeating the Ten

Commandments, getting stuck on number five: "Thou shalt not kill." But wasn't I questioning the suffering? If Richard Wilson were an animal in pain, there would be no question; it would be the humane thing to do in everyone's mind. Did human beings deserve less than other animals?

I looked back at the porcelain god and remembered the little brass Buddha sitting on the shelf over my stove. I addressed them both aloud. "Okay, you enlightened guys, what do you think? Is it okay to ease someone out of suffering toward death? Would either of you mind very much?"

I was answered by a noise the chapel door made when it opened. Two black women entered and sat down in the first pew without noticing me.

One was older than the other and quite obese. The young one was thin and pretty. With her wide, high cheekbones covered by light satin skin, she was the female version of Richard Wilson.

The older woman knelt and started to rock herself. "Oh, Lord, help us." She said it only once.

The younger woman bent over and put her head on the mother's shoulder. Her voice was soft. "It's all right, Mama. It's the best thing. Everybody's suffering is over now." In her words there was great resolve.

Other than a few prayers and some soft weeping, I heard nothing more.

The girl's voice saying, "Everybody's suffering is over now," played like a broken record in my ears as I sneaked back through the hallways and into the conference room thirty minutes later. Hunched over a piece of paper, I was recording my thoughts when Miss Telmack came in and stood over me with her arms crossed over her chest, just as my mother would have done when I was nine years old and in trouble.

"Mr. Wilson just expired. . . ."

She said it as if it were some kind of victory on her part.

I displayed no emotion. Although I'd already guessed as much from the scene in the chapel, the news saddened me and gave me a sense of relief at the same time.

". . . and you are in a heap of trouble." She finished her sentence smiling.

"Okay." That was all I could think of to say. I could tell Miss Telmack expected more, but she went on anyway.

"First of all, the head nurse on the ward is furious you let

Mr. Wilson go unmedicated for so long and has asked you not be placed on her floor again.''

She stopped to see the effect this obvious disgrace had on me. My father had taught me everything there was to know about poker faces when I was five.

"Second of all, I am going to write an incident report against you and put it in your student file.''

As if I were a prisoner going to the gallows she asked in a somber, melancholy voice, "Do you have anything you would like to say?''

I thought for a second, got my bearings, and mentally squared my shoulders. "You're right about not letting the patient suffer, but I am not prepared to take on that responsibility right now. You were also right about this being a problem I'll face again, and I need to handle it better, but heavily medicating a person like Mr. Wilson isn't anything I would ever want to be comfortable with. I'm glad I find it so difficult. At least I know that if and when I ever do put someone out, it'll be a decision made with a lot of thought behind it.''

I paused, remembering Janey's words at lunch.

"Thank you for giving this patient to me, and I'm sorry it didn't work out right for either of us.''

Miss Telmack was not to be moved. "Very pretty speech, Heron, but you still haven't come up with enough to assure me you won't let the next patient suffer for hours while you're putting 'a lot of thought' behind medicating him.''

I stood up and shook my head. That certain righteousness which caused most of the trouble in my life reared itself up against Miss Telmack's hard crust.

"Miss Telmack, I don't feel great about today, either. Did you ever think of that? I can't stand to see people suffer; it makes me crazy. Maybe after I've medicated a few people out of their pain and into another world, I'll be as comfortable with it as the rest of the nurses on the wards appear to be, but for the last time, Miss Telmack, until I've had time to think this issue over, and experience a time when it'll be right for me to do so, you can't push me to do what you want me to do by writing notes against me or getting me kicked off wards. I'm sorry. I think you meant for me to succeed, but I just have to go at my own pace on this one.''

After gathering my books and coat, I went to the door,

feeling daring, brave, and a bit dramatic. "I'm leaving now. I can't handle this place anymore today. I'm going home."

Miss Telmack, to my surprise, didn't protest but, rather, waved me out of the room, saying, "Fine, Heron, do what you want, I don't care."

Walking down the hall, I felt bad about Miss Telmack, but worse for Richard Wilson. I turned the corner and ran into the morgue wagon, the deep gurney with a false bottom which inconspicuously held dead bodies while they were transferred from the bed to the basement. It was coming from the direction of Richard Wilson's room.

When the orderlies pushed it past me, I tapped on the top and watched it disappear into the elevator.

"So long, Richard," I whispered. "I'm sorry I couldn't help you, but there *was* a point; the next time I'll remember you."

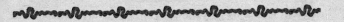

EIGHT

THE WHEELCHAIR and its owner came to an abrupt halt in front of bed one.

To set the brake, I leaned over the old bag lady, known throughout the county as Wheelin' Wilma, and two things happened: I saw her hair, looking very much like an abandoned winter nest, *move* by itself. Then I smelled her.

Without giving thought to how it looked to the other patients, I put my hand to my mouth and backed away, gagging. The rancid smell of her filth stung my nose, making my eyes water. I turned my face to the wall and breathed in a gulp of untainted air, hoping the childhood ability to hold my breath for long periods of time had not left me.

I scrunched up my eyes, to clear away any momentary hallucinations caused by some foreign crustation on my contact lenses, and moved closer to stare once more at the back of Wilma's head.

No! Yes, there it went again; I wasn't losing my mind. The top layer of the matted clump of hair which rested heavily on the old woman's neck actually (my stomach did not want to hear the word) *swarmed*.

"What's yer problem, girlie?" Wilma shouted testily. "Whaddaya doin' behind there anyway? I want some service!"

I finished locking the brakes, and into Wilma's good ear, the one without the hearing aid, I excused myself in the strained voice of one who is holding her breath and backed away from the wheelchair. A few feet away I let out my breath, wiped my eyes, and went in search of someone to confirm what I'd seen.

Despite the sting of Wilma's lingering odor in my nose, I was in excitement heaven. The longest, dreariest winter of my life had followed the inevitable path of nature and ended in spring semester. As far back as January I had begun counting the hours to graduation night; from 2,880 I was down to 201, and 15 hours into the instructors' new brainchild known as the "student forty-hour week."

Since the beginning of March the instructors had hinted there would be a wonderful, mysterious "surprise" for us at the end of the year. In the middle of April each of us was asked to list three areas of medicine in which we would most like to work and indicate the hospitals of our choice.

I figured I'd beat the system and signed up for emergency at Redwoods Memorial as my first, second, and third choices. Janey surprised me by choosing surgery in the Oakland hospital. She said she liked the carefully planned-out nature of the work, bezoars being as much excitement as she could handle.

Most of the other students picked areas Janey and I guessed they might. P.J. was the only one we called completely wrong. Because of her fondness for infants and children, we both assumed she'd pick nursery or pediatrics. Instead, P.J. chose isolation. It was, she said, a place where she'd be forced to stop biting her nails.

In the first week of May, Claudia, our final rotation instructor, handed us our assignments. I was to report for work the following Monday at Redwoods Memorial emergency room under the supervision of Katy Rankin, RN, and Dr. Susan Mahoney.

For reasons as mysterious as the ones for which Miss Telmack disliked me, Claudia favored me and showed concern for my wellbeing every step of the way. After giving us our assignments, she called me aside to ask if I'd thought over my choice carefully.

"It wasn't a very popular choice among the students, you know," she said, looking deeply concerned. "There isn't a lot of slack to relax in that department, and emotional stress seems to go along with the job. Are you sure you want to do this for your last week? I could reassign you if you want to reconsider."

I thought of Amy and for half a second wavered. Then I thought of Tony, and Amy's mother, and the weeping "almost" suicides.

"Nope, I'm sure," I answered with finality. "It's one of the places I'll learn the most while doing the most good."

Inside, I wondered if the week might not cure me of the insane notion that living in a constant state of crisis was what I really wanted in my everyday life.

My first day, however, was slow, giving Dr. Mahoney, Katy, and me a chance for a long and warm reunion. Katy, with her uncanny ability to remember patients, then follow up on them years after she'd seen them just once, gave me the scoop on a few of my star patients from the year before.

Her clear blue eyes sparkled when she told me Tony was finishing his sophomore year as a top honors student. She said she'd seen him several weeks before at a local football game, riding on a friend's shoulders, wearing a bright orange fright wig and a pair of huge fake breasts. "They were being obnoxiously amusing, cheering for the opposing team—you know, typical academically stressed-out type A behavior."

I laughed, recalling the explanation Dr. Menowitz had given when he diagnosed Tony's headache.

"On the down side," Katy added, "Amy's mom flipped out about a month after the accident and ended up in the psychiatric unit. Dad divorced her and then proceeded to lose his job because he was drunk all the time." She squinted in thought. "I'm pretty sure somebody told me Amy's mom finally got it together and now works as a librarian in San Rafael. Anyway, I hope so. She's had enough grief to last her a lifetime."

Dr. Mahoney put in her two cents' worth of information while Katy stopped to think. "You missed one of the biggest news items of the year last December, Ec. The surgeons sent out notices on yellow stationery announcing they'd treated themselves to a present and forced Dr. Drigely to resign."

"You are kidding!" I shouted, clapping my hands.

"I never kid about the antics of my fellow physicians," she replied, mocking seriousness. "Anyway, I guess old Drigely, who was already on probation, was trying out some hand surgery one day when he ran into a few problems he hadn't banked on. He got so wound up, he refused to deflate the tourniquet after the anesthesiologist warned him a few times he was over the time limit.

"Deprived of a blood supply for a bit too long, the patient's hand sustained enough nerve damage to limit its function significantly. It was the last straw on a whole haystack of screwups.

"Of course, I can't remember for sure if the notice was worded quite like that; but it *was* on yellow stationery, and Drigely hasn't been seen since."

Suddenly remembering something, Katy interrupted. "Oh, I know who you might want to know about. Remember Orville Robinson, that sweet old black man with CA of the stomach? He went home, then came back in July to die. He still told people the reason he was sick was that his stomach just got angry at him one day and quit speakin' to him."

"And speaking of nice guys, wait until you see Dr. Menowitz," Dr. Mahoney said, smiling mysteriously. I mugged a sour face.

"Really, Ec, Menowitz's outlook is completely changed now that he's started going to therapy once a week," she said. "You won't recognize him; he's just as sweet as he never was before."

An hour later we were still indulging in the art of gossip when a pretty, slightly overweight woman joined the group. She was introduced to me as Gus, the latest addition to the ER nursing staff. Just transplanted from Tennessee, she'd landed the job after only one year of clinical experience. As stupid as it was, a pang of severe jealousy with its ugly black tarantula legs crossed me.

I liked Gus right off. Besides her enchanting soft southern manner, she had a laugh as infectious as my cousin Ralph's.

One of the few pleasures awarded me as a child was to be shipped off for three weeks to my Aunt Martha's farm. Immediately upon depositing my suitcases, I'd run down the road to the dairy farm which bordered the north end of Aunt Martha's land. There a boy I knew as Cousin Ralph resided.

Together we milked cows, jumped from the rafters of the barn, collected eggs, and, on the very best of those five-star days, were allowed to take turns churning the butter. After a week, when all those things inevitably lost their novelty, making Ralph's life miserable was my favorite pastime. It took him a couple of years, but Ralph finally came up with a retaliation plan straight from the diary of the Marquis de Sade.

Calling on my competitive spirit, Cousin Ralph would engage me in a lemonade-gulping contest to see who could drink the most, the fastest, and with the least amount of swallows. For a half hour or so he'd stick to me like glue until something in his diabolical mind told him the time was right. Then, without warning, he'd tell me every inane joke he knew.

As soon as I let the first giggle sneak out, Cousin Ralph would throw back his head and produce a laugh the likes of which could roust bats from caves. No matter how hard I tried to fight it, I'd end up laughing with such force I would barely make it to the bathroom in time. Of course, Cousin Ralph would have locked the bathroom door from the inside and sneaked out the window. Aunt Martha did more hand laundry in those days. . . .

Gus found out I was as conditioned as Pavlov's dogs; all she had to do was let loose with a Cousin Ralph, and I was holding my sides, headed for the bathroom.

By the end of the day Katy, Dr. Mahoney, and Gus had agreed unanimously to throw everything in the book at me. Even Irene was included in the conspiracy; she was instructed to search me out before anyone else when a patient was ready to be brought back from the lobby.

"No mercy for you, Mountain Noise," said Dr. Mahoney. "You're going to see every patient and assist with or do every procedure that needs to be done."

True to their words, of the twenty-five patients seen between the hours of seven and one-thirty on Tuesday, I'd personally brought back twenty of them and assisted with fifteen different procedures. I helped remove fishhooks from fingers, assisted pulling shoulder joints back into their sockets, inserted nasogastric tubes and bladder catheters, removed sutures, and watched spellbound as new ones were sewn in.

My fascination with lacerations did not go unnoticed, and over lunch Dr. Mahoney took a piece of foam, cut through part of it, and taught me how to do basic suturing. Ever since I'd flunked my seventh-grade sewing class for making a blouse the sleeves of which ended up being attached to the collar, I'd hated sewing, but mending skin was different. I liked the way the jagged shreds could be trimmed and sewn together to look as if nothing had ever happened. Amazingly enough, however, for all its reconstructive beauty, people balked at the idea of being sewn up.

Conditioned adults, who'd long since learned to suppress their natural reactions to pain, often reverted to screaming for mommy at the sight of the suture kit. Children, of course, still followed the tendency to announce their objections loudly no matter how many simple soft-voiced explanations were given. Even with promises of ice cream cones and McDonald's, cajolery rarely worked. Kids aren't fools; no matter how we tried to get them to look at it, "magic mending" still meant needles and pain.

When there was no recourse, we used the papoose board, a contraption made of wood and canvas to render the child motionless while we numbed the laceration and sewed.

Dr. Mahoney preferred the nurses to hold the child down, a job I found hard to execute. As soon as I saw the quivering chins, felt their limbs accelerate in an effort to get free, I had to hide my face to keep from crying. Nonetheless, Katy and Gus demonstrated the various contortions one could single-handedly use to hold down a kicking, screaming two-year-old, be able to speak soothingly to him, and still keep an eye on Mom and Dad if they started looking pale.

During my first attempt at this I lay sprawled limb to limb across the twisting body of a three-year-old while Dr. Mahoney sutured her forehead. Off to the side seven-year-old sister stood next to Dad, looking on, bragging that nothing about blood bothered her. After a few moments of silence I looked up just in time to see the glazed look cross her face, followed by a buckled knee dip. As soon as she passed out, Dad, looking a little gray himself, leaned over to pick her up and, halfway down, followed her example.

Until I leaned over to set the brakes of Wheelin' Wilma's wheelchair, I was sure no rock had been left unturned. Wilma's odor had me singing a different tune.

Irene, like Katy, seemed to know everyone in the county. She could give a synoptic life history of almost every person whose chart she handed me. He was a distant relative of hers or her husband's, or she'd met him twenty-seven years ago while vacationing, or she was the friend of a neighbor's friend who was the dear friend of a friend of hers.

Wilma, Irene told me, was a "repeater," one of ER's regular weekly customers. Sometimes her complaints were legitimate; mostly she was just looking for a warm meal and a little human companionship. Furtively looking around, Irene "confidentially" informed me that after Wilma's husband had died and left her penniless ("Well, actually I'd heard he left her twelve dollars"), her children ("My husband's sister read there was a boy and a girl") deserted her. Unemployable, Wilma took to the streets of San Francisco, taking an advanced course on how to be a proper bag lady. For a few years Wilma did pretty well for herself, living in the lap of bag lady luxury ("Those women make a lot of money off the junk they collect, you know!"), until she'd been hit by a speeding taxicab, which had left her paralyzed from the waist down. ("The papers said she was drunk, you know, stepped right out in front of the car . . . tried to sue the company . . . didn't get a dime.") Tsk-tsk.

Now, as a recipient of the state's generosity ("That means out of our paychecks!"), Wilma lived with her four cats and faithful spotted mongrel in a deserted school bus on the outskirts of Sausalito and in her spare time, which was most of it, took in more stray cats and dogs.

She loved her animals as a mother loves her children. ("God knows her own were failures!"), and with the money from her meager welfare checks, she fed them, groomed them, and turned over whatever was left to a local veterinarian who checked them over and cared for their wounds.

When the animals were restored, Wilma personally found homes for each one of them. It was, in certain sophisticated circles about the county, *très chic* to own one of Wilma's former strays.

While Wilma took excellent care of her animals, she paid very little, if any, attention to her own personal hygiene. On this visit Wilma's complaint was a sore, itching scalp. From what I'd seen and smelled, I believed she had a legitimate gripe.

Dr. Mahoney and Katy were busy pulling a piece of steak out of an inebriated man's windpipe, so I accosted Gus, who was just taking her first bite of lunch.

"Sorry to do this while you're eating, Gus, but would you help me out with Wheelin' Wilma? There's something making her hair move," I said, "and it ain't the wind."

Gus looked past me and waved to Wilma. "Sure. Wilma

and I have a great respect for each other, especially after she bit me the last time she was here.''

Gus moved into the suture room, where she donned a long-sleeved isolation gown, a pair of rubber gloves, and a paper surgical cap over her hair. She waited for me to do the same.

"You never know with Wilma," she explained, "living in that truck out there in the swamps with those animals and no water or facilities; I wouldn't touch her without protection if I were you.''

I put on the gloves but couldn't go to the extent of the isolation gown and cap. "That's going to make her feel terrible, Gus. She's going to feel like some kind of freak leper if we both go over there looking like that.''

"That's up to you, Ec," Gus said, shrugging her large, rounded shoulders. "As for me, I've got two more hours of contact with other patients, and then I go home to my husband, two kids, and one dog, and I'll guarantee you none of the aforementioned need whatever Wilma's got. By the time you finish dealing with her, you'll wish they made condoms big enough to fit your whole body into.''

I considered what Gus said, and a few minutes later we both approached Wilma looking like something from outer space. She glanced first at me and then at Gus. I expected a caustic remark. Instead, she just shook her head and clicked her tongue. "That bad, eh?''

Gus nodded, and holding our respective breaths, we picked Wilma up out of the chair and put her on the gurney. Our neck veins bulged with the effort; for someone who reportedly didn't have enough to eat, Wilma was keeping up on her weight.

Not seeming to mind the rank odor as much as I, Gus drew the curtains around the gurney and was soon breathing normally.

"For God's sake, Wilma, why don't you take a bath? You smell awful.''

Gus had a rare quality to her tone of voice, which, when combined with her southern accent, came out sounding kindly and maternal no matter how harsh the words or how stern the reprimand.

"Aw, come on, Gussie, you know I don't got no water or washtub at my place, and them public showers aren't made for wheelchairs.'' Wilma sniffed. "Besides, the animals don't care, and I quit goin' to all them fancy dignitary dinners a long time ago, ya know.'' Wilma's cackle sounded like the scream of a wounded peacock.

Gus and I removed the top layer of Wilma's various coats and sweaters.

"That's no excuse, Wilma," continued Gus. "If you can take care of those stray animals, you can clean yourself."

Without warning Wilma jabbed a dirty, discolored finger into Gus's shoulder. "Just do your job, sister, and take care of my head!"

Gus ignored Wilma's jabs and continued what she was doing without comment, but I took exception to the incident. There was a certain hostility in the old woman's demand that disturbed my initial impression of Wilma as a "character," eccentric but likable.

After removing a third coat, we got down to Wilma's shirt. Stiff with soil and any number of caked-on substances, the material tore easily under our hands.

Naked to the waist, Wilma's skin looked like a work of modern art, covered with splotches of different-colored dirt and grime. The areas under armpits and around her neck were red and irritated. I handed Wilma a patient gown and told her to put it on. She shoved it back at me.

"You do it," she said indignantly. "I'm tired!"

Rather than hassle with her, I slipped the thin piece of cotton over her arms, feeling a small dose of resentment creep into my throat.

Gus pulled the exam light over to Wilma's head. From a fair distance she studied the old woman's hair and then the skin of her neck. Involuntarily she shuddered and stepped back. Pointing at the back of Wilma's head, she mouthed the word *"lice."*

I leaned closer to look. The small gray-white parasites crawled at a steady pace through her hair and in the folds of her neck. An innocent, subconscious curiosity caused me to pick up the matted bun so I could see Wilma's scalp.

A shiny brown cockroach dropped to the floor and scurried under the bedside cabinet with the greatest of insect speed. Gus, half laughing, half screaming, jumped up against the wall. I clung to the far end of the curtain, whimpering. Cockroaches were to me what the rats in room 101 were to Winston in George Orwell's *Nineteen Eighty-Four*.

Immediately my head began to itch, and I was sure I felt something crawling on my scalp over my left ear. I moved to scratch my head and realized I was about to touch myself with the same hand that had just touched Wilma's hair. I froze, and my arms started to feel crawly. I glanced over at Gus; she was scratching the side of her face with her shoulder.

"Wilma, you got a bunch of creatures taking up residence on you," said Gus, briefly blotting her perspiring upper lip with her shoulder.

"Well, hell, get 'em off me. That's what I came here for!" Wilma said, scowling.

Gus moved around to face Wilma. "I think you've got to let us cut that wad of hair off so we can see why you're sore underneath. I'm sure Dr. Mahoney will send you home with some special shampoo and soap, and you'll have to wash all your clothes and linen. Can you do all that?"

We watched Wilma while she chewed on the idea. After a minute she stared at us, wearing a belligerent expression. "Naw. Sounds like too much work for this old crip."

Gus gave one of her more expressive sighs. "Okay, Wilma, in that case, I think we've got to get county services involved. Maybe they can find you a temporary place to stay and somebody who can help you, but we really can't let you wander around in public like this, spreading these critters all over the place."

Wilma was stunned by the unexpected turn of events, and her eyes filled with tears. "What about my animals? I got a new kitten that needs to be eyedropper-fed every few hours; who's gonna take care of him, huh?"

Gus knelt and looked kindly into Wilma's face. "I'll make arrangements with the ASPCA to take care of all your animals until this is over, but from now on, Wilma, I want to see you take better care of yourself. You've got to promise you'll do something about the way you're living. People won't be as nice to you if you don't try to help yourself; you know that, don't you?"

Still tearful, Wilma nodded her head reluctantly in agreement.

Gus left me to shear off the infested chignon alone. Taping one side of a plastic trash bag to Wilma's neck, I opened the top, and readied my bandage scissors.

I wanted to get the bugs contained as quickly as possible, but after making one cut into the thick gray hair, I stopped abruptly. The sound of the hair being cut brought me to the edge of a dark memory. Skirting around the unpleasant thought, I made another cut, and the sound again roused a hazy memory picture.

Disregarding my conscious wish, my mind rebelliously stepped into the cold fruit cellar of the house where I grew up. Sitting on a high wooden stool, I sat quietly weeping while my mother placed a bowl over my head and sheared off the ends of my already short hair. Vanity in a girl of thirteen, she told me sternly, was a sign of shamelessness and a most grievous sin.

I released Wilma's hair from the grip of the scissors.

"Whaddya stoppin' for?"

Snapping to, I finished cutting off the clump and let it fall into the bag. The newly exposed section of Wilma's scalp was raw and infected from her scratching.

"God, Wilma, you've scratched yourself raw." I showed her the mess of infested hair before I tied off the bag with a piece of string.

Wilma looked at the matted stuff dubiously and shrugged it off. "Lookit, sister, don't bother me with the gory details. It's your job to take care of it."

Fury hit me like a twenty-foot wave. I felt used. The woman was a taker, and nothing anyone could do for her would ever be enough; she would always expect, *demand* more.

I swallowed, gritted my teeth, and let go. "You got that wrong, lady!" The statement came out of me with such sudden force and volume that Wilma jumped, and her watery eyes widened with surprise. "It's not *my* job. It's yours, damn it! You come off with this I'm-a-cripple attitude and that we're some subservient group of butt wipers, obligated to take care of your whims. If you really want to know, Wilma, you are so far off base, it makes me sick! There're a lot of people worse off than you who have really done something for themselves. Stop expecting other people to pull you up. Work a little, Wilma. Struggle a little; go for something better than just surviving."

Self-control grabbed me by the throat and choked me. All of a sudden I was in the throes of remorse. Surreptitiously, I looked around the curtain to see if anybody besides Wilma had heard me.

Dr. Mahoney, standing by the next gurney, looked up from the wrist she was examining. "Subservient butt wipers?" she mouthed, raising her eyebrows. I shrugged, my face burning with embarrassment, and closed the curtain.

Wilma had started to cry and hyperventilate at the same time. She tried poking her finger at me, but I moved out of the way. "You git somebody else to take care of me, somebody who's nice, you dirty-mouthed snot! I got my rights! Git that other nurse back here, or I'll sue you for malpractice!" Wilma blew her nose and wiped her eyes on the hem of her gown.

She looked away from me and muttered, "Little snipe! Treating a poor cripple like that . . ."

The conflicting emotions of wanting to scream at her and pity triggered an instant fantasy in which the basic Wilma, meticulously manicured and dressed, sat in a clean and cozy living room, reading a book on flower arrangements. At her feet lay a snoozing spotted mongrel and four cats; there was not one flea among them.

"Okay, Wilma, just relax," I said. "I'll have Gus come back." Plaintively I sealed my gown and other protective paraphernalia in a plastic bag and left the woman alone.

I was in the middle of explaining to Gus why Wilma had "fired" me when the triage buzzer sounded once. I signed Wilma's chart over to Gus and walked to the lobby.

The couple was highly visible from the other side of the lobby. Both walked barefoot, he dressed in something all white with fringe, she in a floor-length purple dress. Both wore several strands of bright orange beads.

In the man's arms lay a feverish boy of about ten whose face was flushed with pain. The child attempted to keep himself from crying out by puffing up his cheeks and biting down on his lower lip. In the hand that rigidly protected his belly, he gripped a small orange book which his mother urged him to kiss from time to time.

As soon as I escorted them in, Dr. Mahoney, who was in the middle of examining Wilma, rapidly discarded her gloves and gown and turned her attention to the boy. She asked the parents a few pertinent questions about the child's symptoms, examined him, and ordered lab tests.

The man and woman watched everything Dr. Mahoney did with interest, asking all the appropriate questions, yet I had the distinct feeling they were somehow removed from what was happening to their son.

When Dr. Mahoney received the results of the boy's blood work, she told the parents she was ninety percent certain their son was suffering from acute appendicitis.

The man looked abstracted for a moment, then began aimlessly wandering around the room. Ignoring his strange behavior, Dr. Mahoney followed behind him, explaining why the boy needed immediate surgery. She spelled out all the grave consequences of a ruptured appendix, defining peritonitis and the process that could lead to death. No matter what she said, the man did not appear to be interested. Stopping at Irene's counter, Dr. Mahoney picked up the phone and prepared to dial.

"Since you don't list a private physician, I'd like to have Dr. Bell, one of the surgeons on staff here, take a look at your son."

The man took a step in Dr. Mahoney's direction. "Don't you do that!" he yelled menacingly at her. Then, regaining his composure, he added, "My son will not need surgery."

Dr. Mahoney put the phone down and looked at him in complete astonishment. "I beg your pardon?"

"Our son will be taken care of by God. We cannot, under the teachings of our religion, allow surgery on our child. God will heal him."

Although Dr. Mahoney spoke in a soft, monotone voice, I wasn't fooled; I knew the earmarks of a slow, hot temper better than I knew the back of my hand.

"You obviously don't understand what I've said, so I'll repeat myself," Dr. Mahoney stated evenly. "I am almost certain your son has acute appendicitis. The appendix will rupture if it is not surgically removed very soon. If the appendix ruptures, your son may very well die from the infection that could follow." Dr. Mahoney did not take her eyes from the man's stony face. "Do you understand now?"

The woman stepped forth, haughty and domineering. "No, Doctor, it is *you* who do not understand the ways of our Lord. Through our prayers, the Lord will see that one of His children is sick. He will send His healing power to my son. God, not surgery, will heal the boy.''

Dr. Mahoney looked down at the sick child and then back at the parents. ''Why did you come here if you weren't going to let us take care of him?''

Obviously pleased with himself, the man picked his son up. ''We had to make sure the boy was really ill. We didn't want to bother the Lord for a simple case of gas.''

Dr. Mahoney calmly stepped out of the way for the family to pass.

''Thank you for your help, Doctor,'' the man muttered as he walked by her, ''and may the Lord bless you.''

Susan Mahoney glowered at the man. ''Before you leave . . .''

The man and woman stopped in their tracks at the tone of command in Dr. Mahoney's voice. In the same emotionless monotone a police officer often employs when informing a criminal of his rights, Dr. Mahoney spoke up. ''Before you leave, you or the boy's mother must sign a legal document saying you release me and the hospital from all responsibility for injuries or death occurring to your child as a result of your refusal to obtain the advised necessary medical treatment for him.''

She took in another breath and continued to recite, apparently from memory. ''I also need to inform you that what you are doing by refusing medical treatment could be interpreted under the law as child abuse. We will contact the Child Protective Service immediately, and you may face having your child forcibly removed from your custody. Under the laws of California, in the event that your son suffers serious or fatal injuries as a result of your actions, you run the risk of being indicted for homicide.''

She gestured toward me and Katy. ''Miss Heron and Miss Rankin are witnesses to what I've just informed you. Please sign the against medical advice form.''

Irene had the paper stamped and ready. The man smiled knowingly and signed it without hesitation. ''God will protect my family,'' he said softly, walking out the side door. ''Our faith will keep us well.''

Disdainfully Dr. Mahoney watched the couple leave and called out after them, ''You'll need more than protection; you're going to need a miracle.''

She turned her attention to Irene. "Would you kindly put a call into the Child Protective Service, please?"

"Dr. Mahoney, how can you let them take that kid home?" I whispered in alarm.

A touch of temper tenaciously hung on the edge of her words. "I can't forcibly stop them, no more than you can force Wilma to clean herself up and make her stay that way. I'll talk to the Child Protective Service; that's all I can do."

Dr. Mahoney looked at me. "For chrissake, don't look so *worried*. They'll be back! I swear, they'll be back!" She shuffled some papers on the clerk's counter. "You can't live with these people; it wouldn't matter anyway. They'll go right back to their old mind-sets soon as you stop holding their hands."

"But doesn't that get to you?" I asked, refusing to believe she could be so cool after the scene that had just taken place.

"Not like it used to." Dr. Mahoney smiled a little and stared at her hands. "You should have seen me when I was the crusader physician of Berkeley; talk about righteous! Whew! I still get a little hot under the collar, but not righteous anymore . . . takes too much out of me. Listen, do you realize we have a list of eighty-eight patients who can't be treated in this emergency room, unless it's a life-threatening situation, just because they abuse us or the system? You've got to go upstairs to the general medical floors if you want to deal with the nice, nearly normal people who come in with normal, legitimate medical problems, like pneumonia or a clean coronary."

She flicked a few stray hairs out of my eyes. "If you really want to work down here someday, you've got to learn to get a handle on your feelings and control them; otherwise, you'll be a whitehaired, unhappy lunatic of no use to anybody.

"See, doctors rarely have that problem; from day one of med school, we're all conditioned to be scientific about everything, to be always right. We don't really deal with people on the same level as nurses, and sometimes that's unfortunate. But if I walked around here crying or getting pissed-off at every turn, I'd be . . . an unemployed wacko inside a week.

"It's a balancing act of a lot of different factors and emotions, and you are your own master juggler."

* * *

Other than Gus's coat and purse sitting on the back table, I saw no other evidence of human life. I checked the clock: 7:30 A.M. Wednesday. Only seven days to graduation.

The percolator perked and spit, filling the room with a rich aroma of newly made coffee. From the other side of the wall the classic, unmistakable sound of a toilet flushing heralded Gus's appearance. She reminded me of a country-western singer with her long mass of curly brown hair. Beaming, she skipped up to me with outstretched hands, palms up and executed an interesting Al Jolson knee bend.

"Hey, hey, Eckie, baby! How goes it for you on this fine San Francisco Bay Area morning?"

Gus was the only person I currently knew who could be revved up and onstage at seven-thirty in the morning. I guessed she must have had at least two cups of coffee with the night shift while getting report.

She touched my hair admiringly. "Boy, that lice shampoo really made your hair shine, didn't it?"

A Cousin Ralph laugh escaped, and against my will I honked out a hard guffaw.

"Well, Eckie, honey, today's emergency staff consists of Dr. Mahoney, me, you, and whatever float nurse we can beg, borrow, or steal. Katy Finkface called in sick at five and told night shift the only known cure for what she has was to spend the day in Big Sur with her boyfriend. We're wounded but still able to keep the doors to the public open; we'll make Florence so proud of us she'll turn in her grave and spit a wooden nickel!"

At the end of Gus's animated monologue Irene came in, moving languidly, but not without some purpose, toward the coffee. Greeting us, she poured a cup and leaned against the sink. Her eyebrows knitted tightly together, she sipped her coffee with a certain amount of delicacy.

"You know," she said uneasily, "I think I should tell you two there was something very suspicious going on in the parking lot when I came in just now." She stopped for an uncharacteristic pause, then went on. "I overheard, only briefly, mind you, an argument in the big light-colored car that's parked right out in front to the lobby doors. It wasn't any of my business, of course, but when I passed by, I heard a woman say something like 'I'm hurt; you've got to help me.' Now I could be wrong, but—''

Gus and I left Irene talking to herself and went to the parking lot. Just as Irene had said, there was a big light-colored car parked by the doors. Cautiously moving closer to the auto, we heard a man yelling and stopped to listen.

"Hey, asshole, didn't you hear me? I said I'm *not* taking you in there! You did it yourself! Get out and walk yourself!"

Reactivated by the abusive language, Gus hurried around the car and knocked, none too gently, on the driver's window. A moment passed. Gus raised her hand again when the window rolled down with a high-pitched mechanical whir. A large, red-faced man in his sixties focused with difficulty on Gus's white uniform and name tag. Weaving, he looked back at the passenger.

"Here! Here's a nurse. Get her to help you." He turned to Gus. "My wife has had an accident with a cigarette"—he slurred the words—"and she wants to talk to you." Gripping the steering wheel, he stiffly pushed himself back into the plush seat so Gus could see the passenger.

Peering around the man's head, Gus froze, then jerked her head up. "Get a gurney!' she screamed. "Stat!"

I raced into the trauma room and grabbed the gurney. Irene looked at me questioningly.

"Find Dr. Mahoney. Tell her we're going to need her for"—I realized I didn't know what was in the front seat of the car—"for something stat!"

When I got to the parking lot, Gus was standing just inside the opened passenger door. Hearing the squeak of the gurney wheels, she turned around, looking wild.

"Quick, Ec! Help me get her up."

I situated the gurney as close to the passenger door as I could and got a whiff of what smelled like a smoldering campfire.

"Thank God she's as drunk as he is," whispered Gus. I glanced down at the passenger.

The only things I recognized were a huddled human form, a pair of half-melted slippers, and the sleeve of a quilted plaid houserobe. From those starting points I was able to put together the charred figure.

My eyes traveled from the slippers to the head, which was like that of a hairless mannequin painted glossy black. Sticking out over her ears were straggling wisps of burned hair. I leaned closer trying to discern the nose and mouth, when two blue eyes opened and stared into my face.

"Hi, honey, I'm Estelle," she said in a voice that could have belonged to Froggy in *Our Gang*. Her teeth were badly stained with nicotine, and her breath was loaded with booze. "Could you get me a hanky so I can cough up some of this crap from my throat?"

"Sure, sure," I answered, feeling nervous as a cat; my experience in dealing with burns of this magnitude was nil. "Let's get you onto this gurney first, and I'll get you all the Kleenex you can use in just a sec, okay, Estelle?"

Her head wobbled drunkenly, and she laughed a little. "Okey-dokey, pokey."

The woman couldn't have stood more than five feet and weighed less than a hundred pounds. Easily we lifted her onto the gurney. As soon as we were clear of the car, the man slammed the door shut from the inside, gunned the motor, and squealed out of the parking lot. The woman didn't look in the direction of the car but raised her voice. "You miserable bastard! I hope you run into a pole and break your goddamn head!"

As we sped through the empty corridor into the trauma room, Gus told me the only information she'd got from the man was that his wife had fallen asleep smoking and woke up in flames. He couldn't, however, remember how long ago that had been.

As we flew past Irene's desk, she caught a glimpse of the burned form and pivoted away from the sight.

I grabbed a box of Kleenex and, in my nervousness, took out too many, spilling half of them on the floor. The spindly right arm and hand, the only unburned part of her, came up to grab the tissue. With a wet, rumbling cough, she brought up a glob of gray mucus streaked with black.

Gus grabbed my arm. "Oh, shit!" she said under her breath. "Her airway is involved. We've got to move fast." She placed a two-pronged oxygen cannula in the woman's nose, being careful not to irritate any of the burned skin, and turned the flow to high.

Irene hurried to the door. "Dr. Mahoney is in ICU reintubating a patient. She said to hold down the fort as best you can and she'd be here as soon as she could."

I shot a look at Gus. "Help!" I said, panicking. "I don't know what to do. I've never seen anything like this before. You're going to have to walk me through there."

"Sure," she said. I could see her mind was racing. "Sure. It's okay, don't worry, we can do it. The airway is the main thing, but that's okay for right now, so you get her vitals and I'll start the IV."

I cut away the scorched sleeve of Estelle's right arm and took her BP and pulse, while Gus assembled the IV equipment.

We were so intent on what we were doing that when the woman suddenly spoke, we both started. "Yeah," she said loudly, "I tried to get that son of a bitch to bring me in before, but he was too drunk." The woman giggled. "Of course, he wasn't as drunk as me. . . ."

Gus applied the tourniquet to Estelle's arm and sponged off the skin with an alcohol wipe. She picked up the large-bore angiocath. "What do you mean, 'before'? When did this happen?"

Estelle ignored the question and pulled her arm out of Gus's grip. Tentatively she touched the top of her head and pulled off a clump of the burned hair. Her hand wove as she tried to study it. "Yeeech! What a mess! I must look like hell," she murmured.

I wondered if she knew the irony of her statement.

Gus gently pulled her arm back down and probed for the large antecubital vein. Finding it quickly, she slipped in the angiocath and released the clamp, letting the IV solution run in wide open.

Together we cut away what was left of the robe. Pieces of black cotton, mixed with strips of what must have been a flannel nightgown, lay in a small heap on the floor.

In the fastest mathematical calculations I'd ever done, I added up the percentage of Estelle's body which had been burned, using the rule of nines. Her chest, a mixture of third- and second-degree burns, accounted for eighteen percent; her left arm added another nine percent; the head nine percent, and so on, until I came up with a total of seventy-two percent. From the burned pattern of her clothes and limbs, I guessed the fire had started at her feet and spread upward. Besides her right arm, which must have been under something or outstretched, her buttocks and upper back, which had pressed against the chair, had also escaped harm.

Gus tried to ease off Estelle's right slipper and had to cut around the plastic that had melted into the skin. When I removed the left slipper, four of her toes were missing. Checking inside the slipper, I found the remains of the woman's foot mixed with a gob of plastic and nylon.

We covered her with two sterile sheets and doused them down with saline. Halfway through the second quart, Dr. Mahoney appeared.

While we gave her the scanty information we had, she quickly listened to the woman's lungs and checked over the rest of Estelle's body. Looking concerned, she stepped over to the door and spoke rapidly to Irene. "First call respiratory for intubation; then call lab. I want a paramedic ambulance in ten minutes flat and put in a call to the San Francisco burn center; say we're sending them a female with more than seventy percent burns. I'll give the details when you get them on the line."

Dr. Mahoney brought her face parallel to Estelle's. "How do you do. I'm Dr. Mahoney. Can you tell me how and when this happened?"

"Hi, honey, I'm Estelle." After that Estelle seemed to forget the question and closed her eyes.

"Estelle, wake up for a minute and tell me what happened. You can go to sleep later."

Estelle coughed, bringing up more of the black sputum. "Oh, I got potted with my old man last night and got into a fight. I was so mad at the bastard I drank more than usual and passed out with a cigarette in my hand."

The woman was becoming short of breath. Dr. Mahoney turned up the oxygen flow and called out to Irene to page respiratory and find out what was taking so long.

"When I woke up, I was on fire . . . tried like hell to put out my robe, but couldn't."

"What time did this happen, Estelle?"

"Oh, I dunno, I think maybe about five."

Dr. Mahoney shot an incredulous glance at me and Gus. "Estelle, it's almost eight now. What have you been doing for the last three hours? Did you pass out?"

Estelle waved her hand in the air. "I know, I know . . . I begged that bastard to bring me to the hospital, but he said I deserved it, and it was my fault for burning myself up. He got really pissed and said I had to wait until he sobered up before he'd give me a ride."

"Why didn't you call the paramedics?" I asked, unable to believe the woman had waited in the condition she was in.

Estelle snorted. "Are you kidding! That old fart would've killed me if I'd made a scene with the sirens and everything. We're in enough trouble with the neighbors as it is now."

Irene called Dr. Mahoney to the phone, and I gathered the supplies I needed to catheterize Estelle.

"What did you do while you waited for your husband to bring you here?" Gus asked.

Estelle looked off into the distance, straining to recall. "Oh, honey, I was so drunk I can't remember. I think I tried to clean up the mess in my room, but I couldn't stand up long enough."

The respiratory tech hurried in and stopped short at the sight of Estelle. Moving quickly, he set up suction, opened a clean oxygen bag pump, and made ready the intubation instruments.

Dr. Mahoney returned and touched a small, unburned piece of Estelle's arm. "Okay, Estelle, let me tell you what I want to do now. I'm going to insert a tube down your nose into your lungs; it's going to help you breathe better. I'll make sure you're really sleepy so you won't feel the tube go down, and when you wake up, you'll be in San Francisco at a hospital that takes care of people who've burned themselves." Dr. Mahoney waited a moment. "Is it okay with you if I do all that?"

Estelle seemed to be losing consciousness. "Everything's okey-dokey, pokey," she slurred.

"Are you having pain?" asked Dr. Mahoney.

"Nope. Sleepy, just sleepy."

Dr. Mahoney saw the puzzled look on my face and answered the question before I could ask.

"There's no pain because she's in shock, plus the alcohol is still in effect, and last but not least, when someone has full-thickness burns to the extent she does, the nerve endings that would normally pick up the pain have been destroyed."

After Estelle had been sedated and intubated, Gus wrapped

her like a mummy in sterile gauze strips soaked in saline, then spread blankets over her in an attempt to conserve what little body heat she might have been generating.

I brought the sterile supply tray to the gurney and prepared to insert a silicone catheter into Estelle's bladder. Gently spreading her legs as best I could without disturbing the wrappings, I brought the lamp closer.

Like the surprise one feels upon finding some barely recognizable melted object in the ruins of a burned house, I was appalled as I gazed at the area where her genitalia should have been. I shook my head to clear it, then searched the severely damaged tissue until I found the grossly inflamed and swollen meatus. Gingerly, I inserted the catheter and was rewarded with a few drops of mahogany-colored urine.

Gus gave her a small amount of morphine, and in less than forty minutes after she'd arrived, Estelle was en route to the burn center. Without missing a beat, the rest of the morning went on as usual.

Over lunch we discussed Estelle's chances for survival.

"They're practically nonexistent," said Dr. Mahohey. "She was over seventy percent burned, her airway was involved, there was a delay in getting help, and I seriously doubt whether she was in great shape to begin with. I'd guess she won't make it past the end of today."

"I hope she doesn't," Gus murmured sadly. "What kind of life would that be for her with all the pain, not to mention the disfigurement?"

"What about the husband?" I asked Dr. Mahoney. "Will he be arrested?"

Dr. Mahoney looked surprised. "No. On what charges would he be arrested?"

"I don't know. What about something like 'unwillingness to aid'?"

Dr. Mahoney sat down. "Unfortunately, my naïve girl, there's no such law. We have good Samaritan laws and malpractice laws, but if you walk by on the street and see someone bleeding to death and don't help him, you've not broken any law; maybe some moral ones, but nothing you could be arrested for."

"But what that man did is basically stand by while his wife

suffered and do nothing. That's got to be negligence or something!''

Dr. Mahoney shook her head and laughed at my disbelief. ''No, believe me, Ec, it isn't. Now if he'd set her on fire or knocked her unconscious, yes, but as it stands now, he's done nothing wrong.''

That evening I found I could not shake off the visions of the burned woman or the scene in the car, no matter how hard I tried to concentrate on the simple pleasures of being home, safe and sound with Simon.

I waited until after dinner and called Janey to tell her what had happened.

''That's why Claudia offered you a chance to reconsider your placement, Echo.'' There was just a hint of uncharacteristic impatience in her voice.

''Now, take me, for instance; I had a nice, quiet, sterile day in OR. In every case we saw, there was a definite beginning, a middle, and a clean, well-sutured end—nothing left over to bring home as a midnight snack for my ulcer, nothing to agonize over.

''You, on the other hand, chose to work in a nut house where you see talking crispy critters and fight off hostile old women and cockroaches. I know you've got a soft place in your brain for all that fast, wild, and crazy stuff, but, Echo, you can't let it get to you.''

''Have you been talking to Dr. Mahoney by any chance?'' I asked suspiciously. ''She's been telling me the same thing ever since I met her.''

Neither one of us said anything for a while after that, and we entered one of those comfortable silences which occur during phone conversations between good friends, each party getting lost in sidetracked thoughts or doodles.

''Oh! I forgot to tell you I picked up two application forms for us in the nursing office today.'' I threw back my head and laughed, remembering how the clerk behind the nursing administration reception desk had visually picked me apart head to toe before handing over the applications.

''Applications?'' Janey asked blankly.

''Ah, Jane? I think somebody slipped a few sutures in your brain when you weren't looking. Applications for *jobs*, Janey, you know, what you do to get those green rice paper slips that exchange nicely for all sorts of things, like food, heat, rent, new shower curtains.''

"Ah, yes! Now I remember. We can actually earn money for what we do, can't we? I'd forgotten there was another reason besides insanity we went into this.''

Another long silence ensued, and I continued my sketch of a cat, using the inside seam of my jeans for a canvas.

"Echo?"

The whiskers weren't right. "Ummm?"

"Do you think we'll pass the boards and be real nurses?'' Janey's voice had gotten very small, the way it did when she was worried.

I stopped and pulled back to look at the finished picture; an artist I was not. "If we don't, Janey, I may have to retire to a small farm in Bakersfield and raise chickens, how about you?''

"Sounds okay, except chickens make me nervous.''

"Don't worry. If you can be a nurse, you can get to like chickens.''

"See you at graduation in exactly one hundred and sixty-seven hours, Echo.''

"Right!''

Later on, lying in the dark of my room, I stared at the ceiling, surrounded by thoughts of Estelle and her husband. I'd run into the question which, in one form or another, had kept me lying awake a lot of nights since I was a small child. I was trying to figure out just how people were able to do what they did to one another and themselves. After a lifetime of my playing witness to people's inhumanity it still affected me to the point of losing sleep. To put all the broken pieces back together was partially why I'd chosen nursing. I never had figured out what went on in a person's mind that allowed him to feel nothing as he watched or caused the suffering of another person. On my "Man's Inhumanity to Man" scale it ranked alongside mass murder and child abuse.

Around midnight I finally dozed, drifting on a 1950 memory where I rode through the dark of another night in the front seat of an old Buick.

Curled next to my father, I'd been sleeping when I was awakened by a roar which hurt my ears. I focused on the eerie orange and red light reflecting on my father's face and timidly peeked over the rim of the window. In the distance a barn burned furiously, while a handful of men ran in and out of the flames, trying to save any piece of equipment they could.

Even from where we were parked, I'd felt the heat. Then, somehow, my father became one of the men running toward the flames.

Terrified, I waited, scarcely able to breathe until I saw him reappear out of the flames, leading a young horse with a rag wrapped about its eyes. The horse whinnied and pulled frantically on the lead rope while my father spoke softly, trying to calm it.

Later, miles away from the flaming monster, he pinched my nose, his way of saying everything was all right. "It's not right any creature should suffer like that," he said. "We need to look out for those that can't fend for themselves."

Without warning, the memory metamorphosed into a nightmare where I was running in slow motion through a raging fire, holding Simon in my arms. In wild frustration I looked down to see why I couldn't run faster and saw my feet melting into huge puddles of plastic.

Gasping, I woke up in a pool of sweat, my skin burning.

I did not need to look at the clock to know the time to the minute. It was 4:00 A.M., the hour I experienced nightmares, anxiety, and, at times, soul-wrenching flashes of truth.

We started off Thursday morning treating a San Quentin prisoner with a stab wound to his chest. We all thought it might be an omen of how the whole day would go, but after we'd transferred him back to the prison infirmary, the rest of the day dragged like snails carrying lumber.

Katy, fully recovered from her mysterious illness, spent a portion of the morning describing the wondrous beauty she'd found on the California coastline.

Dr. Menowitz was working the day shift. Despite all the glowing reports I'd heard, he still seemed on edge, although I could tell at times he was straining to be nice.

Gus, I noticed, was somewhat subdued; Cousin Ralph had gone into hiding. I cornered her at one point in the morning and asked what the problem was.

"I didn't sleep all night. I kept having bad dreams about burned hands coming at me from out of the walls."

For more than an hour we exchanged dreams and tried to analyze them with our amateur Jungian analysis skills. Even though it was after the fact, it was comforting to know I hadn't been alone in my 4:00 A.M. nightmares.

We continued to be slow through the noon hour. Lunchtime brought none of the usual food preparation accidents or lunch break casualties. Gus and Katy occupied themselves with shoptalk while Dr. Menowitz sat by himself at his counter space, reading.

Once, when I walked past him, he glanced up, and in that instant I caught a glimpse of a distinctly unhappy man. As soon as he realized I'd seen him off guard, he forced a smile, and the screen went up between himself and the world. On an impulse I pulled up a chair next to him and sat down.

"Are you happy, Dr. Menowitz?"

He stuttered at the confrontation. "I, ah, relatively, I suppose." He leaned back in his chair and crossed his arms over his chest; then, aware of his body language, he relaxed and leaned forward with his arms resting at his sides.

"For chrissake, why did you ask me that?"

"I don't know, I guess because you don't seem very happy to me."

He shrugged. "I'm not unhappy. I'm just like everybody else, I suppose."

He shifted in his chair and smiled, then discarded what he'd said. "Now, if my therapist were here, he'd laugh at that statement; I'm supposed to aim for honesty and not fall back into the comfortable old lies." He brought up his hand to make a point. "Let me put it this way: I'm not really unhappy. I'm a discontent loner at heart, fearful of interaction with people, and totally disgusted with myself."

"Oh, my God!" I laughed. "And you chose this profession?"

Dr. Menowitz laughed, and his whole face changed; it opened him and cleared away the scowl lines. He nodded his head side to side and shrugged. "It's all Uncle Arnold's fault," he said. "My uncle Arnold was a doctor. He liked kids, but he never married, so when I was born, Uncle Arnie more or less decided I was the perfect surrogate son. As I grew up, he gave me everything a kid could want, but in return I had to be what Uncle Arnie wanted me to be.

"So, when I reached high school, he made a deal with my parents that if I followed his footsteps into medicine, he'd pay for my education. That was a deal no Jewish parents in their right minds would have turned down. Nobody ever consulted me on what *I* wanted to be, of course, and off to med school went unhappy Morton Menowitz to become a good Jewish doctor."

Dr. Menowitz stopped, scrutinizing my face for any sign of uninterest.

"I don't like being a doctor," he resumed. "I never did. People come in here expecting me to be God. I am supposed to fix them and change their lives forever, but I'm really not interested in saving humanity from itself. I don't want to be subjected to the guy who's been smoking two and a half packages of cigarettes a day for twenty-five years who gets angry at me when I tell him his x-ray looks suspicious."

Dr. Menowitz put one foot up on the rung of my chair and rested his chin in his hand. "Do you realize that for a month in advance I know what every day of my life has in store for me? That alone will put me in my grave faster than if I smoked four packs a day. I want more. I want to be shocked or come alive with surprise at least once a day, even if it's a tiny surprise."

Dr. Menowitz leaned back and stretched. "I want to be doing other things, but I'm such a coward." Embarrassed, he chuckled and added, "Do you know what I really wanted to be?"

I shook my head, certain I'd be surprised.

"Believe it or not I always dreamed of being a forest ranger and a writer, off in the woods by myself, writing poetry about the trees."

Dr. Menowitz's flood of information about himself touched off a twinge of guilt that I hadn't bothered to look past his icy exterior before this.

"Do you remember when I chewed you out last year?" I asked. "God, I thought you were the world's biggest jerk!"

He smiled. "You had every right; a lot of people did. I was so angry at myself that the anger would periodically get out of control, like a snowball rolling down a hill, picking up more and more snow until it was this huge boulder running over everybody.

"My therapist said I was on the brink of a 'survival shift'—great term, huh?"

"Do you know what you need to do?" I asked, suddenly excited over the prospect of rearranging Dr. Menowitz's life for him.

He shook his head.

"You need to take a year off and find a cabin in the mountains and think, write, discover who you are and how you want to spend the rest of your life."

Dr. Menowitz laughed. "I think at forty-three I'm too old to run away."

"That's not true! And you aren't running *away*; you're running *to*. Mom, Dad, or Uncle Arnie told you you weren't supposed to wiggle around in your cocoon, and you bought it. There're a lot of bitter eighty-year-olds sitting around nursing homes who never knew who they were or what they really wanted either. It's not too late for you. What's a year out of your life?"

Dr. Menowitz held up his hands, as if to ward off my enthusiasm. "Hold on already! It's not so simple. I have other things to consider, like an expensive wife who hates hiking and any kind of isolation from parties. Tearing her away from the luxuries a doctor's salary can afford would make her a miserable human being to live with. I also have a large house with a pool that needs to be paid for and two big dogs that've flunked obedience school three times."

For a moment Dr. Menowitz seemed lost in his listing of obligations. Then he spoke up again with another insight.

"See, when I started therapy, I was looking for a quick way to extricate myself from all that, you know, looking for the 'magic pill.' Then I discovered that wasn't the way it works. I've still got to find a way to pull out the stops and reemerge as the person I want to be without disrupting other people's lives." He finished with his face set in an expression of misery.

"So what you're telling me is that you're uncomfortably comfortable in a well-established unhappy security." I shook my head sadly. "That's one of the all-time most agonizing forms of self-torture I can think of. But . . . you sound as if you're at least thinking in the right direction."

Dr. Menowitz stared into my eyes. From his expression I knew what was coming.

"Would you like to go hiking with me on Saturday?" he asked, confirming my fears.

Sabotaging my cool exterior, I turned into a blushing maniac, scrambling for a way to frame my answer without hurting his feelings.

A movie flicks on in my head, where Dr. Menowitz and I rest on a hill overlooking the ocean, reading our poetry and tending to each other's hiking wounds. I even call him Mort.

Suddenly a title flashes on the screen over the picture of a menacing, sinister-looking man: "THE SUBTLE DANGERS LURKING BEHIND MID-LIFE-CRISIS MALES."

I blinked myself back into reality.

"I don't want to hurt your feelings, but no."

Dr. Menowitz's face fell, and I saw whatever fantasy he'd been dreaming of, fly away.

"Maybe someday, if Mrs. Menowitz ever changes her mind about hiking, we all can go together, except by then you'll be living in the forests of Oregon, writing beautiful poetry for the world."

Dr. Menowitz smiled sadly, looking more like Harpo Marx than ever. For a moment I lost my sense of propriety and put my hand on his arm.

"Oh, I only wish." He sighed. "But if wishes were horses . . ."

When Friday came, I was melancholy, ecstatic, and nostalgic all at once. One hundred and twenty hours away from graduation, I felt like the sprinter who madly breaks away just before the finish line. On this last day I would be totally in command. With strength and confidence I would meet every challenge as a weathered veteran of the nursing wars, perfectly balanced between my emotions and my intellect.

Of course, with that resolve, nothing came in all morning, and I sat in the back, reading up on emergency care, while my strength and confidence twiddled their thumbs.

At noon Dr. Mahoney yawned and said she was going to the doctors' room to relax; Gus and Katy restocked the rooms while being entertained by Irene, who read the gossip columns aloud.

Half an hour later I'd sunk as low as filing my nails when Irene asked me to take some reports to medical records. I jumped at the chance, knowing the minute I was out of the department, someone was bound to come in. It didn't matter what; even a fecal impaction would be welcomed.

When I returned, the beds remained empty. Discouraged, I started working on the next nail in line when, sensing profound silence, I realized I was the only one in the department.

I went to the bathroom door and knocked, calling for Gus. When I didn't get an answer, I called out Irene's and Katy's names; the department was like a tomb.

I went to the back feeling a bit uneasy and occupied myself by reading the articles on the bulletin board. Halfway through my second reading of the one about penile frostbite in cold-weather joggers, the buzzer went off twice.

In frozen animation I ran toward the door, thinking of Amy, trying to jump-start my brain cells. *Okay, Echo, just remember the basic ABCs; A, open the airway; B, breathing, mouth-to-mouth; C, cardiovascular, the heart, CPR.*

While I was sweating bullets, the door swung open, and I stopped short.

In front of me stood Dr. Mahoney, Irene, Katy, and Gus, holding a cake. On the top, between the pink sugar roses and two candles, it read: "Happy Graduation, Nurse Heron."

I stood still, a blank expression on my face while my mind ground gears, going from its adrenaline-rushed state into the celebration of the moment.

Not too sure how to read my silent expression, they looked at each other. Gus spoke up. "We were going to wait until three, but we thought it'd be better to do this now since we're so slow and so close to lunch."

My smile thawed my mind, releasing me from shock. "Jesus Christ on a bicycle, you creeps! Do you realize I could have had a coronary?"

All of us began talking at once, right there in the lobby. Outpatients and visitors stopped to watch the goings-on, craning their necks to read the cake; everyone walked on with at least a smile.

Irene talked the people in the kitchen into sending us a quart of ice cream by telling them we had four diabetics having insulin reactions.

The sugar rush and the sense of celebration left us giddy. Between Dr. Mahoney's and Gus's senses of humor, we were brought to the brink of incontinence more than once.

At two, the pneumatic doors opened at the same time the buzzer went off. The hard, squealing howl of a baby reached our ears.

"At least we know this child is not in respiratory distress, a good sign," said Dr. Mahoney as we rushed, single file, toward the noise.

All of us came to a halt in front of a giant of a man in overalls, holding the squalling child as if it were some faintly disagreeable foreign object.

Shyly he handed the baby to Dr. Mahoney and we all moved, as if chained together, to the nearest gurney. She removed a large blue bandanna from around the baby. The little girl was covered with scrapes embedded with road dirt.

The man took the soiled piece of cloth from her apologetically. "Sorry, ma'am, but I didn't have anything else to wrap it in."

Dr. Mahoney felt the baby's skull, looked into her eyes and ears, and ran her expert hands over the miniature body while the man spoke.

"My name's Paul Jepson, and I'm a driver for a trucking company out of L.A."

Mr. Jepson followed Dr. Mahoney over to the sink. She lined the bottom with soft towels and ran in warm water. The baby's crying died down to a soft whimper as she played with Dr. Mahoney's glasses.

"I was driving my rig along the highway . . . just coming into San Rafael, when I noticed this passenger car about a quarter mile in front of me start slowing down and weaving off to the side, like it's got trouble.

"The next thing I know, this lady sticks the top part of her body out the back window, screaming like she's getting killed or something, and throws this thing out onto the road. At first I thought it was a bundle of rags, but then I see this kid fall out of the middle of the bundle. I pulled off and ran to pick it up as quick as I could; I was afraid somebody might think it was just a doll or somethin' and hit it.

"Anyway, I left the rig there since it's one of those big piggyback jobs and flagged down the next car. It seemed to be the fastest way to get the baby to the hospital."

Silently we all watched the baby splash at the bubbles as Dr. Mahoney gently soaked off the road dirt.

Two minutes later she picked up the child and wrapped her in a warm flannel blanket. "Well, all I've got to say is it's a good thing these little people bounce. There's no damage that I can see other than the road burns."

Irene was leaving to pick up a bottle of formula and some flannel sleepers from the nursery when two California Highway Patrol officers came in to ask about the baby and the truck driver who had picked her up.

Relieved his truck had not been cited, Mr. Jepson gave his statement and was allowed to go.

The officers helped themselves to the cake and hot coffee while they filled in the blanks of the story.

"The baby's name is Phoebe. She's six months old. Our unit in San Rafael picked up the mother about fifteen minutes ago hitchhiking along the freeway, spaced out of her mind on something, looking for her child.

"According to her, she and the baby's father were out for a ride when they got into an argument over drugs. The father said she threatened to kill herself and the baby but decided to throw just the kid out and let it go at that."

Dr. Mahoney stopped playing pattycake with the baby and looked over at me. "Remember the other day when I was telling you that I didn't let things get to me anymore?"

I nodded my head.

"I lied. This makes me sick."

The county hot line phone rang, and Katy answered, then handed the phone to the officer. He listened for a minute, then covered the mouthpiece and spoke to us all. "The officers feel the mother needs to be medically cleared before they can book her." He paused. "They want to bring her in here."

In unison the four of us yelled, *"No!"*

"Sorry, chief," said Dr. Mahoney, "I don't think we could treat the woman with any kind of objectivity. Better take her to Brand X Hospital." Brand X was what the staff of Redwoods Memorial called Madison General, a small hospital less than five miles down the road.

Phoebe was admitted for observation overnight and then

released to the custody of the Child Protective Service until a more permanent foster home could be found.

Six months later we were informed, though we never understood why, that the court had awarded custody of Phoebe back to her mother.

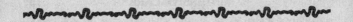

NINE

GRADUATION CEREMONY was only two hours away.

With my waist-length hair wrapped around empty frozen orange juice cans, I bounced through the house like a gazelle in a state of extreme anxiety and absent-mindedness.

Earlier in the day, while I was still thinking somewhat levelly, I'd arranged for Simon to spend the afternoon with Patrick; it would have worried him to witness my various displays of distraction. So far I'd put the milk carton into the hamper, placed my blouse in the freezer, locked Mooshie in the closet, and searched frantically for my white stockings when they were on my legs the entire time. Every time I caught myself in the middle of one of these acts, I'd glance furtively around just to make sure no one was peeking through the windows.

I'd applied and removed my make-up countless times, the results going from bad to worse. With my last effort the lipstick made my teeth look like loose Chiclets, and the blusher more like second-degree burn than glow. I gave up. Nothing, I decided, was going to make me look like Jacqueline Bisset.

After I'd spent four hours shopping, at one minute to closing, the very last white uniform on the rack revealed itself to me as the perfect graduation dress. The first thing I did when I walked into the cottage was to throw the old blue pin-striped sack into a Goodwill bag. Slipping the soft cotton dress over my head, I looked at the transformation.

The nurse in the mirror was really me. Just to make sure, I pinched myself.

At six I received a call from P.J., saying the class had

suddenly decided we all should wear our caps for graduation. Frantically I searched through closets, drawers, and attic trunks. At six-thirty, when the white piece of cardboard remained unfound, it dawned on me to look in the least likely place; immediately I found the slightly crumpled cap under Simon's toy chest, between a broken music box and a plastic baseball bat.

The old Chevy must have sensed my state of derangement and switched on its magic automatic pilot device because as I pulled into a parking space, I realized I couldn't recall the drive from my house to the campus.

I entered the Tower Auditorium via the back door and checked my watch for the last time; out of all the hours there were ten minutes left to wait.

A first-year nursing student presented me with a half-opened rosebud. Enviously the girl pinned the flower on my shoulder, chatting excitedly, alive with dreams of the ideal nurse. I looked at her and nodded, knowing that within a year's time, the innocence would be replaced by an invaluable reality.

Janey appeared out of nowhere and stood next to me. She was glowing, her silken blond hair attractively framing her face. She smiled and hugged me.

I pulled back to look at my trenchmate, shaking my head. "Janey? Do you realize I've never asked you why you decided to be a nurse?"

She shrugged. "It seemed like a good idea at the time. Bringing up a son by myself made me realize I needed to do more in life than be the PTA bake-off queen. I wanted to be really *worth* something in this life."

Daintily nibbling one freshly painted fingernail, P.J. quietly joined us. Waiting for our cue, we didn't say much to each other and leaned up against the banister to watch the rest of the class gather in the stairwell behind the stage.

We were a breath-taking group in our white uniforms with a red rose pinned to every shoulder. I detached myself and listened to the nervous laughter and disjointed conversations no one would remember in an hour. How much in measures of time and anguish had been sacrificed by each of us to begin here, waiting to become humanity's caretakers?

At 7:00 P.M., zero hour, the music started. Two by two,

forty-eight of us walked slowly into the auditorium. I was
dimly aware of a small aching lump in my throat.

In the front row of the audience, among my friends and
neighbors, I caught a glimpse of Simon sitting on Patrick's
lap. Breaking through the solemn silence of the auditorium,
his little hands clapped, and like the spark that sets off a
roaring dry grass fire, the rest of the audience burst into applause. "There's my mama!" he screamed over the applause,
pointing in my direction. "That's *my* mother!" Laughter rip-
pled through the audience.

I passed by the end of the row, and a woman I vaguely
recognized gave me the okay sign and winked. I winked back,
forcing my mind into dusty corners, trying to remember
where I'd seen her before.

When I turned to take my seat, I glanced up at the auditorium full of people gathered in our honor. Warm affection
glowed from every face.

The magic of the moment caused the lump in my throat to
swell, and I started to tear. Janey caught the look and, in
exasperation, pulled me into my seat. "For God's sake, not
yet!" she whispered fiercely into my ear.

"But, Janey, I'm just so happy. I'm so—"

Tessie, the mistress of ceremonies, cleared her throat and
tapped the microphone. She wore an ear-to-ear grin.

"See, you guys, we told you you'd make it!" she said,
speaking directly to the class.

While we laughed, she stepped back to adjust the mike to
her level and addressed the auditorium in full voice. "I can't
speak for everyone, but to these ladies in white I must say:
You all look absolutely beautiful, and I for one am very, very
proud of you!"

A wave of hard, confirming applause swept the audience.
A tear broke loose, rolled down my cheek, and dropped onto
Janey's arm. Startled, she glanced down at the wet spot and
rolled her eyes. "Not yet, Ec."

Tessie waited until the applause settled into quiet.

"A week ago our director informed me I should make a
brief speech this evening. After looking up *brief* in the dic-
tionary, I told her, in light of my multiloquent nature, *brief*
rarely had anything to do with my speeches. I warned her the
minute I saw this microphone and was placed in front of an

audience, she was taking a chance that none of us would get out of here for days."

We all giggled. Everyone was aware of the fact that Tessie's classes usually ran late as the result of her tendency to get carried away during her lectures.

"So we decided it was best to drop the speech. Instead, I thought I might tell you some of the basic truths about nursing and yourselves."

Tessie paused and scanned our faces, one by one. "You have chosen one of the most honorable professions in the world. I have a right to say that because over the years I have worked with, and come to know, thousands of nurses—women and men from every walk of life. It is from them I've learned firsthand what truly incredible people nurses are.

"To those you care for, a nurse is a person of many faces: You are a warrior against death and suffering, a technician of the highest degree; you are a mother, a sister, a best friend, a psychiatrist; you are a teacher, a magician, a sounding board, a secretary, a fortuneteller, a politician, but most of all, you are a loving human being who has chosen to give that love in one of the best ways you can.

"You are also courageous. You willingly expose yourselves to sickness and at times to physical harm every day with little or no recognition for your efforts. You work long, hard hours, striving to heal, knowing that death is always there, threatening to undo everything you've done in a moment. Yet here you are, smiling and hopeful.

"The foundation on which this very special profession is based can clearly be read in every one of your faces right now. It is the most important thing in the world, because, my dear, compassionate ladies, the foundation of nursing is love."

Tessie paused. The auditorium was perfectly silent.

"If each of you were to ask me for the best piece of advice I could give, I would say, Try never to lose sight of the ideals you have today. And the best way I know of how to do that is keep your eyes open, use your brain, but never stop working from your very special heart."

Tessie stepped back from the microphone and smiled. This time, the applause was deafening.

Taking advantage of the noise, I lowered my head and

sobbed. Janey squeezed my hand and swallowed hard. "Not yet!" Her voice was tremulous.

After a few minutes Tessie held up her hand to interrupt the applause. "I will now call up the members of the class, two at a time, for the presentation of their class pins and the pinning ceremony."

Fifteen minutes later Tessie called Janey's and my names. I managed to get the pretty gold and green circle attached to Janey's left lapel without sticking her. Janey, however, was taking forever. I crunched my chin down into my neck to get a better look at what she was doing. Shaking out of control, she couldn't blink the tears away fast enough to focus on what she was doing. "Not yet, you sentimental fool!" I whispered. "Wait till we get back to our seats."

Janey managed a weak giggle, closed her eyes, and finished the pinning by feel.

When the ceremony was over, audience and graduates tore through the crepe paper barriers, eagerly headed toward each other. The common joy could not be ignored; everyone hugged aunts, grandfathers, cousins, and children they'd never seen before.

The young woman who'd winked at me from the front row hugged me warmly. I looked into the golden eyes, and my mind flipped back a year. Slim and healthy, Marie, the pre-eclamptic woman I'd taken care of in Burl's rotation, stood before me. Taking her hands in mine, I opened her arms and leaned back to look at her. "You look wonderful. How did you know about tonight?" I asked.

Marie fidgeted with a small hand that was pulling on her dress from behind. "I thought about you a lot since Jesse was born, so when I finally called the school for your address, they told me you were graduating tonight. I thought since you were at my big event, I should be at yours, plus I wanted you to meet the thriving result of your efforts."

Marie moved aside, and a duplicate pair of twinkling golden eyes peered shyly from behind her skirt. I coaxed the little beauty over to me. Nothing I observed about the bright child betrayed any hint of his difficult birth. I shook his chubby hand and introduced him to Simon.

"My mama won the award!" he yelled, beaming with pride. "Did you see my mama win the gold award?"

"I sure did!" Marie laughed, holding Jesse up so he could see the sparkling pin.

Simon tugged on my hand and motioned me down to his level; it was time for a whispered message. I stooped down, and he cupped my ear. "Mama, I'm more prouder of you than anybody else." He whispered so fast all the words ran into one another.

I kissed him in the middle of a clump of curls. "Thank you, sweetie, and I'm proud of you, too, for working so hard to help me."

Simon indicated he needed to whisper again. Whispering would be the only acceptable way to communicate for the next three days.

"Mama, if you need me to help you some more, I can go to kindergarten later."

The honesty of the tender offer left me in tears again thinking, *Not yet . . . not yet.*

One week before the state nursing boards, Janey and I pooled our scant savings and checked into a quiet old hotel with two small bags of clothes and four suitcases full of books. With our children safely tucked away under the care of the indispensable commodities known as natural fathers, we prepared to cram with fierce intensity.

Our master plan was to dedicate one day and night to each of the five sections of the test. Wednesday we covered psychiatric nursing; Thursday, pediatrics; then came medical, followed by surgical. On Sunday we finished with obstetrics.

Monday was, ironically enough, Independence Day. After packing away the books, we swam in the ocean, went to three movies, had a late dinner at the hotel, and, over a bottle of champagne, drank ourselves into giggling fits. Only when Janey came back from the ladies' room with a paper toilet seat protector caught on the back of her skirt did we know it was time for sleep.

We both automatically woke up at seven on Tuesday, too nervous even to think about the scenic hike we'd mapped out. By eight we'd unpacked the books and were sprawled out on the floor of our room, shooting questions back and forth like spring-loaded Ping-Pong balls.

By three we were driving toward Sacramento through the

wiggling, invisible waves of heat which slithered off the highway and into the sky. The heat numbed the pretest paranoia
just enough that we were able to talk about the two-day ordeal
we were headed for without activating our ulcer pains. Self-
protective mechanisms allowed us to discuss the megatest as
if it were something that wasn't happening to *us*; it was out
there, happening to our classmates and thousands of other
people.

"I think most of the people will pass, don't you, Janey?"

"Probably. If they don't, they can always work as unlicensed graduates and retake it in January."

I sucked in my breath. "God! Can you imagine any one
of those poor bastards having to go through this twice in one
lifetime?"

Janey shook her head, staring blankly at the road. The circles under her eyes deepened a shade with the question. "It's
a real possibility, though; I heard they've made this year's test
almost impossible to pass because there're too many grads
flooding the job market."

I was the one who had passed the rumor on to Janey. "Well,
the way I chose to look at that is: Either you pass it or you
don't; it's too late now to sign petitions."

In response Janey opened the glove compartment and removed a bottle of antacid. Shaking, she unscrewed the top
and took a long swallow. "Yeah, I suppose."

Several miles of the yellow farmland went by before either
of us spoke again. I held off my anxiety by reverting to a
childhood traveling game in which I imagined the hills and
flatland as part of a humongous giant, and we were moving
over it the way a flea crawls over a dog. The trees and grass
were body hair, and the houses and ponds were birthmarks
and blisters. The fences were, of course, old scars. The fantasy was good for the first mile. After that I became heavily
involved in a fantasy in which I picked out the nicest farm I
saw and imagined myself as the woman in charge of the place,
like Barbara Stanwyck in "The Big Valley."

Just as I was about to perform a dramatic emergency Cae-
sarean section on my prize cow, Janey's voice yanked me out
of the barn and back to the cabin of her ancient Volkswagen.

"What if somebody throws up all over her test? Do you
think she'd have to take it all over?"

"Probably not," I answered, calmly considering the horrendous situation. "She'd probably just have to take over the pages she messed up."

"Whew," she said, genuinely concerned about the possibility. "That's good to know. I'd hate to have to start all over."

It was five by the time we drove into the capital city. Two blocks from the convention center, the place where we'd undergo temporary personality changes for two days, we found the motel we'd booked a year in advance.

The motel's neon sign jutted out over the street: NURSES OF CALIFORNIA WELCOME—NO VACANCIES.

"You were lucky to reserve early," said the bespectacled runt behind the counter. "This is the most graduates we've ever had. There's not a room to be had for love or money in all of downtown Sacramento." Janey and I glanced at each other out of the corners of our eyes and between us came up with fifty new paranoid fears.

Several groups of women from our class had booked rooms on the floor above ours, and P.J. and two other nurses from our group were already settled in the room next door.

We were dragging the suitcases of books from the car to the room when P.J. staggered to our doorway, drink in hand, slurred speech on tongue.

"Hey, you old buddies, everybody's gonna party in room 207 starting an hour ago. Bring your own, but bring a lot." She wove and laughed hysterically.

I set my jaw and shook my head. "No thanks, P.J., we're going to study and get some sleep. If I were you, I'd—"

"Aw, c'mon, c'mon, you got to party. Forget 'bout the test, you old sticks-in-the-mud, don't be 'diculous." She staggered out the door, tripping over the mat, and went on to the next room.

I closed the door and double locked it against the craziness in room 207, glad I had Janey on my side, good old level-headed Janey. "After dinner, Janey, I thought we could go over the therapeutic modalities for arthritis. What do you think?"

Janey had pulled back the curtain and was peering out across the pool toward room 207. A few of our class members danced on the balcony outside the room to the loud rock-and-roll music belching from a radio.

Oblivious of my question, she kept staring wistfully. "You

know, Ec, it might not hurt to relax for just an hour. Maybe we *are* old sticks-in-the-mud, you know?''

The fear that Janey was going to defect to room 207 left me no choice but to philosophize. ''Well, you can if you want''—I sniffed—''but just remember this, Janey: Sticks-in-the-mud may not always have fun, but they never blow over.''

After dinner I was interrogating Janey on the fine points of degenerative joint disease when a particularly shrill scream of delight and raucous laughter drifted across the pool. A pained, faraway look came to Janey's eye.

''You know, Ec, if we went over and had just one beer and maybe danced a little, we'd sleep a lot better tonight.''

I gave the potential traitor a look that knocked her back into her chair, cringing. As a follow-up, I reiterated my thoughts on the importance of a full eight hours' sleep and threw out several impromptu, rather fantastic statistics on how many brain cells could be destroyed by alcohol and dancing.

At 10:00 P.M. we closed our books and turned on the air conditioning to drown out the music and laughter from room 207.

While Janey watched the news, I went into my night-before-a-big-day ritual—fifteen minutes of stretching exercises, a hot bath, a cup of warm milk heated in the coffee-maker—and while Janey showered, I numbed my brain by watching one of the mindless shows harvested from the vast wasteland of television.

At eleven-thirty I was lying on my back, staring at the motel ceiling, which still managed to sparkle through the dark.

''Janey?''

''Yeah?''

''Janey, I can't sleep. What if I don't get to sleep and screw up on the test tomorrow?''

''You won't screw up. Don't worry, you aren't the only one; lots of other people in this town won't be sleeping to-night, including me.''

''Janey, I'm so scared. What if I fail it?''

Janey yawned. ''You'll take it over again in January, just like a lot of other people, including me.''

''But I don't want to take it over in January!''

''Then concentrate on passing this time and go to sleep.''

''Janey?''

"Ummm?" Janey sounded sleepy. The thought of being left to worry alone, worried me.

"Janey, how can you be so calm at a time like this? How can you act so normal, knowing what's facing us in the morning? I mean, I don't get it. I don't—"

"Shhhhhh," Janey mumbled. "Just relax. Just . . ."

A few minutes passed. I tried to relax my muscles and joints and started thinking about gout.

In a panic I sat bolt upright; I couldn't remember anything about the disease. "Janey! Janey, wake up! I forgot the treatment for gout. . . . Janey?"

There was no answer. I leaned over and took the pillow off her head. She was drooling.

I listened to the regularity of Janey's breathing for a while until the sound of the air conditioner started grating on my nerves. I tried to imagine what would be worse: to be stifling hot or to live with the sound of an eighteen-wheeler in the room. Using Dale Carnegie tactics, I turned the noise into something positive and imagined myself the driver of a huge semi, hauling tractors to Reno. There really wasn't a test tomorrow, and I really wasn't a nurse—this was all just part of a truck driver's idle fantasy.

Around five I drifted into a light sleep while going over the signs and symptoms of rheumatoid arthritis.

When the alarm went off at six, I unglued my eyes and saw Janey sit up and yawn. "Whew!" she said, stretching her arms over her head. "I didn't get one wink of sleep all night!"

The true utilitarian dresser, I closed my eyes again and fumbled for my basic jeans and T-shirt, which I put on under the covers. I stuck a few bobby pins in my hair and did the half-awake shuffle into the bathroom. In front of the mirror Janey was curling her hair, applying make-up and whistling all at once. I could barely brush my teeth successfully. By the time I finished washing my face, Janey was trying on her third outfit.

"Janey, would you like to tell me what the hell you're doing?" I tried to effect my best Miss Telmack voice. "We are about to be subjected to a grueling and torturous eight-hour test, and you are preparing for the Miss America finals."

Janey blotted her lipstick. "I know that, Ec, but if I make the newspapers, I want to look nice."

As I feared, my mind wasn't up to par. "Newspapers?"

"You know"—Janey held up her hands to frame the imaginary headlines—"the one that reads: 'Nursing Student Goes Berserk During State Exam.' "

For breakfast Janey had a three-egg cheese omelet, a large orange juice, and an order of flapjacks. I forced myself to drink a small OJ and tried desperately not to watch her. Where was the *justice*, I wanted to know. A full night's sleep and a meal fit for a normal person; it wasn't fair.

Following the crowds, I trudged to the convention center, just barely holding on to my OJ, while Janey tried to decide where we should go for dinner that evening. We entered the center through one of the twelve sets of double doors.

The room was roughly the size of a football stadium, or perhaps three. At the long tables thousands of women and men were already seated, most of them staring blankly ahead of them, most of them pale. I wondered if they were just worried about the test or if it was the soon-to-be-flooded job market which bothered them.

Janey and I found our assigned seats on the right-hand side of the auditorium next to an exit. At least, I thought with relief, if I needed to freak out or throw up, I was only a few steps away from the door. All I'd have to worry about was making sure the door was closed behind me before I started screaming.

I sat down and folded my hands in front of my face, concentrating on keeping the panic at a manageable level. During my third Act of Contrition I heard an IV pump alarm. I mentally sorted through all the information cards I had on auditory hallucinations, but when the sound persisted, I realized I wasn't the only one hallucinating; a hush had fallen over the entire room.

Following the general gaze, I saw a hospital bed in the very front of the room. Squinting, I could make out a woman in traction. She had a couple of IVs running and was nervously tapping a pencil on the bedside table placed over her lap. An attending nurse turned off the alarm and replaced the empty IV bag with a full one.

The woman, I later found out, was a nursing student who'd been in a car accident two weeks before and had made special arrangements just so she wouldn't miss the test. I never found out her name, but she changed everything for me. It was as Tessie said: We were a courageous lot of people, we nurses.

We'd all been through two, three, or four hard years of this learning business. One more test shouldn't interfere with the plan. The sick nervousness left me, and I started anticipating the challenge of the monster test with a degree of pleasure. Free from the nervous juices that bound it, my stomach growled, demanding to be fed. Lunch was four hours away; it would have to wait.

Along with the standard number two pencils, the rules were issued: No bathroom privileges unless accompanied by a proctor, no communication was to go on between any of us after the tests had been handed out, and when we finished, we were to leave by the nearest exit doors and not reenter the room until it was time to begin the next one.

Janey sat in front of me, already biting through her pencil.

"Pssst! Hey, Janey! Talk to me!"

Janey started and pivoted around. Dismayed, I saw that her happy glow was gone and had been replaced with the pale Twilight Zone zombie look. "Oooomygod, I'm scared, Ec."

I saw the proctor at the end of Janey's row, handing out the tests, one at a time.

"Don't be. You are going to pass this test, and so am I. I guarantee it."

Janey blinked. "Are you sure?" she asked doubtfully.

"Positive. And, Janey?"

The proctor was two people away.

"Yeah?"

"I love ya."

"You, too," she said, and smiled just as the proctor handed her the test.

When the starting signal was given, we made the thumbs-up sign and began.

That evening, over dinner, we reviewed hundreds of questions. "What did you put for Wilms's tumor? What range did you choose for normal ABG's? Can you believe there were so many questions about rheumatoid arthritis? What did you put for the cause of . . . Did you get the question about . . ."

By nine Janey and I were having yawning contests. I forfeited the stretching exercises and the warm milk and, barely able to keep my eyes open, climbed into bed. Just before I lost consciousness, Janey propped herself up on her elbows and addressed the blank TV screen. "Echo?"

"Ummm?"

"I think we can put away our books on chicken farming."

The next morning we dawdled over breakfast, then walked slowly toward the convention center, enjoying the warmth of the early sun.

"Only two more sections to go." Janey made the statement sound like a warning.

"Yeah. I just hope that girl in traction is still there; she's definitely the best good-luck charm I've ever had."

Janey laughed one of her best laughs. "Only you, Ec."

We were entering the center when Janey got quiet on me. I directed her to look at the girl in traction. She shook her head. "It's not the test," she said. "It's just that I don't know how I'm going to adjust to a normal life after this."

On the way home Janey turned up the car radio, and I undulated and swayed to the various beats, uninhibited by the strange stares from people in passing vehicles.

When Janey dropped me off at the pink cottage, I floated across the parking lot. Reaching into my purse for my keys, I heard the distant ringing of my phone.

Once . . . twice . . . Where the hell are those keys? Three . . . four . . . Ah! Gotcha!

Like a maniac, I jammed the key into the lock . . . five, six . . . On the ninth ring (it *had* to be somebody who really wanted to talk) I answered, out of breath.

"Hello?"

"Hello yourself," answered the only other voice in the world that was identical to my own.

"Hey, Stormy, how are you? How's life?"

"Echo, I'm wonderful, and life is just fantastic!"

My sister was dying to tell me something, I could tell, but with Storm, one had to proceed at her rate.

"What's up?"

"Oh, this and that."

She was going to be difficult; I was going to have to bait her.

"How're the children?"

"Oh, wonderful, just wonderful. Everything is just . . ."

"Wonderful?"

"Oh, yes!"

I was getting closer; her respirations were picking up.

"So! Tell me, how's your job at the bank?"

"I quit!"

Bingo! "Oh?"

"Are you ready for this?" She giggled, and I could see her jumping up and down in Chicago.

"Ready."

"I've just been accepted into nursing school. I start in August, and I want you to tell me everything about it!"

Taking in a deep breath, I sat down in the window seat and settled in for a long, long conversation.

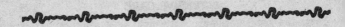

TEN

NIGHT SHIFT AT REDWOODS MEMORIAL was getting to me.

Night shift got to everyone eventually. No one really liked it, and the night people who claimed they did were, for the most part, pale and reclusive. They were people one might imagine doing strange and perverted things to their toes in the dark.

I started work on my birthday to the tune of $5.85 an hour; that was in the front part of June. It was now the back end of July, and it felt as if several years had passed. There was no time for anything other than working and sleeping. My appetite went out for an ice cream soda one day and never came back; I was losing weight as fast as I was losing my sanity.

I missed Simon more than anything else. I was given every sixth day off. Outside of that, I got to see him for only a few minutes each day when I would pick him up from Patrick's apartment at seven-thirty in the morning, give him breakfast, then walk him to the day care center a few minutes from the cottage. Stumbling back home, I'd make it to the bed and, without taking the time to undress, become immediately unconscious. Patrick would pick Simon up in the afternoon, and I wouldn't see him again until the next morning.

Besides all that, I just didn't fit into the night shift mold and the others knew it. Not only was I a rookie, but they sensed (with that special intuition only night people seemed to have) that I was a natural-born day shift rookie to boot. Thus, onto me they unloaded the heaviest assignments, then

pretended I was invisible. In my first week I discovered the
night people suffered from intermittent deafness, not only to
my pleas for help but to my patients' call bells as well.

In the back room where report was usually given, I sat,
half-asleep, wondering what in God's name I had done wrong
in my life to deserve working such unnatural hours. I laid my
head on the warm surface of the table, mildly disappointed
at not finding any relief from the heat. Closing my eyes, I
reviewed for the one millionth time the interview wherein I'd
landed this nightmarish job.

When I walked into the personnel office, I recognized the
clerk as the same person who'd given me the job application
during my student forty-hour week. She regarded me with
suspicion when I announced I was there for an interview with
the director of nursing personnel. "What position?" she
asked curtly. I flinched under the cold, officious stare; it
kicked right out of me whatever lightheartedness I may have
felt.

"Well, to be honest, I'm not really sure *what* position I'm
being offered. I'm a new UGN and I received a letter saying
to be here at this time for a job interview with a Mrs. . . ."
I couldn't remember the interviewer's name and riffled
through my purse to find the letter.

"You're an unlicensed graduate nurse? Are you *sure* you
have the right hospital?" The clerk spoke loudly enough to
make the other people in the waiting room look up from their
magazines.

This woman was in the wrong job; she would have made
the perfect druggist's clerk. She was the type who'd snare
folks into whispering what they needed, then scream over the
loudspeaker, "Hey, Joe! We got any of those double-strength
hemorrhoid pellets left? The lady in the red coat needs a few
packs *right* away!"

I found the official-looking letter and handed it to her. She
held it by the tip of one edge and read it over. When she was
done, she pointed to the far corner chair. "Very well, sit
over there until Mrs. Miller is ready to see you."

After slinking to my corner, I'd just started an interesting
article on growing your own prunes when amazingly enough,
a woman whose face resembled an albino prune came out of
a plush royal blue office and gave me a tight smile. I wondered if it hurt her to stretch out all that wrinkled flesh.

Her faded orange and silver hair was swept up into one of those upside-down bird's-nest creations, and her starched white uniform looked so much like cardboard that I was tempted to reach over and poke it just to see if it would dent.

"Miss Heron, I presume?" Her accent was English, distinctly London.

I extended my hand; the woman seemed alarmed it might touch her. "How do you do?" I said, in my most formal American accent: unmistakably Schenectady. Briefly she touched my hand with her moist fingers. It was not an agreeable sensation to either of us, I was sure.

"I am Mrs. Miller, the director of nursing personnel here at Redwoods Memorial. Do come into my office, won't you?"

Seated opposite her at the large mahogany desk, I checked out the decor of the room while Mrs. Miller shuffled papers around. Over her head was a watercolor of two rosy-cheeked children playing with some ducks in a typical English garden. Below the picture was a butler's table on which sat a china tea set of white, edged with delicate blue flowers.

Mrs. Miller cleared her throat, and the prune mouth stretched and pursed several times before she spoke. Her expressionless gray eyes stayed glued to my face.

"We've done a bit of checking up on you, my dear." She started pleasantly enough. I shifted uncomfortably in my seat, wondering if Wheelin' Wilma had made good her threat to speak to the administration about me.

"We understand you were graduated top of your class, and several of our nurses here at Redwoods Memorial who've observed you in action recommend you quite highly."

"Oh?" I nodded, and smiled slyly: good old Katy and Gus.

"Since the Redwoods Memorial nursing department prides itself on hiring only the *crème de la crème*"—Mrs. Miller twittered, and I almost bit my tongue off to keep from laughing—"I'm offering you a temporary full-time night position on the isolation ward." She beamed quietly the same way Michael Anthony used to in "The Millionaire" just after he'd given away a check. She might as well have just told me Simon had been chosen for execution.

"Nights? I—I can't work nights! I'm not a night person; I fall asleep at nine o'clock, and I have a son who's just starting kindergarten, and I'm a single parent, and I have no relatives in the area. I—"

"As an unlicensed graduate nurse you really don't have many choices available to you," she said tersely. Her prune wrinkles pulled tighter, and her eyes narrowed. "It's night shift on isolation ward or nothing. Really, I should think most young nurses would be tickled pink, given this opportunity."

What opportunity? I wondered. *The one to become a certified midnight zombie?*

She picked up a piece of paper and scanned it. "Let me see . . . ah, yes, you're scheduled to start next Wednesday, June the fifth, I believe."

I winced. "But that's my birthday," I whined. "I'd prefer not to work on my birthday. Could I start the next night?"

"No. It's next Wednesday. It says right here in the schedule, see?" She pointed to the June 5 slot with a bony, well-manicured finger. My last name, misspelled with two *r*'s, was penciled in.

"I'm sorry, but the schedule can't be changed now. It's too late." She rustled the paper and placed it back into the drawer.

"Were there any questions, Miss Heron?" she said, folding her hands in front of her.

"What time do I—"

"Be here at eleven P.M. sharp!" She looked at my hair. "And of course, you'll have to cut that mop before then."

"I have to cu-*cut* my hair?" My upper lip broke out in a sweat.

"Well, at least put it up and keep it off your collar." She sounded as if she were making a huge concession. "And no hair ornaments, no perfume, of course, no jewelry. Uniforms must be white and clean, and only a light application of cosmetics will do." She had a second thought and reached back into the magic drawer. For a moment my heart soared; perhaps she remembered she'd made a mistake and was going to tell me there was a day shift available after all. Instead, she pulled out a small red booklet and handed it to me. The title was embossed in black: "REDWOODS MEMORIAL HOSPITAL—RULE AND POLICY HANDBOOK FOR NURSES."

"Keep this with you always when you work, Miss Heron. Live by it, and you should have no problem getting along." Mrs. Miller blinked twice. "Was that all you wanted to know,

Miss Heron?'' I was afraid to ask anything more; ignorance, I decided, was bliss.

Anyone who's lived long enough and is even minimally aware knows that bad things happen in clusters—like bunches of rotted, moldy grapes on the vine of life.

I dialed Janey's house from the pay phone outside the personnel office. The clerk peered over her counter and raised one eyebrow when Janey's sweet savior voice answered.

''Hi.'' I moaned. ''My world's falling apart. I got the job. Ready for this? *Nights* on *isolation* ward, starting on my *birthday.* I dare you to say something cheerful.''

I could hear Janey smiling. ''Okay, since you asked, are *you* ready?''

I nodded and held my breath.

''I just got an acceptance letter for a six-week surgical nurse training program that starts in two weeks. As soon as the program is over, they've promised me a day position with full benefits and a salary that knocked my socks off!''

''Oh, my God, Janey, that's great!''

''Ummm . . .''

''Isn't it?''

''Well . . .'' Janey sucked in her breath, and a dark shadow passed before my eyes.

''Well what, Janey?'' My heart started to skip every other beat.

''The hospital that offered me the job . . .''

''Yeah?''

''It's in San Diego.''

I sat down on the small wooden bench and pressed my forehead into the silver coin box. A man with a briefcase tapped on the glass of the booth and raised his eyebrows questioningly. I growled and motioned him away.

''I couldn't turn it down, Ec. I said yes before I thought about the moving and leaving-everybody-behind parts.'' Her voice lowered a full octave. ''Don't worry, Ec, I'll be up to visit, or you can come down there. It's supposed to be hot all year 'round just the way you like it. . . .'' She trailed off.

I kneaded my temples with my knuckles, feeling sick. ''When are you leaving?''

Janey hesitated. ''A week from tomorrow. I've got to pack

everything, hire some movers, and find a place to live all in one week.''

For a moment there was silence. The man with the brief-case pointed to his watch, looking irritated.

"Do you need some help packing?" I stood and turned my back on him.

"You mean it?" Janey let out a sigh of relief. "I thought you'd be angry."

"I am. I just want a chance to get at your best dishes."

"Tssssss. Boy, I sure am gonna miss you!"

"Yeah," I said, choking down the strangulating throat lump, "me, too."

On the morning of departure, Janey and I stood shivering and crying in front of her old house. Her small car was loaded down with boxes, plants, and a rocking chair strapped to the top.

I jammed my toe into the side of her tire. "You creep! I just don't believe you're really going to leave." I blew my nose and made a mournful, whimpering sound; I was hoping to give her the going-away gift that would keep on giving: guilt.

I was successful. Janey went into an acute outbreak of sobs. "I didn't think it'd be so hard to leave."

"Jesus, Janey! How could you not know it was going to be devastating? We've been through the war together. Don't you ever watch the old movies where it's D-day and the two army buddies are saying good-bye?"

"Yeah," she said, wiping away the tears, "except one of them's usually just been shot; it's got to be easier that way."

When phone bills brought us to the point of bankruptcy, we resorted to writing long, poignant letters full of complaints, gentle advice, and humor. I carried hers with me for a quick dose of moral support whenever things got too rough.

According to her letters, Janey was doing great. Her first day there she'd found a cozy little cottage right on the ocean; she loved her job, was making twice as much money as I, and was sleeping normal hours. To put the cherry on her life, by the end of the first month of training she'd found Mr. Right

in the form of the chief oncology resident; all I'd found were
the bags under my eyes.

The door to the report room opened, and the swing shift
nurse came in, looking tired and short-tempered. I sat up
straight and checked the clock; it was eleven-fifteen and the
air felt like an electric blanket turned to the "10" setting.

The medical units were stifling hot in summer. Administration insisted it was not "structurally possible" to install
air conditioning in the patients' rooms. This did not explain
why the administrative offices were fully air-conditioned, but
no one had deemed it safe to ask.

Last to receive the assignment sheet, I saw I'd been given
eight of the nineteen patients, all of whom needed to have
vital signs and a physical assessment done before twelve-
thirty. Five needed dressing changes, two of which were complicated and time-consuming. All but one patient were to
receive medications at midnight and 6:00 A.M., and just to
spice it up, one of the eight was confused, one was dangerous, and one was just plain crazy. It should be, I decided
halfway through report, one hell of a night.

The other two nurses on the floor were regular night shift
personnel, and I could tell by the warning looks on their
ghostlike faces I was not to interfere with their evening.

When report was over, I remembered the Dale Carnegie
courses I'd taken many years before and, in a surge of positive thinking, set a goal: Within one hour I would have all
eight vital signs completed, have physical assessments on the
patients who really needed it, and have dispensed midnight
medications plus sleepers and pain relievers. I took in a deep
breath, grabbed the automatic thermometer before anyone else
got to it, and set off.

In room 402 was a nineteen-year-old schizophrenic who
had been transferred up from the psycho ward for a tonsillectomy four days earlier. Mr. Bonowski was my "easy" patient. Healing without complications, he was scheduled to be
transferred back to the psych ward in the morning; unfortunately, not soon enough for me.

Walking into the room, I could see he had rearranged the
furniture again. Mr. Bonowski rearranged furniture everywhere he went: doctors' offices; department stores; even the
lobby of the Federal building. It was part of a profound regression that was typical of his psychosis. Looking at Mr.

Bonowski, I could see his regression had gone beyond profound.

Hanging monkeylike from the trapeze frame of the bed, with matted blond hair arranged in spikes about his head, he held his eyes wide open as if in perpetual, wild surprise.

"Won't you come down now?" I asked, removing the bedside chair from the desktop.

Mr. Bonowski made an unfamiliar jungle noise as he dropped to the mattress.

I explained I needed to check his temperature and pulse, then give him some pills. In response, he climbed back up the trapeze and once again assumed the hanging position.

Getting into the swing of things, I coaxed him down with promises of bananas and was allowed to take his temperature and blood pressure only after he had sniffed and tasted my stethoscope to his satisfaction.

Mr. Bonowski rubbed his stomach and pointed to his mouth; it was midnight snack time in the jungle. In the kitchen, I managed to scrounge up a glass of milk and a ripe banana, and hurried back. I tried not to notice that his bedside table had been moved to the closet. Mr. Bonowski was sitting humanlike on his bed, looking just a little mischievous around the eyes. Without further incident he took his pills, peeled the banana, and bit off a piece. The rest he carefully rubbed into his eyebrows.

Tucking him in, banana brows and all, I headed for the door and spoke before I had a chance to fight off the temptation. "Good night, Tarzan."

As the door clicked shut, a perfectly normal male voice answered, "Thank you, Jane."

One down. The stumbling block at the starting gate wasn't so bad. It was only ten minutes after midnight, and the perspiration rings on my uniform were still at a minimum. Sailing into 404, bed one, I was the cool white version of Florence Nightingale on the loose.

Lying in total composure while reading a thick, intellectual-looking book was every woman's fantasy. The thirty-seven-year-old postoperative hernia repair was absolutely one of the most handsome men I'd ever seen; he was Mr. GQ himself, lounging in his one hundred percent cotton dust blue patient gown, with rounded collar. Immediately I turned into

a stumbling, babbling idiot who shouldn't be allowed to care
for houseflies, let alone human beings.

"I'm going to take your sital vines—I mean, your vital
signs now." I giggled and nonchalantly pulled the blood
pressure cuff out of its basket on the wall.

Bad went to worse as the expanding coil which attached
the cuff to the meter on the wall snapped at the connection
and hit the GQ man in one of his sparkling blue eyes made
even deeper blue by the tinted contact lenses.

Rushing to check his eye, I tripped over the wide base of
the ancient bedside table, spilling a glass of ice water into
his lap. He threw me a look that made me feel like a member
of the laundry staff disguised as a nurse.

Apologizing profusely, I flew to get fresh linen, a new
gown, and an ice pack for his eye. In a record eight minutes
I'd made the bed, finished his vitals, checked his eye, and
assembled the equipment I needed to change his dressing.
Mr. GQ refused to let me touch the fresh postoperative site
by shrugging one of his well-developed pectorals and rolling
his baby blues to the ceiling. He gave me a bored look and
sighed. "Come back later. I'm not quite ready for my nighty-
night tuck-in yet." The man didn't crack a smile.

"Nighty-night tuck-in?"

"You know, milk and crackers and a long, luxurious back
rub. Let's say, in half an hour?" He yawned and rolled back
to his book. It occurred to me that pretty boy here was one
man who believed nurses, maids, and whores all came from
the same egg.

My watch read twelve-forty. I was a bit behind schedule,
but I could do it, said Dale Carnegie, thinking positively.

Room 404, bed two, was my seventy-eight-year-old
"pleasantly confused" TUR, or transurethral resection of the
prostate, three days postop. I pulled back the curtain which
separated his part of the room from Mr. GQ's side. Mr.
O'Reilly was stark naked, quietly struggling to free himself
from his Posey jacket.

The Posey jacket was one of nursing's finest inventions to
keep confused or agitated patients from falling out of bed or
wandering off the ward. The small mesh vest had two long
ties which, after being laced up the back, could be tied to the
side rails and thus "gently remind,' the confused patient that

he or she was in bed. In truth, it was an abbreviated strait jacket that bound the patient to the bed, period.

Mr. O'Reilly had one foot on the floor, while his other foot pushed desperately against the side of the bed. From the waist up, his body was entangled in the Posey. Taking a firm hold of the vest, I managed to slip the jumble of ties and mesh down away from his face.

"What are ye do'n' here, lass?" he asked innocently as he made a bee line for the door. Quickly grabbing the tangled Posey, I ran after him and tripped over one of the trailing ties.

Mr. GQ was taking in the whole scene. The minute he saw me come close to the end of his bed, he drew his knees up and shrank back. (Dear God, *please* don't let her come near me.)

I tackled Mr. O'Reilly's arm just as he reached the door to the room. The nurses at the station looked up in time to see me make a grab for the naked old man with the Posey vest wrapped around my ankles. They gave me a look of distaste and proceeded to ignore me. No surprise there.

After slamming the door, I put Mr. O'Reilly back into his gown and guided him to the bathroom. "Is this what you wanted, Mr. O'Reilly?" I asked, pointing to the toilet.

Mr. O'Reilly looked bewildered for a moment and then covered his mouth with his hand. "Oh-oh," he said, wide-eyed, just like a child.

I puzzled over the expression until I felt something warm splash up and then trickle down my left leg in rivulets. Of course, this *would* happen on the one night I had decided to break rules and not wear stockings. My shoe made a little squishy noise as I stepped to the side. Embarrassed, Mr. O'Reilly nudged me out of the bathroom and closed the door behind himself. "Go away, lass," he yelled through the door. "I'll be talkin' to me solicitor for a time. Come back later."

I tried to keep out of bed one's view while I washed off my leg and stuffed paper towels in my shoe. I figured I could run to the next patient, do vital signs, and be back before Mr. O'Reilly was finished.

The two other nurses sat at the station, drinking coffee and chatting. Seeing me, they stopped long enough to tell me Mr. Dickson in 410 had had his call light on for more than an hour. An hour! I glanced up at the clock. To my horror it read one-thirty.

Mr. Dickson, a forty-six-year-old convict, had been shot in the leg while attempting to escape San Quentin. He'd been with us for more than three weeks because of an infection in his wound that did not want to go away no matter what we treated it with. Encumbered with a long history of drug abuse, Mr. Dickson had no problem becoming dependent on the Demerol shots we gave him for pain control.

Mr. Dickson was under maximum security: two guards at the door and one in the room at all times. The first time I took care of him, I'd plied one of the guards with doughnuts and coffee in an effort to find out why Mr. Dickson was on death row. I was sorry I'd asked. Mr. Dickson also known on the streets as "Killer Man Dick," had two counts of first-degree murder, one kidnapping, and four counts of rape under his belt.

Flying into his room, I made sure the guard was right behind me before I approached him. Through clenched teeth he demanded his pain shot and told me it had better be a good one to make up for the delay.

In the medicine room I checked the order for Demerol only to discover that just this very evening Mr. Dickson's doctor had halved the usual dose in an effort to start weaning him off the narcotic.

Wearing a fake smile, I returned to Mr. Dickson's room with the shot hidden in my pocket. I took his vital signs and, while he was searching the ceiling for the imaginary spider I'd pointed out, injected him.

"How much was that?" he asked in a gruff voice, eyeing me suspiciously. It was, I knew, one of his Seven Patient Rights to know the answer.

I casually washed my hands and mumbled the dosage over the running water, hoping he wouldn't hear me. Mr. Dickson had hearing better than sonar.

"You m-----f-----g c---!" The man gave me a straight-line intensive dagger look that tore through my eyeballs. "I want the rest of my dope, bitch, or you is one dead nurse."

I froze. The guard, the same one who I'd bribed with the doughnuts, pulled me out of the room and told me that if I was done, it was a good time to leave. I looked back over my shoulder and saw Mr. Dickson write something on a piece of paper next to his bed. He shook his pen at me and yelled that he'd put my name in his funeral book. Perhaps, thought the Dale Carnegie part of me, he'd written UGN as my last name.

A sneaking suspicion crawled into my stomach, and I checked my clipboard; Mr. Dickson was one of my more complicated dressing changes. I wondered if maybe the day shift nurse could do it instead. Looking back at him, I was *sure* she could.

As I backed out into the hall, the emergency bell went off over room 404. I raced down and found the other two nurses standing in front of the bathroom door, yelling over Mr. O'Reilly's screams.

"Get me out o' here, lass. I'm wantin' to get out now! Would ye be wantin' to keep an innocent man locked in the johnny?''

Mr. O'Reilly couldn't unlock the door, the emergency bell could not be turned off from outside the bathroom, and he was as deaf as a doorknob—especially since his hearing aid was lying on his pillow.

I ran to the crash cart, where the rusty emergency bathroom key was kept. Jamming the key into the lock, I twisted it a full 360 degrees. At once, it became immovable. Not to be outdone by some inanimate object, I applied a touch of force. After the first clanking noise there was a sound similar to that of a turkey wishbone being broken. Pulling the key from the lock, I discovered the end had been sheared off. I marveled at my own strength and chalked up a game point for the inanimate-objects side. The night engineer was called to bring his tools.

When I returned from the phone, Mr. O'Reilly had worked himself into a frenzy. "For the love of Mike, lass, let me out o' here, or I'll be suffocatin' to me death waitin' fer ye." His voice cracked a few times.

After ten minutes, and six different tools, the engineer was still unable to get the door open. There was, he said, one more tool he hadn't tried and he'd be back as soon as he found it.

I felt dizzy and leaned against the door. The other two nurses had deserted me again. I could see them busily stuffing sterile cotton balls into the emergency bell and then into their ears.

I began sweating profusely when Mr. O'Reilly had been silent for almost a full five minutes. What if he was having a cardiac arrest? It certainly was possible for a man his age, especially after all this stress . . . Like a crazy woman, I pulled at the door. Did I feel the lock begin to give way? I pulled again, harder, putting all of my one hundred pounds into the tug of war.

From behind, the GQ man appeared. "I'll do this," he said, looking determined in his cool, macho man-about-town way. Before I could stop him, he'd pushed me aside and attacked the door as if it were some personal affront to his masculinity. I had grabbed for his waist, trying to explain why he wasn't supposed to exert himself so soon after surgery, when a final loud crack ripped through the door.

The door, all cockeyed, hung sadly on one hinge. Mr. GQ stared in disbelief at the loose doorknob in his hand, and then at the stark naked Mr. O'Reilly, who stood in the doorway, grinning.

"Top o' the mornin' to ye, lads a' lassies!"

I looked up and saw the nursing supervisor peering in from the hallway—of course. She looked from what was left of the bathroom door, to me, to the GQ man, then to Mr. O'Reilly before she slowly shook her head. "Heron, I hope to God for your sake the incident report you write up sounds better than this looks."

Leaving the GQ man sitting on the edge of his bed, I guided Mr. O'Reilly back to his, dressed him in a new gown and Posey, and tied him down, using my special Houdini method.

When I got back to Mr. GQ, he was still holding the doorknob, terrified he was going to bleed to death; his stitches, traumatized by the exertion, were oozing. Checking the surgical wound, I assured him that it took a long time to exsanguinate and that he had only disturbed the stitches, not pulled them out.

After prying the doorknob from his grasp, I re-dressed his wound and told him I was too busy for a nighty-night tuck-in of milk and graham crackers, but I'd check on him in a couple of hours to make sure he was still breathing.

Still feeling a little dizzy, I glanced at the clock; I was two hours late on midnight medications. The incident reports were going to take me forever to write. Desperate for help, I brought tears to my eyes and threw myself on the mercy of the younger, less jaded of the two nurses. After fifteen minutes of my bended-knee begging, she agreed to dispense the late medications for me on the condition I would work a weekend shift for her in exchange.

I walked into room 406, convinced Dale Carnegie knew nothing about nursing.

Mr. Vasconcelos was a fifty-three-year-old who, two months before, found a boil on the back of his neck. In order to "get the core out," his wife tried some at-home surgery, cutting it open with a steak knife. It became infected two days later, and more at-home remedy was employed in the form of Mrs. Vasconcelos's "secret formula" poultices.

It was time to go to the doctor, they decided, when his temperature hit 102.5, and his neck was yellow and purple with a raging staph infection. It had taken well over three hours of surgery to remove the necrotic tissue.

The heavy, sickening odor of staph almost knocked me over when I opened the door. Mr. Vasconcelos was sitting in the dark facing the window. A large bald man with tattoos of a snake and a dragon on each arm, he reminded me of a New York City policeman or an insane ax murderer.

I said hello and got a grunt in return. His vital signs were normal, and I told him so, thinking that would make him feel better and perhaps elicit some conversation. Instead, another grunt erupted from somewhere inside the giant abdomen.

His wet to dry dressing change was a complicated procedure designed to debride dead tissue from a moderately large wound while it healed from the inside outward. Using long-nosed sterile tweezers, I pulled the old gauze packing from the gaping hole which, at one time, had been the other half of his neck. "My, my, my, what a big dressing," I said through the nausea. Mr. Vasconcelos gave a double grunt.

Next, I packed gauze pads, soaked in a sterile medicated solution, into the hole. On top of those I placed damp and then dry gauze. I finished by wrapping a long strip of gauze around his neck, like some flimsy winter scarf.

"There we are! Now, how about getting some good, solid sleep, Mr. Vasconcelos?" Mr. Vasconcelos moved slowly around in his chair to face me. Raising one bushy eyebrow, he pointed to the door and grunted.

Onward to the next room. I'd made progress. I could feel it in my tired and aching bones. Was it time to go home yet?

I wondered? No, of course not, the night was still young. It was only two forty-five.

Room 408 was going to be easy; comfort measures only. Mrs. Daughn was a sixty-five-year-old terminal lung cancer patient who had been in a coma for two days. The room was dimly lit, and by the night light I could see her profile. She seemed very aristocratic and peaceful. There was no sign of pain on her face.

I tried not to disturb her. "Hello," I whispered in the lowest of whispers, "I'm only taking your vital signs, and then I'll let you rest."

Using my flashlight, I found the blood pressure cuff and slipped it around her arm without moving her.

"It was a lovely day today," I said, thinking my voice would sink through the curtain of her coma and be soothing to her. "It was such a blue sky!"

I pumped up the cuff.

"I remember warm nights like this when I was just a kid. . . ."

I didn't hear any pressure. I tapped my stethoscope and readjusted the earpieces.

"I remember on nights like this I used to sneak down to the river and . . ."

Still no pressure. I picked up the woman's wrist and instinctively jerked my hand away from the ice-cold limb. I pulled the overhead light cord.

I estimated she had been dead for at least three hours. The relaxed pose told me she died peacefully, thank you for that.

While I washed her body and wrapped it in a cotton blanket, a vision of Dale Carnegie cheerfully reminded me I now had only seven patients. I knew my moments of positive thinking were numbered when I told him to shut up and leave me alone. I looked down at my feet and wondered if they were really mine or if they'd been replaced with burning lead blocks while I wasn't looking. I stifled a jaw-popping yawn and blinked back the aborted yawn tears, refusing to acknowledge the clock, which stared me in the face, screaming three-thirty.

Entering 410, the room of one Mr. Leroy T. Love, I got the creepy feeling I was being watched and looked back toward the nursing station. Leaning over the top of the counter, straining on the tippy toes which supported their piano legs, were both my fellow night nurses, giggling and wishing me luck.

Night people had limited senses of humor.

The snoring Mr. Love was a twenty-five-year-old circumcision and my first penile dressing change. I didn't know exactly how to go about it, but I figured it couldn't be too complicated.

Very gently I shook the big lump under the bedcovers. Emerging, and then emerging some more, came a groggy Mr. Love, six feet seven inches of hulking black man.

"You must be Mr. Love!" I said, watching the giant unfold. In reply, he nodded; he was indeed the very same one.

Explaining who I was and what I needed to do, I waited with bated breath, expecting some kind of argument. Instead, he fell back into the pillow, sound asleep.

I checked his vital signs and set to work. Timidly inching back the covers, I was surprised to see the man's penis covered in several layers of gauze, propped up between his thighs on what appeared to be a miniature hammock.

From the far left field of my mind came the thought that perhaps I should offer it a glass of lemonade. That proved to be too much, and before I could slap my hand over my mouth, a deep hysterical laugh escaped from my throat.

Mr. Love started and opened one beady eye. "What you laughing at, girl?" he asked gruffly.

I wondered what the proper etiquette was in this matter and decided honesty was the best policy. "I'm laughing at this little sling thing here. It looks so funny!" There was a pause. "Ah, don't you think it's funny?"

Mr. Love didn't laugh or smile but opened the other eye (also beady) and said, "I think I'm going to be watchin' you while you're foolin' 'round down there, girl."

Obviously this was not a joking matter to Mr. Love. I cleared my throat. "Yes, of course, no problem." I unwrapped the old dressing, careful not to rock the hammock, as it were. The stitches were clean, and the surgical site was healing well without any sign of inflammation.

"Looks good to me!" I said, beaming.

Mr. Love's eyebrows lifted up to where his hairline began.

Immediately I heard my own words and got the feeling that was not the thing to say. I squirmed. "What I meant was, it

looks very nicely healed . . . no infection or anything like
that, there's no . . . ah, I mean, it's not red or anything.''

Uh-huh.

Mr. Love, true to his word, continued to watch every move
I made. Carefully (very carefully) I applied a new dressing
and tried to engage the man in conversation. Gnawing at me,
my curiosity threatened a sleepless day unless I asked the
obvious question: "Say, Mr. Love, if you don't mind my
asking, how come you're having this done at your age?" I
didn't dare look up from what I was doing.

"Do lots of diving," he answered.

Oh? (*Dear Janey, You'll never believe this one. . . .*)

I sensed either Mr. Love was a man of few words or he
was too sleepy to elaborate. I decided to let the answer stand
as it was. Someday, perhaps when I wasn't so tired, I'd know
what he meant.

I put the freshly dressed appendage back in its hammock,
covered the man it belonged to, and went to the next bed.

In the private room at the end of the hall was Mr. Eugene
Landau, the forty-one-year old paraplegic with a badly infected sacral decubitus ulcer, more commonly known as a
bed sore.

I felt sorry for Eugene, although I found it hard to deal
with him. He was loud and verbally abusive to anyone who
tried to help him, especially the nurses. When he wasn't curs-
ing us out, he was making flagrant sexual advances toward
us. Rebuffed and scolded numerous times, Eugene seemed to
have changed tactics of late; his most recent trick was to put
on his call light, and when the nurse answered, he uncovered
himself and began masturbating.

The situation had progressed to the point where the female
staff avoided his room and often ignored his call light. I'd
repeatedly left anonymous notes on the front of his chart
stating the problem and requesting his primary physician to
call in a psychiatric consult, but they'd been ignored.

As if he needed to announce his existence to the world in
any way he could, Eugene's television was cranked up so loud
he didn't hear me come in. Marijuana smoke hung in the air
like a heavy velvet curtain. By policy, I was obligated to write
up the odor as an incident, and although none of us ever did
so, we were putting ourselves on the line by letting Eugene
repeatedly get away with smoking dope in his room.

I touched his arm.

Mr. Landau started and cursed at me for deliberately trying to scare him to death. Ignoring the colorful phrases and names, I told him I needed to take his vitals and debride his decubiti. Eugene, in turn, ignored me and told me I could sit on his face.

He'd picked the wrong night to mouth off. Angry and under more than a little stress, I screamed he was not to talk to me that way, and he wasn't to smoke dope in the hospital room.

While I turned off the television and opened all the windows, Mr. Landau glared. Armed with the military presence I had learned from Miss Telmack, I brusquely took his vital signs, avoiding eye contact. When I tucked the blood pressure cuff back into the wall holder, Mr. Landau pulled the covers up to his shoulders and informed me I was a scuzzy slut bag and to leave him alone.

I sighed. "I'm sorry you feel that way, because we're only half done. Now it's time to debride and dress your ulcer. C'mon, Eugene, cooperate with this. You're two hours overdue as it is."

Eugene refused flat out, and I responded with a Telmackian steel edge to my voice. "Turn over!"

Turning off the light, Eugene called me a name I haven't heard or seen since the subway walls in New York City.

I turned on the light and reasoned with him as the emotional two-year-old he was and the one I was rapidly becoming. The name of the game was Control and Power, and I was so tired I wanted to scream.

From down the hall I heard the emergency bell go off again; Mr. Landau had won by default.

The "emergency" was in Mr. Dickson's room. Of course, how could I have missed that? His pain shot was five minutes overdue.

Drawing up the full dose of Demerol, I headed into his room with enough steam and bad temper to match his. All three guards were asleep in their chairs—oh, wonderful.

Purposefully I tripped over one of the guard's legs, hoping to wake him. He didn't move a muscle.

Mr. Dickson opened his mouth, ready to hurl verbal diarrhea, but I showed him the syringe before he even had a chance to pass a whisper of wind.

"Not one word," I warned, "not one word, or you won't

get your fix." Mr. Dickson shut his mouth and turned up his hip, looking almost docile. Pulling back the plunger, I sent happy dreams into his gluteal muscle.

My bad temper seemed to have a life of its own. When I sailed back into Mr. Landau's room, I snapped on the lights and threw back his covers.

With new, demonic energy coursing through my veins, I rolled him onto his stomach, removed the old dressing, and swabbed hydrogen peroxide around the infected area. Slowing down only for an instant, I cleaned away the dead tissue from the sides of the ulcer. Eugene cursed, but I knew by his dampened tone he'd seen the light in my eyes.

Finished with his dressing, I pulled the light cord, but the room remained bathed in light. Startled, I looked out the window. The rising sun played peek-a-boo with my eyes. My watch read six-thirty.

Riding the wave of one last adrenaline rush, I got through the dispensing of six o'clock meds posthaste and returned to the main desk. There, my patients' charts were lined up, like little soldiers. I calculated at least an hour or more of charting to be done, plus two incident reports.

Both the other nurses looked fresh and well rested. Finished with their charting, they were ready to give report and go home. They smiled at me, and somehow I refrained from shouting loud and uncharitable things at them.

The old, familiar pinging sound of the time clock made my ears ring. It was 8:15 A.M. Instead of calculating my overtime pay, I pointed out to myself that there were only fifteen hours before I had to come back to this place. In one last burst of positive thinking, I figured I could sleep for eight, and with the other seven, I'd try to find a way to get off night shift.

San Francisco was experiencing a perfect blue-skied Indian summer, and I was missing it, along with the rest of life.

The day after Labor Day I'd managed, with superhuman effort, to pick Simon up from Patrick's as usual, go back to the cottage, make breakfast, comb his hair, tie his new shoes, give him the rundown on what his first day of school would be like, walk four blocks, show him where to wait for Patrick when school was out, and gently push him through the bright orange door into the wondrous world of kindergarten.

On the way home, I sat down on the curb to loosen the ties on my nursing shoes and leaned against the tree behind me. A daydream about Simon took me through misty mental images of watching him graduate from Stanford summa cum laude. Two hours later I woke up still sitting against the tree, only slumped to the left and drooling. A pleasant-looking sandy-haired policeman was kneeling next to me, shaking my shoulder.

"You okay, lady?"

Wiping the drool off my chin, I made a pretense that sleeping on curbs was normal business.

"Oh, hello, Officer. Nice day."

The man laughed. "Hi. I'm Officer White. I was just driving by. We don't see too many people sleeping on curbs dressed in nursing uniforms. Graveyard shift, huh?"

I blinked stupidly, then laughed at myself. "Yeah, I walked my son to school and just stopped to fix my shoe—"

"Listen, it's okay, no explanations needed. I worked graveyard for six years; I never got used to being a night person either."

"Yeah," I said, suddenly feeling I wanted to cry; I'd been emotionally labile lately. "It's too much for me."

I stood up and almost fell over. I stretched. "Well, thanks a lot. I gotta get home before I fall asleep in the middle of the street and get mistaken for a speed bump."

Officer White tied my shoelaces. "Be glad to give you a ride home," he said jovially.

I could just see my neighbors peering out of their windows ("Ten-thirty in the morning, and the police have to bring her home . . . still in her uniform. . . . What do you think she's done now? Tsk-tsk!") "No, thanks. I've only got a block to go. I promise I won't stop until I'm safely tucked into bed."

The second and third days of walking Simon to school went without incident; I just promised myself I wouldn't sit down on any curbs. On Friday the two of us held a family conference and agreed he could walk by himself. The cats noisily demanded their breakfasts while we said a cheerful good-bye at the door. My bed was waiting for me, all snuzzy warm and soft. . . .

Simon got to the end of the steps and turned. "Bye-bye, Mama. Have a nice nap time."

I smiled, holding on to the door for support. I leaned over and untied one shoe.

At the end of the driveway Simon was still waving, walking backward. His steps slowed a little. "Bye-bye, Mama." I continued waving with my left hand while I untied the other shoe. Slipping both shoes off, I backed away from the door a step. Simon was still waving as he turned the corner onto the main street. "BYE-BYE, MAMA, I LOVE YOU," he yelled in a pitiful, cracking voice. He was crying.

My first reaction was to go to him and finish walking him to school. Then I realized he had to go on his own someday; it might as well be today.

I closed the door halfway and heard his high-pitched emergency scream: "BYE-BYE, MAMA. I'M OKAY."

"Bye-bye, Simon. I love you."

Still smiling, I closed the door, fed the cats, and crawled into bed. Two seconds later I was heavily involved in one of my vivid full-color morning dreams.

At first I was being chased through a dark underground cave by Mrs. Miller. I wound up in the front of the cottage, watching Mr. Bonowski, who was attached to the top of a phone pole by a huge rubberized string, bouncing back and forth between the clouds and the concrete. Every time his head hit the ground, it made a sound like someone knocking.

Through the molasses dream state, I realized someone *was* knocking . . . at the front door. I looked at my watch; it was 9:00 A.M. Groaning, I rolled off the bed, fell to my knees once, then groped my way to the front door.

Officer White stood in front of me, holding a teary-eyed Simon on his shoulders. "This your son, ma'am?" He laughed.

Dumb with sleep, I squinted. Was it? I wondered.

"I found this tyke sitting on a curb about a block from here, crying . . . says he got lost. I had a feeling you might be his mom; curb sitting runs in the family, eh?"

Simon squirmed to get down from the man's arms and took my hand. "Don't be mad, Mama, okay?"

Snapping out of the fog, I smiled and knelt next to him. Questioningly I looked into his face. "What happened, love?"

Simon's chin quivered, and he put his arm around my neck. "I got scared. I couldn't find the orange doors, and I thought I was in the wrong school. A big boy told me to go back to the baby school, so I ran away."

Ten minutes later I yawned and opened the orange doors to his kindergarten room. Instantly he ran toward the flurry of activity taking place around a caged rabbit, stopped, and came back to reassure me. "It's okay now, Mama. It was just a minor setback." I laughed at his use of the adult phrase and wondered where he'd heard it; he was growing up fast, and I was afraid I was going to miss it all.

Going through the morning mail one night, I came upon an envelope with "Consumer Affairs" printed in the corner. Thinking it was an advertisement, I threw it into the wastebasket. The only place I ever did any consuming anymore was the all-night corner store down the street. The piece of mail landed face up, and I glanced again at the return address: "Sacramento, California." Hmmm? I cleared my eyes. "Board of Registered Nurses."

Jumping up like a shot, I grabbed it, tore open the top, and skimmed the contents. The letter was printed in script type.

"CONGRATULATIONS! You have been successful in the examination . . . you may now practice as a registered nurse . . . give your license to your employer as soon as possible . . ."

I hugged the letter to me and squeezed my eyes shut. "Thank you, dear lady in traction," I whispered. "Thank you."

On Thursday I found a memo from Mrs. Miller on my time card asking me to stop by her office after work the following morning. "How's it working out for you in isolation, dear?" she asked, looking calm and well rested from a full night of sleep.

I stared deliberately at her with troubled eyes and pointed to the dark purple bags under them. "It isn't. I am not a nocturnal bird, Mrs. Miller. I want to see my son grow up. I want to return to the land of the living."

I don't think Mrs. Miller expected such a direct answer, because she hedged it. "It has made a better person of you, Miss Heron. It says here in your evaluation you are quite a capable worker." She expelled some air through her narrow little nostrils and smiled; her teeth were large and straight, like tombstones.

I knew the night people had written that so they could keep me around. They needed someone to torture.

"But now that you have joined the ranks of full-fledged registered nurses"—Mrs. Miller twittered again—"I have an offer for you to think over."

I pulled myself to the edge of my seat, maintaining poise with some difficulty.

"There are six new positions opening in our coronary care unit. A two-week training session will begin next week. Four people have signed up thus far, and I wondered if you might not like your name added to the list."

My mind went into shock. It was like winning a million-dollar jackpot in Las Vegas. Coronary care? The hospital was actually offering to train me in coronary care? I opened my mouth, then snapped it shut again. Suspicion wound its black reptilian body around my heart, sniffing out the loopholes.

"Wait a minute, Mrs. Miller. What shifts are we talking about?"

While I held my breath, Mrs. Miller shuffled the papers on her desk, hesitated, then picked one up. "Ummm, let me see. Ah, yes! We have one on-call evening shift and one full-time night position available. Since you've had time to adjust to nights, perhaps you might like to stay on that shift?"

Was Mrs. Miller deaf, I wondered, or did she have a mean streak a mile wide? "Ah, no. That's okay, Mrs. Miller, a P.M. on-call position is just fine; put my name down . . . one *r*."

Training for CCU in two weeks was like trying to stuff a bale of hay down the throat of an ant in twenty seconds. Annie, the feisty head nurse of the unit, was our instructor . . . or, to be closer to the truth, our baby-sitter. Seven of us, all brand-new grads, sat in the cramped back room of the CCU lounge, trying furiously to learn the complexities of diseased and ailing cardiovascular and pulmonary systems.

Annie somehow managed to cover everything and still make

us eager to come back the next day for more. At the end of the fourteen days she insisted we were ready to take whatever information we could retain and begin our on-the-job-training.

On my first scheduled evening shift I pulled my time card from the slot. Pinned to the top was my new name tag. I stood, transfixed. Next to my name was "RN—CCU." The small bit of plastic suddenly made it vividly clear that everything I'd struggled for was very much mine. I was living out my dreams, and for the first time in my life I felt unashamedly proud.

"Hello. Did they spell your name wrong or something?" I jerked around to see a tall, striking woman with long black hair watching me with concern. I estimated her to be about five feet seven inches tall and to weigh maybe a hundred pounds at the most. Shyly, she took the tag from my hand and read it.

"So, you're the new person with the weird name," she said, smiling and nodding her head. "I'm Jan Tobin, your team leader on swing shift, and I'm pleased to have you with us." Her voice was well modulated, and she spoke with a kind of soft deliberation, making it sound as if there were a slight pause between each word.

After we had shaken hands, Jan bashfully shuffled her feet and started to say something but stopped and nervously wrung one of her long, skinny fingers. I could see her hipbones through her uniform.

"Jeez, doesn't your mother feed you?" I asked finally, gently pinching her arm; it was like pinching a skinny chicken wing. Jan opened her mouth in surprise, then burst out laughing. Her hand fluttered up to her mouth, and she looked out from under her long dark lashes.

"Well, yes, yes she does," she said timidly, "and I still get gold stars for eating all my vegetables."

The CCU was as exciting as the emergency room but in a well-controlled kind of way. The unit was divided into two sections by a set of double doors. Arranged in a semicircle around the monitor banks, the acute CCU, known as the ACCU, was made up of four large glassed-in rooms. These rooms were the sites of miracles.

Here critically ill cardiac patients were given full benefit of advanced cardiopulmonary technology in the form of pacemakers, echocardiography, electrosensitive intracardiac wires, respirators, and administration of new and powerful cardiac drugs, all designed to keep failing hearts working.

The nurse working in ACCU was required to exercise her judgment and expertise more than any other nurse in the house. Caring for the patient on a one-to-one basis, she was responsible for knowing not only the physiotechnical aspects of all diagnostic and life support equipment, but also every dynamic of the patient's illness and all possible complications.

At her discretion a nurse working ACCU gave drugs and initiated certain procedures. She was with the patient around the clock, recording every change, and always on the lookout for the insidious, more subtle changes which usually meant disaster. These nurses were often referred to by the cardiologists as their second pair of eyes and hands.

The intermediate CCU, also known as the ICCU, housed the central monitor desk plus seven two-bed rooms. Reserved for the survivors of the acute side and for patients with chronic or stabilized cardiopulmonary problems, the intermediate side had a slower, less frenzied pace, although all the patients were considered potentially ready to go down the tubes any second.

More often than not, it was the CCU nurse who determined which patient was acute and which one was stable enough to be intermediate. Most of the CCU nurses were so experienced all it took was a quick glance to categorize the borderline patient properly.

Jan took personal charge of teaching me the finer points of cardiac nursing. Patiently she instructed me on everything from interpreting EKGs to doing the most thorough cardiac assessment. She was, without a doubt, one of the finest cardiology nurses I would ever know.

Jan also had a knack for pulling the best out of people without doing anything other than just being herself. Although she seemed to be made up of a strange mixture of grace, tact, naïveté, kindness and practicality, I sensed she loved being shocked by the outrageous.

During my clinical training Jan and I developed a kind of mutual understanding and respect for each other; we were opposites who balanced each other quite well without a great deal of effort on either of our parts. Situations continually came up where I forced her out of her shell, and when I became too flippant, she instilled in me a certain controlling calm.

One evening Jan observed me while I completed my physical exam on Mr. Viscousi, an elderly gentleman admitted for a mild bout of congestive heart failure.

Mr. Viscousi not only suffered from heart failure but also had a bad case of FMPS, or fluff-my-pillow syndrome. He was one of those patients who, when the nurses entered their rooms, would stop watching TV or whatever they were doing and begin to moan, claiming total body pain and weakness. He played up every twitch and bubble of gas as life-threatening in order to extract as much sympathy and attention as possible.

Jan stood by, being her cordial and proper self, correcting me on the small details of the assessment that I'd forgotten or been too casual about. At the same time she was extremely sweet to the man, catering to all his pseudo aches and pains.

When I pulled back the covers to check his legs and feet for edema, it was more than apparent that he had been incontinent.

"Don't worry, Mr. Viscousi," Jan cooed with a forgiving lilt to her voice. "We'll change your bed and make you comfortable again."

Mr. Viscousi knew a sucker when he saw one and took full advantage. "Oh, oh, dear," he bleated, "I'm much too weak to move myself. How will you make my bed while I'm still in it?"

I put a hand on my hip and rolled my eyes. "How 'bout if you levitate?"

Jan's eyes flashed a clear message of "livid" as she motioned me out to the hall. "We don't do that here," she said. "It's tasteless humor at the patient's expense. I don't want to hear it from you again."

I interrupted to tell her I'd seen Mr. Viscousi just an hour ago coming back from the kitchen, walking faster than I, loaded down with enough sherbet and graham crackers to kill a moose.

"It doesn't matter. The man is sick enough to be here. He needs the attention for some reason. Maybe he's lonely or maybe he's really feeling sick. In this unit always give the benefit of the doubt, and don't be so fast to judge how the patient feels. Sometimes the CCU patient is like a time bomb: From the outside he looks fine, and the next minute he's in a full code. Don't forget, he's the one in that bed with a diagnosis, not you.''

I thought about what she said and realized she was right—to a point—though I was beginning to think Jan took her job too seriously. I decided she needed lightening up.

The chance came two nights later, after a hellish shift with five admissions and one code. Jan had let me solo while she held down the fort with her usual grace and diplomacy. Where I or anyone else might have been short-tempered during the thick of the confusion, Jan always found a moment to explain to family members the meaning of a certain blood test result or tactfully tell a doctor why one of his patients had to be bumped to the medical floor.

By eleven the five of us who'd been working with the patients were so exhausted we were silly. We decided Jan needed to get silly, too.

I'm not positive who gave birth to the idea, but after several minutes of whispers and passed notes we left the station one by one and rejoined down the hall, just out of Jan's range of vision.

There we silently formed a human pyramid—three of the younger nurses on the bottom, the unit clerk and I in the middle. As soon as the formation was stable, I called out for Jan, heard her mumble about leaving scopes unattended, and where was everybody, anyway?

When she came around the corner and saw us, we all went into hysterics. Instead of scolding, she looked around, took off her shoes, and scrambled to the top, completing the pyramid.

Mrs. Cervecki, a pacemaker patient, came to her door to see what all the laughter was about. From atop the five other human bodies, Jan stuttered, trying to remain poised and calm while inventing a logical reason for what we were doing.

With a devilish gleam in her eye, Mrs. Cervecki laughed and took off her slippers. All 193 pounds of her headed for our triangular work of living art. She'd just put one foot on someone's rump and started to hoist herself up when the girls on the bottom went down on their elbows. Six of us landed

on the floor, laughing until we wheezed. By the time we got
to our feet, all the patients who were ambulatory were standing in their doorways, applauding, laughing almost as hard
as we were.

At the end of my formal ICCU training, I coaxed Jan into
going out after work to an all-night diner near the hospital.
While we waited for the blue plate special, I told her my life
story. I could have gone on forever pulling stories out of my
closet if just for the joy I felt as I watched her eyes light up
with vicarious pleasure every time I hit upon some outrageous detail. By the time dessert was served, I was just ending the monologue with the story about Mr. O'Reilly in the
bathroom.

"So, tell me about you. I've talked your ear off, and all
you've done is sit there, taking notes. Will the real Jan Tobin
now step forward and offer a little scandalous information
about herself?"

Jan hesitated, looking unsure and nervous as if she were
about ready to walk a tightrope over the Grand Canyon.

"Well, compared to you, I've led a really dull life. I—I
don't know what to tell you, except I had a normal childhood,
although I've always been introverted—"

Jan stopped. I leaned forward expectantly. "And?"

She twisted her fingers one by one, as if she were trying
to remember the rest of the story. "Ummm, let me think. . . .
I, ah, always wanted to be a nurse, I'm stubborn, and a per-
fectionist, just like my father. I love watching movies, listening to all kinds of music, wearing sapphires, and the smell
of yellow roses. Someday I'd like to go to a real stage play,
learn how to cook, and go to Italy." She shifted and stared
into her coffee. "And . . . I . . ."

"And you what?" I asked.

Jan sighed plaintively and looked up. With her high cheekbones and dark almond eyes, she reminded me of the white
man's version of a perfect Indian maiden.

"And, I've got Hodgkin's disease." She wore the same
look Simon did when he'd done something wrong.

My heart stopped. "Well, should I cancel your subscrip-
tions now or wait a month or two?" I laughed, while my
insides flipped over.

Jan sighed as if I'd just saved her from disgrace. "I knew
I could count on you to say something like that. Hardly any-

body knows about it; it's the world's most guarded secret, you know.''

"Why? I would think you'd want people to know, for the emotional support and all that.''

She shook her head. "It doesn't work that way. When people know you have cancer, they treat you differently. Some avoid you; others stare at you like you're a freak in a side show. The ones that got to me the most were the people who walked on eggshells around me. I remember once going to a restaurant with three friends who knew what was going on, and I opened this package of saccharin to pour in my coffee. That was when the saccharin-causes-cancer scare was at its peak, remember? Well, you'd have thought I'd poured cyanide the way they all shut up and stared. 'What's the matter?' I asked. 'Afraid I might get cancer?'

"I meant it to be funny, but they sat there looking like basset hounds. One started to cry and ran off to the ladies' room. . . . God, it was ridiculous.'' Jan smoothed her bangs over to one side. "People have such a morbid curiosity about someone who's dying. The funny thing is, though, everybody else is dying, too, except most people don't know when.

"What's important to me now is living the best way I can until my biological time alarm goes off, and then all I ask for is to die in my sleep right away so I won't be a burden to anyone.''

Silently, we both stared at the small glob of melted ice cream in the middle of my place mat. Casually, I traced a flower pattern around it with my knife.

"So, when did you find out that you—I mean, what happened?''

"Two years ago I'd started feeling generally crummy, and there was this lump in my throat that didn't go away, so after a few months of that I finally went to my doctor. I remember he came in and sat behind his big desk.'' Jan drew her chin into her neck and mimicked an old man's voice. " 'Well, Miss Tobin, you've got Hodgkin's disease. I'd say you have anywhere from six months to two years to live . . . but don't hope for much; we've caught it at stage three B.' '' Jan rolled her eyes. "Well, I was absolutely infuriated. 'Like hell I'm going to die,' I said. 'I'm only twenty-three years old!' '' Jan laughed but looked sad. "As if being twenty-three were going to save me, right? Anyway, I kept waiting for somebody to tell me it was all a mistake; but nobody ever did, so I decided to make a liar out of the guy, and here it is two years later, and I'm still in remission. Now my fantasy is that I'll pick up the newspaper one morning and read that someone's found a cure for it, and I'll live to a ripe old age of forty or maybe, if my luck holds out, forty-five."

She turned her head to the side to look at the ice cream flower on the place mat. "It's a good thing you weren't working in the unit back then. God, I was such a tyrant! I lived with this internal shadow that colored everything black."

"So what happened? I don't see your co-workers cower when you enter the room now."

Jan giggled. "Believe me, they used to. But that all changed after I took care of this one man who was waiting around for a heart transplant." Her eyes sparkled, and excitement filled her voice as she remembered.

"You would have loved that guy; he was so special, so full of life; he reminded me of a Jewish Leo Buscaglia. In one shift he managed to get through my iron wall with this very simple message about living with courage. He told me people who knew they had short appointments here had a choice between being pissed-off and despair-ridden or spreading around a lot of love before they signed off."

She sighed. "Anyway, I'm tired of living like a sheltered old lady. I'm ready to crawl out of my protective shell and take off for the sky while I'm still in remission."

"So why are you still working? Why don't you quit and do all the things you've always wanted to do? Go wild."

Jan wrapped an empty sugar package around one of her pencil thin fingers. "No. I love my work. Taking care of people keeps me alive; it gives me a real purpose. When I say I want to fly a little, I don't mean I want to run away. I just want to get out and experience some of the things normal people do, like go to a play and not worry that the person sitting behind me is going to see my radiation marks or not be afraid to ride a cable car on a rainy, foggy night because I might get a cold. Those things are just normal everyday occurrences to you; to me, they're adventures in living dangerously."

I waited for the waitress to clear away our plates.

"Okay, Jan, you got me. The epitome of my unrest will now lie in getting you out to all the best museums and plays and hiking trails. It will be my personal duty to keep you well supplied in adventure."

Jan gave one of her enigmatic Mona Lisa smiles. "Good! I'm ready to take on almost anything, but you should think about the fact that I'm not going to live for a long time; I could go out of remission tomorrow, and there you'd be—stuck with spoon-feeding me my strawberry daiquiris and carrying me up hills to catch the cable cars."

"You know," I said, cocking my head and squinting at her, "for a skinny person who doesn't say much, you sure have a way of dropping bombs that warms my heart. Just give me fair notice when I need to hire the organist."

"Oh, ha-ha, very funny. Listen, I'm just warning you about the pitfalls of being a friend of mine; I don't want you getting all smarmy and weak-kneed on me if I drop dead during one of your 'little' hikes."

"Don't worry. I'll deal with those things only when they reach out to stop me."

Simon loved Jan. She was, he said, like a kind and pretty fairy with a voice like mashed potatoes.

After making the rounds of most of the museums and a few of the easier hiking trails on Mount Tamalpais, the three of us started going to plays. Jan loved everything from Ibsen to Neil Simon. In the dark theaters she sat spellbound, watching the actors weave fantasy around her, her eyes sparkling with childish delight through even the most tragic of plays.

On one blustery, rainy night, as we were leaving a theater in San Francisco, Simon frantically grabbed hold of Jan's hands and pulled her back into the lobby.

Puzzled, we stared at him. "What is it? What's the matter, Simon?" she asked.

"The wind," he said, worriedly pointing outside. "I'm afraid it's gonna blow you away."

A shadow passed over her face, and then she laughed. "Well, if you and your mom hold on very, very tight to each of my hands, the wind won't be able to get me."

Simon brightened up with the idea. "We won't let the wind get her, will we, Mama?"

Between the two of them they were the essence of what the "good" people of the earth were made of. I slipped my arms around them both and pressed them to me. "That's right, we'll hide her so the wind won't ever find her."

ELEVEN

THE OLD MAN'S HEAD fell into the nest of his pillow like some white bird tired from too long a flight. Squinting, I tried to reconstruct a younger face over the thin, blue-veined skin covering his skull. He took my hand in his translucent fingers and held it to his heart; I wondered if the strength of my body could seep into his by some strange osmosis.

His mouth wrinkles spread out smoothly in a smile, and with that we understood each other completely; his ancient eyes told me he was a wise and tender sort, a frail and delicate shell being held together by only the core of his spirit.

To him I was a kind of angel of mercy who would change his linen and give him pills, foolishly trying to fight off what he already knew was inescapable. He hoped I was not too young to know eighty-four-year-olds were still human.

"Hi, Mr. Turk. Remember me? My name's Echo. I took care of you briefly when you first came in."

"Please, call me Turk," he said in a voice that was pleasantly rough after a lifetime of words flowing over the same cords. "Glad to see I didn't scare you away the first time, Ethel."

I chuckled at the common mistake and bent down to speak directly into the old man's ear. "Not Ethel, Echo—like up in the mountains."

"Oh, my, how unusual," he said. I watched his red-rimmed and rheumy eyes dart around the ceiling for a second. "Of course, you're too young to know the song they wrote about you." Weakly he cleared his throat and held up

202

a trembling, arthritic finger. In his wobbly old man's voice he began singing "Little Sir Echo," a tune people had been crooning around me since the day I was born. I sang along with him to the end of the first verse when he let out a wheezing crackle.

"What's so funny?" I asked. "Am I off key?"

Turk shook his head and smiled a smile that was veiled by memory. "Oh, no, you reminded me of someone when you started singing, your voice and the way your hair goes all fluffy by your neck there." He pointed to a few stray wisps of hair that had fallen from the knot on the top of my head.

I watched the gleam in the man's eyes and thought about how much I'd come to like old people. They were such treasuries of astonishing stories if one just took the time to pay attention. So few people listened to these walking, talking history books, except, of course, the children. In their brief time of wisdom, children knew the value of what the elderly had to say.

"And what was the lady's name?" I asked, reaching over to smooth the covers away from his chin.

Turk's gaze was drawn to the ceiling again. Mulling over my question, he unconsciously rubbed the timeworn ring on his right hand. Gently I held it to the light to study it more closely. On the gold dome was etched an intricately detailed eagle's head. It was easy to see the handwork belonged to the era when people valued craftsmanship over mass production.

"Her real name was Nettie, but I used to call her Ned 'cause she really wasn't like a girl at all." Turk watched me inspect the ring and looked at it more closely himself for something he might have missed. "She was one wild filly for back in those days, I'll tell you. That girl could ride a horse and throw a rope as good as any of us boys . . . And stubborn?" Turk let out a long whistle and shook his head. "Lord, what a stubborn mule she was! Once that girl made up her mind, *nothing* could get her to change it."

Without disturbing Turk's legs, I broke one of nursing's numerous rules by sitting on the edge of his bed. He looked at me questioningly.

"I'm getting comfortable for this one," I said, adding firmly, "And I want the *whole* story, Turk. Don't leave out one word."

Pleased and embarrassed, Turk waved his hand. "Oh, I

don't know, a young girl like you wouldn't be interested in all that. It's all just an old man's prattle.''

"I beg to differ with you there, sir," I said, pretending to be indignant. "How many people nowadays have the opportunity to hear stories firsthand from someone born in 1896? I've always thought if I could go back in time, those are the years I'd want to live through."

Wagging his finger, the old man cocked his head to the side. "No, you wouldn't, angel; they weren't like now with your autos and spaceships, I'll tell you. Back then, when the country was just learning to walk, it was a hard life. The TV plays it up as a romantic, fancy time, but it wasn't like that for the common people."

I put my chin in my hand and crossed my legs. "I know it was difficult, but I still would have liked it, I think. It sounds exciting to have to live by your wits; no plastic money, no highways, no smog. Do you realize you are one of a minority who's actually seen what's under all this concrete?"

Turk turned slightly toward me with sparkling eyes and shook his head. "Mercy, she was like that, too—always dreaming about other times."

"Well, then, that does it," I said. "Now you've *got* to tell me the rest of the story."

Turk licked his lips and for something to do with his hands, adjusted the bedcovers. He laid his head back in the pillow, allowing me to watch his Adam's apple move up and down. At length he began.

"Ned was about my age. While we were growing up, she was the farm girl tomboy, so of course, none of us boys really paid much attention to her; we thought of her as the tag-along pest, if we thought of her at all.

"Then, one year—I guess we were sixteen or so—she stopped wearing braids and turned her overalls in for dresses." Turk redirected his gaze out the window, where the gray air was busy with an unseasonal outburst of October rain. Staring abstractedly, he softly started again. "Lord, what a beauty she turned out to be with that gold hair hanging down her back and a waist no bigger than a fence post. All of us were like a bunch of lovesick mangy dogs the way we moped around her." Turk rallied, smiling to himself. "Things couldn't have gone on like that for long, or we'd have killed ourselves just trying to outdo each other showing off.

"Eventually she picked me over the other fellas because she said she liked the way I talked to the animals, as if they had feelings, and"—Turk blushed—"because she said my eyes reminded her of an eagle's. She had a lively imagination, that one did, used to say I was her 'gentle eagle' when we got to be alone."

Unmindful now of my presence, Turk fixed his eyes on a faraway point. "I remember I was allowed to court her once a week on Saturday nights. After dinner I'd sneak into my mother's dresser and steal a drop of the lavender toilet water she wore to church on Sundays and rub it in my hair. I'd go out of the house smelling like a fancy women's shop. My brothers used to run out into the yard to tease me." Turk extended his arm, pointing at the memory of himself and re-creating the singsong child's taunt "There goes Nellie Al . . . . all prettified for his gal." He smiled and stayed lost in the memory until I spoke to him a few moments later.

"So what happened? Did you get married?"

He shook his head. "Nope, but we should have; we were thick as thieves." Turk's eyes smiled. "She was my first and I was hers." Lifting one eyebrow, he wagged his finger with a look of remonstration. "You young people think you invented all those things you do in the back seats of cars? Ha! We had it all over you. Let me tell you, nobody ever improved on romancing on a bed of fresh hay in a warm loft.

"We were an adventuresome pair for a couple of hicks. After we got engaged, me and Ned decided the first thing we'd do when we were married was work our way to Europe on a steamboat, all 'cause she saw a picture of the Eiffel Tower in a picture book and decided she couldn't rest until she saw it first hand. Then we were going to California and mine gold and then move to Florida and buy a little house right on the ocean with all the money we'd make from mining." Turk lay back on his pillow, and his eyes sought out the rain again. I stayed silent, sensing an unhappy ending to his story.

"She was crazy as a loon, but Lord, she took my breath away. Then one day, about six weeks before the wedding, a friend of her father's was passing through, and she and he kinda took to each other. . . . Three weeks later they ran off together."

Turk fingered the eagle's head. "Lord, I thought losing out

with her was the end of the world, but I managed to survive somehow—at least long enough to meet my wife about six years later while I was going to school.

"Grace is dead now. Died in 1963 . . . cancer of the stomach. She wasn't any great beauty, but she was a good, practical woman and a devoted mother to the boys. I never had to worry that she'd even look at another man. . . .

"I always wondered, though, if I didn't lose the better part of living sometimes by not going off to find Ned." Turk motioned for me to move closer. "I loved Grace and the boys, and I gave them everything they needed and all; but I'd think of Ned at some of the craziest times, like in the middle of a Christmas dinner or when Louis was born, times like that . . . damnedest thing."

"What happened to her?"

"Aw, I don't know . . . never asked," he answered simply enough. "But life wouldn't be any fun without a little mystery, would it?"

Turk suddenly looked small and worn-out, like a deflated white balloon, and I sensed it was time to change the subject.

"Your sons seem very devoted to you."

Turk straightened his back as if the act would rid him of Ned's shadow. "Oh, yeah, fine boys . . . well, they're men now, but they've always been my boys. Louis is like his mother was: very practical, good business sense, too. John's more like me: sentimental and soft. Both of them married well, and all their kids are in college or married."

Adjusting his position again, Turk trailed off: "Good men, both of them."

Turk grimaced, and I noticed he seemed paler than earlier. On the monitor a certain segment of his EKG complex was taller and larger than it had been a moment before, indicating he wasn't getting enough oxygen to his heart.

"Turk, are you having pain? Tell me what's going on."

He strained to take in a deep breath. "Not pain, just a little pressure here." He pointed to the middle of his chest.

I checked his blood pressure, which was higher than usual, and gave him a nitroglycerin tablet to dissolve under his tongue. When it failed to relieve the pressure, three milligrams of morphine made him not care if there was pressure or not.

I decided to hold off on doing his physical assessment until he was pain-free. I waited with him, sitting on the edge of his bed and holding his hand until he grew sleepy and began to nod.

At the monitor banks I turned off the alarm hold. Immediately, beeps and buzzers sounded through the room. The control board's two screens were lit, revealing Turk's rhythm; above them the date and time flashed, accurate to the second. Most people walking in off the street would have viewed the high ceilings and glassed-in effect of the room as something created from sets left over from an old Flash Gordon movie.

Sitting down, I looked around; Alonso Turk and I had the entire acute side to ourselves. After a year of on-the-job CCU training, I'd completed my certification requirements to work on the intermediate side. But Jan wasn't satisfied to have me stop there. Priming me for charge nurse duties, she took it upon herself to teach me all the complex skills I'd need to work the acute unit. In three painstaking, frustrating months, she had me ready for my debut into the real world of critical care and then consistently assigned me the sickest of the acute patients. Turk's admission marked the end of my second year in CCU.

Because Turk's heart was irritated, I was alert to the possibility he might have an increase in arrhythmias. Alternately, I looked from the monitor to him.

In the middle of the softly lit glass room, the elderly man lay surrounded by a jungle of IV poles, wires, and plastic tubing. He raised his hand to scratch his nose, and it dawned on me this eighty-four-year-old man had survived a stormy course of illness many people younger than he might not have made it through.

Two days prior to his admission, Turk suffered from what he'd diagnosed as a simple case of the flu. The initial runny nose and diarrhea decreased but left him with a persistent, nagging cough, a tight chest, and a feeling of nausea that never went away. An independent man, Turk had little use for, or patience with, doctors and stubbornly refused his sons' offers to take him to one. He proceeded to treat himself with aspirin and small quantities of lemon-grass tea prepared with honey.

On the morning of his admission he awoke feeling a strong pressure in the middle of his chest. He took two aspirin with a cup of tea but vomited before they were halfway down. Not to be sent to his bed so easily, Turk decided to settle his stomach and relieve the chest pressure with a swallow of peppermint oil. Reaching up to open the spice cabinet, he felt his heart "stumble over itself" and take off, racing. Immediately he became sweaty and dizzy, vomited once more, and lost consciousness. An hour later John, his younger son, found him collapsed on the floor halfway between the kitchen and the living room, clutching the phone between his knees.

Overriding his father's protests, John called the paramedics, and an hour later Turk was admitted to ACCU in the process of infarcting the inferior wall of his heart. Dr. Purdy, Turk's semiretired physician, called in Dr. Joseph Cramer, the newest and best cardiologist on the block.

After a week, Turk was just barely tolerating his hospitalization. Not used to the invasion of privacy and lack of control over his own life, he was grinning and bearing it good-naturedly, but it was clear he was becoming more depressed each day. Using IV propranalol, a drug given to lower the blood pressure and control cardiac pain, Dr. Cramer had managed to break the continuous pain cycle, but Turk was still considered too unstable to be transferred to the intermediate side.

Jan peered through the double doors and waved. I waved back. "Everything okay?" she asked. "You look so tiny all alone in this giant cave."

"The bears and I are fine, thank you, ma'am."

She jerked one of her long skinny thumbs in the direction of the entrance doors. "Mr. Turk's sons are in the waiting room and want to visit. Is it okay if they come in?"

I felt tentative about letting anyone disturb the man's rest but knew if I didn't allow the visit, there'd be repercussions, especially from Turk's older son.

Most of the problems with family visits stemmed from the two-visitors-at-a-time and the ten-minute-limit rules, but visitor's tempers also heated up over other regulations such as being asked to leave the room so the patient could rest or being made to wait in the waiting room while exams, procedures, or personal needs were taken care of. So much of our time was spent smoothing ruffled family feathers, playing policeman, or trying not to get pulled into family politics that it made it hard to remain cordial.

I nodded reluctantly. "Okay, but tell them before they get

in the door, they can stay for only a few minutes. He had some chest pain a little while ago, and I'd prefer it wasn't aggravated.''

No one could say Louis and John weren't devoted to their father; they came to the hospital twice a day, every day, and stayed as long as the nurses felt Turk could handle the stimulation.

Louis, a joyless, stout man in his late fifties, was the type of family member I'd come to know as a ''malpractice hound.''

He watched everything that went on with a strict eye, demanding to know how and why each procedure was done, all the while taking notes on every drug given and every word said. He kept a small notepad in his hand from the time he walked into the room until the time he left.

Usually nurses welcomed and encouraged family members to ask questions, but with Louis, one got the feeling whatever was said would end up being quoted in a courtroom. He'd further managed to intimidate us by taking all our names, demanding to know how long we'd each worked in CCU and what our qualifications were. Curt and insistent, Louis made a barrage of small demands, mostly for things Turk did not need or want.

At first the demands were easily met: Vaseline for Turk's lips; drops for his eyes; straws for his beverages; four pillows instead of two. The day after Turk's admission, however, Louis, over his father's protestations, got to the point of insisting his father be spoon-fed by the nurses.

Patiently we explained to him how overdoing the caretaking could demoralize his father and rob him of all feelings of independence and, in fact, make him worse, but Louis bore a grudge against anyone who didn't follow his orders, complaining that we weren't doing enough for his father. Over the course of only a few days most of us dreaded his visits.

John was younger than Louis by at least five or more years, and just as Turk had said, he was sensitive and kind to everyone. Often he helped us turn and bathe Turk, placed and removed the bedpan, or assisted with changing the bed linen. At first both father and son were shy and self-conscious while John tended to his father's personal needs, but after the initial nervousness had been conquered, a tender connection of giving and receiving was made.

Louis walked in and nodded at me. "How is he?" he asked. John patted me on the shoulder and squeezed my arm, and from the way Louis looked away, I could tell his brother's display of affection disturbed him.

"He's been having some chest pain on and off today and this evening. I gave him some nitro and morphine about forty minutes ago, so he's dozing now."

"How much morphine did you give?" Louis asked.

"Three milligrams," I answered, highly conscious of the spiral notebook sticking out from his pocket. "Enough to take the edge off the pain."

With the malpractice look written all over his face, Louis had started to ask another question when John hooked his arm through his and led him into Turk's room.

"Thank you, dear," John said over his shoulder. "We'll stay only a few minutes."

Through the glass I watched John take his father's hand and kiss his forehead. Turk attempted kissing him on the cheek, missed, and awkwardly got his chin instead.

Louis stood sternly at the end of the bed, saying nothing.

I started at the sudden buzz of the intercom.

"A mysterious young male caller is on line one, waiting for his mother to say good night," said Jan at the other end of the phone.

"Thanks, boss." I laughed and pushed the blinking line.

"Hi, Mom." ("Mama" was no longer acceptable; it was a "baby" word, not allowable for first graders.)

"Hi, darling. Are you ready for sleeps?"

"Yep. Dad said I could have some ice cream before I went to bed if I brush my teeth, okay?"

"Okay, but only one scoop."

Simon fidgeted and sighed a few times, winding up to ask his usual list of questions. It was a ritual we went through whenever he called me at the hospital.

Considering he was the product of divorced, working parents, Simon spent more quality time with each of us than most of his friends who lived with both parents. With my on-call position, I often had three or four days a week to spend with him, while Patrick gladly took over on the evenings I worked. After two or three days of separation, one of us was always excited to see him and catch up on all the latest happenings of his life.

"What's wrong with your patients tonight, Mom?"

"I have only one patient, an old man named Turk who had a heart attack. His heart keeps making those bad beats I told you about, but mostly his chest still hurts."

"Does he have asthma, too?"

Ever since Simon was diagnosed as having asthma, he'd somehow gotten the idea into his head that all hospitalized people suffered from the pulmonary disease no matter what else ailed them.

"No, he wasn't lucky enough to have asthma. He has worse things."

"Is he—is he going to d-die?"

"I hope not. He's a nice old man, but I'm afraid his heart is just worn-out."

Simon covered the phone and directed his yell to the background. "Hey, Dad! Mom says her patient's heart is all worn-out." In the distance, I heard Patrick sound appropriately dismayed.

"Hey, Mom? Are you going to work tomorrow?"

"Nope. I've got three days off in a row this weekend, so we can go up on the mountain if you want, or maybe we can ask Jan to come to dinner and then go to a movie, or if you insist, we could even clean your room. I saw a pair of socks crawling out from under your bed today before I left for work."

Simon giggled. "Let's take Jan to a scary movie tomorrow, and we'll all get scared and shaking, okay?"

Out of the corner of my eye I saw two ectopic beats in a row and leaped for the printout button. Louis noticed the graph light flash on his father's bedside monitor and looked out at the desk, alarmed.

"We'll talk about it when you get home from school tomorrow," I said hurriedly. "Gotta go, honey. See you tomorrow. I love you."

"Love you, too, Mom."

I counted to three from the time I placed the receiver on the cradle to the moment Louis walked to the desk with John close behind. Louis put his face anxiously near mine, and for just a second, I thought I smelled alcohol on his breath.

"What were those funny-looking beats on my father's monitor just a second ago?"

I showed him the strip of the two aberrant beats. "These?" I asked nonchalantly.

Louis nodded.

"We call these PVCs, or premature ventricular contractions, also called ectopic beats. All it means is that the heart's electrical system sometimes goes haywire and beats before it should. If the heart is irritated enough or if a beat comes just at the wrong time, it can set off a whole run of those beats.

"The reason we pay such close attention to them is that when they fire off, the heart isn't really beating or pushing any blood around at all; it's shooting blanks more or less."

John stepped forward and studied the strip while biting his thumbnail. "How do you stop them?" he asked in a tone much softer than his brother's.

"Remember I told you your father has two drugs in his IVs called procainamide and lidocaine? Those suppress the ectopics. Most people usually only need one of those; but your dad's had a big infarct, and his muscle is still irritated, plus his blood pressure's being so high doesn't help."

"And what if he has a whole run of those PVCs and the drugs don't work?" Louis asked.

"In that case, we countershock with so many watts; sometimes that shocks the heart back into a normal rhythm, and sometimes into other arrhythmias."

Louis looked at his father and stood back as if to discount the possibility of anything like that ever happening to *his* father. "My father has always been a very strong man. He can make it out of here if you people do your jobs."

I took the strip from John and proceeded to paste it on the monitor sheet. "Your father is also eighty-four years old and has damaged a major portion of his heart," I said without looking up.

Louis flared. "What's that supposed to mean?"

One of my warning lights went off, and I knew I had to be careful what I said, not only from a legal standpoint but because of a lesson I'd learned while caring for one of my first acute patients. Maintaining a straight face, I recalled the incident with embarrassed amusement.

The patient was also an older man who, like Turk, had suffered a major heart attack. Early in his hospitalization he and his wife agreed there were to be no heroic measures taken if his condition deteriorated. Shortly afterward his rhythm went out of control despite any of the antiarrhythmics we gave, and his blood pressure dipped low enough to be considered almost nonexistent.

The man had stopped speaking or moving and would only occasionally open his eyes for what I called a "location check" (Have I died and gone to heaven yet?).

Dr. Morrison, his cardiologist, came in to see him when I thought the end was near. "He's going to die in the next few minutes," he said after checking the man over. "Just make note of the time he goes, and I'll come back to pronounce him after I see a few of my other patients."

I cleaned the room, turned off the monitor, and opened the curtains so the man could die bathed in the lambent afternoon light. With the appropriate solemn face I trudged into the waiting room to fetch his wife. "He's dying," I said in my most funereal tone of voice. "It will be over in a few moments." Both of us sniffled as I led her into the man's room. She sat next to him, speaking in the low, soft voice people often use in the presence of death. Partially leaning across the bed, she stroked his head.

After forty minutes she stood up and stretched her back, looking at me questioningly. I checked the dying man's blood pressure; it was normal. I turned the monitor back on; his rhythm was the same. By all rights he shouldn't have had a normal blood pressure. I noticed, too, his color was just a bit less pale.

Dr. Morrison tried not to show his surprise when he went in to do his postmortem check of the "body," but I could tell from the way his facial tic kept going off that it really threw him for a loop that the man was still alive. Not wanting to believe his eyes, he assured the wife it was still only a matter of moments—an hour or two at the most. She smiled in the most patronizing way and patted his hand.

By dinner the wife had worked up a hearty appetite by reading most of the Sunday paper to her husband and left for the cafeteria. When she returned an hour later, her husband had started putting out urine and was asking for sips of water despite the awful rhythm showing on the monitor. When I left at eleven-thirty, they both were watching the news.

Two weeks later I walked through the main entrance of the hospital and caught a glimpse of the same man as he gave the transport girl a pinch and got into a taxicab with his wife.

I decided then and there to try never to be too sure of anything.

I cleared my throat. "That means, Mr. Turk, that you need to look at the reality of the situation and not put the entire determining factor as to whether your father lives or dies on us."

John stood up. "Well, I think it's time to go now. You probably have things to do. Come on, Lou, dinner's waiting." Sour and unyielding, Louis walked out of the unit. John hesitated and turned back at the door.

"My brother isn't going to let go very easily," he said apologetically.

I stared at Turk through the glass. "Your father is such a sweet man, John, I understand why you both love him so much."

There was silence, and when I turned around, John had gone.

I walked quietly into Turk's room and gently lifted his left arm, hoping to wrap the blood pressure cuff around it without disturbing his sleep. Turk roused and opened one eagle eye. "Hi, angel."

"Hi, Eagle Eyes, time for your bedtime physical: heart check, lung check, lube, and oil."

Turk looked pale, and I noticed he had his left hand balled into a fist. His blood pressure was elevated dramatically.

"You're having pain again, Turk?"

"It's nothing," he answered.

"Turk, you know you're supposed to tell us when you have even the slightest twinge," I said. "We want to keep ahead of the pain, not let it get ahead of us, remember?"

Turk nodded. "I didn't tell you this time because it's in my back, not my chest."

Turk had pressed my panic button. Back pain in the cardiac patient with a fresh injury was a bad sign. In my short experience I'd seen it twice, and in each case the patient had developed an aneurysm in one of the main vessels of the heart which later tore open altogether.

"I'm going to give you some more morphine and call Dr. Cramer. I don't like all this pain business."

Opening his eyes, Turk stopped me by taking hold of my arm. His fingers were like icicles. "Angel, if something happens to me, promise you won't let them put any hoses in my lungs or put me on those machines that keep people alive."

I started to chide Turk for being silly but stopped. His eyes told me to listen.

"What do you mean? Are you saying you don't want to be resuscitated if anything happens to you here?"

He hesitated a moment before committing himself. "I don't want to be kept alive with machines," he said slowly. "I am eighty-four years old, angel. I raised my kids and saw my grandkids grow up. I worked hard and got everything out of life I was supposed to; now I want to get on, die in my own bed naturally. As far as I'm concerned, all these modern drugs and equipment are just a way of messin' around in God's workshop when His back is turned."

I tousled what was left of his white hair. "I'll tell Dr. Cramer you said so, and he can talk to Louis and John about it. The final decision will be up to them, and to be honest about it, Turk, I don't think Louis is up for letting you go without a major battle."

Turk almost sprang out of the bed. "Damn it! He's not the one laying here. Don't you dare let anybody turn me into one of them bed potatoes who wear diapers and can't even blink."

The old man fought back tears, and I touched him lightly. "It's okay, Turk. I'll tell Dr. Cramer tonight. We'll see if we can't get this all set straight just in case. But knowing you, you'll live to be a hundred."

Turk sadly took my hand and kissed the back of it. "I don't want to live to be a hundred, angel. Lord, don't wish that on me!"

"Why don't you want to, Turk?" I asked.

"I've seen too much. I know too much about . . . things," he said, and closed his eyes.

I'd heard this answer from older patients before when I asked them about their deaths. Because of the look that often went with the pat answer, I'd never pushed to uncover its true meaning but imagined it to be one of the answers in a book issued to all people over the age of seventy entitled *The Elderly's Book of Standard Answers for the Young.*

I gave Turk more morphine and waited for him to doze off before I put in the call to Dr. Cramer.

Dr. Cramer had joined the main cardiology group six months after I'd been working, and most people, including his patients, still didn't know what to make of the man. At a cursory glance, Joseph Cramer was a borderline eccentric who walked stiffly and as straight as a man with a fused spine; he mumbled a lot, laughed at the strangest moments, and spoke to people he didn't know or trust only when absolutely necessary.

From a medical standpoint he seemed a reserved, almost austere man who practiced his cardiology with the precision of a powerful and flawlessly tuned engine. He was one of the few doctors who could run a code smoothly without costing everyone a high depletion in adrenaline levels or, more important, without making enemies. He read the nurses' notes, asked our opinions, and, unlike most physicians, kept his ego on a leash and under control—even when being bombarded with questions, problems, and almost impossible tasks. I figured he must have broken the physicians' code of behavior because he readily admitted when he was wrong.

All that was straightforward and easily read, but it took me two months of carefully decoding his mumbles and watching how he handled the sixty-seven strong-willed personalities of the CCU nursing staff before I realized the key to understanding this unique man was his dry, if somewhat cynical, sense of humor.

Within five minutes the exchange had Dr. Cramer on the line. "Hi, Joe, Echo. I'm taking care of Turk tonight, and I think we're getting into trouble. Along with his usual chest pain, he's started having pain in his back, and the MS isn't holding him. Other than that, his BP is coming off the ceiling, and he's having more PVCs than he's had in days; as a matter of fact, he coupled a little while ago."

Joe spoke with a slow East Coast drawl. "Okay, let's see how well I've trained you; tell me what you want to do from here."

I thought for a moment, then wrote down what I thought I needed. "I want a twelve-lead EKG and blood gases to start, and a potassium level and CPKs with isoenzymes; that'll tell me if he's extending his infarct and why he's having so much ectopy. Next, I want to give him some nitrates to get his pressure down."

Panicking only slightly, I realized, looking at the flow sheet, that Turk's urine output had fallen off dramatically over the last twenty-four hours. "He needs a diuretic, probably forty milligrams of Lasix to start." I hesitated.

"Anything else?" Joe asked, meaning there was.

"A chest x-ray to see what might be causing the back pain."

"Want to venture a possible diagnosis of what's going on with this gentleman?"

"Possible dissecting aneurysm?"

"It's a shame your mother dropped you on your head, Heron, because you just might have made it through med school, given some encouragement.

"Well, I think there still might be hope if you'd give me the address in Mexico of the mail-order place where you got your diploma, Joe."

"Sorry, it went out of business right after I got mine."

I switched the telephone from my left hand to my right and made an okay sign to Turk, who was looking through the glass, searching for me.

"Speaking of going out of business, Joe, there's another problem you need to deal with ASAP."

"I can hardly wait to hear it."

"You have to talk to the sons about Turk's code status. As it stands now, he's a full code, and he just informed me in no uncertain terms he does not want to be resuscitated."

"At eighty-four I think the man has made a sensible choice," Joe said. "I'll talk to the sons when we find out what's going on here."

"And at thirty-four I think you take a hint quite well, but listen to a word of warning: Don't expect much from the older son; he's as stubborn as black snake shit on a white pillowcase."

"Is this the standard Heron criterion for determining obstinacy—the color of reptile feces on pillows?"

"No, it's one of the ones I use to describe the really tough cases."

"I'll keep that in mind. Call me back when all the results are in."

A few minutes later Jan came over, and together we examined the twelve patterns of the EKG, each representing a separate location of Turk's heart. She put in a call to Joe while I checked Turk again and gave him more MS to dull the pain brought on by the ordeal of taking a chest x-ray.

The intercom buzzed once. "And the results are?" asked Joe as soon as I said hello.

"Looks like he's extending to his anterior wall; he's got S-T changes in all of his anterior leads."

"Typical," said Joe. "Do you want the rest of the bad news now, or would you rather not know since you're almost ready to go home?"

I sighed and sat down. "No. Go ahead and tell me now, so I can worry about it for the three days I have off."

"The radiologist just called to say Mr. Turk has a newly developed aortic aneurysm. You win."

I winced. Not only had Turk infarcted two major sections of his heart, but now he was ready to blow a hole through one of its major vessels.

"Oh, wonderful," I said, sagging over the desk. "My ulcer sends kisses."

"Now, Heron, tell me, what's my next step here?"

"Lines?"

"You catch on quickly for someone who slouches."

I groaned. This meant poor Turk would end up having two more wires inserted into him. The pulmonary artery line would be threaded into the right side of his heart to measure the amount of fluid in his body and the amount of force his heart was pumping it around with. The other catheter, called an arterial line, was a shorter wire that threaded into an artery and provided us with a constant readout of his blood pressure.

"It's ridiculous putting lines in an eighty-four-year-old man who wants to be left alone, has had a major infarct, and now has an aneurysm. Where is this going to stop?"

"If what you're saying about the son is true," said Joe, "nothing is going to stop until after I put in the lines. But medically it's clear that he needs them, and soon. Now, if the man really doesn't want the procedure done, I can't force him, but I'd be willing to bet you the sons show up within twenty minutes and exert enough pressure on him to make him consent to the procedure."

"Okay then, what about pushing for at least a change to a modified code? Anything's got to be better than a full one."

I spoke knowing Turk wouldn't approve of that code status either, although with the modified code there was only a partial effort at resuscitation: no intubation, no CPR, and perhaps one or two defibrillations. Drugs were almost always given, but without the pump to circulate them, this was considered a "gesture." It was a way to nullify the guilt of the family and put the patient through only moderate discomfort.

"I'll call the sons now to let them know what's going on and mention it to them. I'll be in to talk to the old guy myself in about forty minutes. Why don't you go ahead and start setting up the equipment?" Joe paused, then added, "And Echo? You might break it gently to him what's cooking, so it isn't such a shock when we all troop in."

Thoroughly discouraged, I watched Turk dozing peacefully. "Okay, I'll do the scut work"—I sniffed—"but I'm really glad I don't have to witness the committing of this crime."

"Good-bye, Sarah Bernhardt," Joe said, and hung up.

A few minutes later I'd gathered all the equipment together in Turk's room and started opening packages. He eyed the equipment with suspicion. "What're you planning to do with all that stuff?"

"Dr. Cramer wants to insert a couple more wires: one to check out how much fluid you have in your body and the other to show your blood press—"

Turk shook his head once. "No, angel. You tell Dr. Cramer to stay home, and just put all that stuff away, because I'm not going to have another damned tube inserted into this old body, I'll tell ya."

It was hard not to tell Turk that if he stuck to his guns, Cramer wouldn't go over his wishes, but I also knew no matter what I said, Louis would talk him into consenting to the procedures in the end. I continued assembling the transducer and the pressure bags.

"Louis and John are coming in to talk to you about it, and Dr. Cramer will be in right afterward. Just remember it *is* still up to you."

Turk shook his head. "This is crazy. All of a sudden in the middle of the night they decide to do this, and Louis and John are coming in? What the hell is going on?"

"Oh, you know medicine, Turk, it waits for no man. We're the people who wake you up in the middle of the night to give you a sleeping pill."

I finished putting together the arterial line and hung it next to Turk's bed and started on the pulmonary artery line. "Dr. Cramer will explain it to you before he does anything."

Turk ran a shaky hand over his skull, looking discouraged. "Aw, nuts!" he said, and sighed.

I gave report to Dana, the senior nurse on night shift, and went in to say good night to Turk. I regarded him with a sense of loss, sure he wouldn't make it until I was scheduled to work again.

He opened one eye. "Why aren't you home and asleep?" he asked.

"I will be shortly." I leaned over and gave him a quick kiss on the cheek. "Be good until I get back. Don't chase any of those other nurses around or I'll be jealous. John and Louis will be here any minute, and so will Dr. Cramer, so rest up now."

Turk took my hand and kissed it. He was trembling.

"Until we meet again, angel, may the Lord bless you and hold you gently in the palm of His hand."

Without warning, I choked up, kissed him again, and fled out of the room. At the door I glanced back to look once more through the glass wall; Turk blew me a kiss and smiled.

Over the weekend Simon and I accomplished the major task of cleaning his room. This was always an adventure in discovery, uncovering all sorts of odds and ends, like the old banana peel under his bed that was so covered with a black, furry mold we both thought it was a tarantula and screamed in unison. By Saturday evening we had seven bags of clothes and slightly maimed toys ready for Goodwill. The results were visible; we'd cleared a path to the door.

On Sunday afternoon Simon, flanked by Jan and me, marched fearlessly into the local theater to watch what had been billed as the scariest movie of all time.

We exited two and a half hours later, squinting at the assault of light, glad to touch base with reality. For the rest of the afternoon we all lived in a state of immediate post-horror-show hysteria. Every small sound caused us to suck in our breaths and listen bug-eyed, afraid that some slimy, repulsive creature would spring from the nearest dark corner.

Simon went to bed with more reluctance than usual, insisting Jan and I look under the bed and search his room for hungry monsters lying in wait for a tender young boy afflicted with asthma.

At nine-thirty he ran screaming into the living room, where Jan and I lazily lounged in front of the fire, sipping hot amaretto; it was his fifth time out of bed. This time he swore he could hear the heartbeat of the creature just outside his window. Cradling him in her lap, Jan stroked his head until he fell asleep.

We both sat mesmerized by the flames as the soft strains of a Bach concerto wafted from the stereo. I'd avoided talking shop, mainly because I was afraid of hearing about Turk. Jan must have sensed it because when I couldn't stand the suspense anymore and finally brought him up, she tried to steer me off the subject.

"Why is it," she said, still staring into the fire, "when two or more nurses get together, the subjects they inevitably end up talking about are shop, shop politics, shop gossip, love, and sex?"

I opened my mouth in mock surprise. "You mean there's something else?"

"Are you sure you want to hear about Turk, Echo? You'll be assigned to him when you get back to work. Why don't you wait till then?"

"Just give me the basics so I can rest easier," I said.

Jan sighed and gave in. "First of all, everyone is up in arms because the older son still refuses to budge on the full-code status. He wants everything done to save his father, even though Joe essentially told him Turk's prognosis was not great. It didn't seem to make a whole lot of difference what Joe said or how much Turk was going to suffer; the guy feels he *has* to keep his dad alive no matter what the cost. The other son, John, doesn't say much; he just walks around, trying to keep the peace. I don't think he ever goes against his brother." She took a sip of her drink before she resumed the story.

"That night, after you left, the sons and everybody showed up, and Turk agreed to let them put in the lines. That went okay, except when Joe pressed the old man for a definite answer on what he did and did not want done, Louis took over and wouldn't let Turk say anything. It was eventually decided to leave everything at a full code status until Louis and Turk could decide on something mutually acceptable, and of course, you can guess what immediately happened.''

I put my head in my hands and felt my stomach go to jelly. ''No, I want to hear it.''

Jan paused briefly, then continued. ''The lines were in by one A.M. By six he was having continuous chest and back pain and his BP was up to two-ten over one-ten. We started him on a nitroprusside drip and lots of Lasix to get his pressure down; but we overshot the mark, and when the stuff hit him, he dropped his pressure to seventy over forty. He started looking dusky and acting confused, so off went the nitroprusside, then we poured in the IV fluids to bring his pressure back up, tipped him on his head, and started a dopamine drip.'' Jan delicately eased herself and Simon back from the warmth of the fire.

''The end of the story is he dropped his blood pressure out anyway and went into ventricular tachycardia. Basically, we ran a full code on him.''

I passed my hand over my eyes and peeked out through my fingers. ''Oh, my God, don't tell me they intubated and shocked him.''

Jan nodded her head. ''Yep; defibrillation, CPR . . . the whole works. The really horrible part about it was he was alert during most of it.

''Dr. Van Buren was called in as a consult because Turk aspirated some emesis before we intubated, and so, on top of everything else, he now has an aspiration pneumonia.''

I listened to the crackling of the fire, then looked at Jan. ''Why is it so hard for us just to let people die when they're supposed to?''

''Oh, you know,'' she answered, looking tenderly at Simon. ''For the docs it's sometimes the whole idea of being defeated or fear of lawsuits. For the family or loved ones it's the guilt or fear of having to face the loss.''

Jan smiled and laughed. ''After what I've seen, it makes me want to go out and have 'No Code' tattooed on my chest so there won't be any mistake . . . not that anybody in a normal hospital would ever let that stop them. I've made my mother and father practically sign a contract saying they won't try to keep me alive.''

Jan spoke casually about her death, and although I was able to support her and listen to the occasional frustrations that cropped up around the subject, I did not want to face the fact that someday Jan, as she phrased it herself, "would no longer be available by phone."

After I'd known Jan about a year, we were lying in the sun one day, watching the bay from atop one of the old bunkers built into the hills along the San Francisco coast. The day was hot, and the long hike up the side of the hill had put us both into a state of dreamy exhaustion.

I remember she'd been cheerfully talking about the cremation versus burial question when I closed my eyes and suddenly felt myself being pulled into a vortex of black nothingness. Jan's voice, the sun on my face, the smell of the grasses—all faded and disappeared. For a second I had a powerful presentiment that one of the states of death would be similar to being under anesthesia, a total nonawareness. I tried to imagine being in that state forever and felt a chilling mixture of fear and depression.

Along with the unpleasant feelings, a memory of the nuns' telling us how long the eternity of death lasted popped up out of one of the forgotten places in my mind. I could see them parading in front of the class, saying, "Imagine a steel ball as large as the sun"—here they paused and held their arms outstretched, revealing the endless folds of their mysterious black habits—"and once every one million years a small sparrow lightly brushed his wing against the ball. For as long as it takes that ball to be worn away to a piece of metal the size of a pin is how long your spirit will remain in heaven with God, or"—here they paused again to give the notorious sinners a long, menacing look—"remain enduring the tortures of hell."

Later, hiking down the mountain, I'd told Jan about my experience and asked her if the thought of death ever made her afraid.

"No," she said matter-of-factly, "and the only reason you fear it so is that you don't think about your own death very often. Your first reaction to the pseudoexperience is to feel the loss of the sensual things and the mental-emotional attachments.

"When you're forced to face your own death every day, you realize soon enough that death is simply the natural end result of having lived. The very nature of the cycle teaches that the important things are beyond the attachments you form while you're alive. As soon as you realize there's a higher purpose to living and dying, you let go easier." Jan softly played with one of Simon's curls. "I've lived with death for a long time; we've made peace. The only thing I do fear is what the process of my death will be. I just pray it's clean and quick—in my sleep, no hospitals, no IVs, no nothing."

I nodded and indulged in some self-induced misery, imagining how much I would miss her. Sensing what I was feeling, Jan put her spindly hand on my back and rubbed. "Don't go off feeling depressed about something that hasn't happened yet. Think about everything you have right now, and be happy." Jan sighed. "I wish you knew how much I appreciate you just being you."

"I do," I said. "We're all cut from the same piece of cloth. Hell, sometimes I even think I know what goes on inside you when you get all introspective and secretive on me."

In his sleep Simon's eyelids twitched, and he smiled, then frowned.

I leaned back against the rocking chair. "God, Jan, I feel so bad for Turk."

"Yeah," she said, "he doesn't deserve to die like this."

Turk's eyes were wild with rage and indignation. I had betrayed him; we all had.

When he saw me, he tried to talk, choked on the endotracheal tube, and went into a spasm of coughing, his face turning red and ugly. Dark purple and yellow bruises covered his arms, and his wrists were scraped raw from his struggles to free himself from the restraints securely tied to the side rails.

Every orifice held a tube: There was the endotracheal tube in his mouth, along with a bite block forcing his jaws apart; a tube down his nose that went into his stomach; the pulmonary line threaded into the external jugular vein; two IVs in his left arm and one in his right; an arterial pressure line in his groin; a urinary drainage catheter running through the urethra and into his bladder; and yet another larger catheter had been pushed into his rectum to aid the draining of liquid stool. It was everything he did not want.

The noise of the respirator alarm and the raspy sound of mucus rattling in the endotracheal tube mocked him as he opened his mouth and made a silent scream. He shut his eyes tightly, and tears ran down the channels of his wrinkles.

The sight made me sick with anger and sorrow. During report, the day shift had repeated the story Jan told in front of my fireplace, adding only that Turk was refusing to respond to his sons or the staff.

I opened the chart to the doctors' orders and checked through to make sure they'd all been marked off. I noted Dr. Purdy had come in at 8:00 A.M. and written several orders for minor things; at 8:20 Dr. Van Buren wrote four orders which canceled all of Purdy's; and at 9:15 Dr. Cramer's five orders canceled out two of Van Buren's and reinstated one of Purdy's.

What a circus, I thought, although this was a mild version of the usual ludicrous state of affairs whenever three or more doctors were called in on a case. The right hand seldom knew what the left was doing, plus with all the political undertones and prima donna personalities, it was often impossible to give the family a straight story. I recalled with a shudder the patients who'd been unfortunate enough to require six or more doctors. The only way to prepare for that experience, I decided, was to see a lot of Fellini films.

I turned to the progress notes next and struggled to decipher the four different handwritings. On the first page was Dr. Van Buren's notes:

9/2, 0800 hrs.—Pt. holding. Alert. ABGs fair, considering recent events. Scattered rales and rhonchi all fields. Chest x-ray showing diffuse atelectasis in both bases with effusions. Dr. Bell to consult for possible surgical repair of aortic aneurysm.
S. Van Buren, M.D.

I looked up at the ceiling. "Oh, my God!" I said aloud. This was a joke. They were actually thinking of doing surgery on an eighty-four-year-old man who had not wanted to be resuscitated in the first place. I went on to the next note:

9/2 0930—Patient still on nitroprusside, lidocaine, procainamide. Alert and obviously not pleased with situ-

ation. Vital signs labile. Hemoglobin and hematocrit
low. Still breaking through with PVCs, some couplets.
At son's insistence, have agreed to call in Dr. Bell for
surgical consult. Both sons apprised of gravity of situation. Eldest son continues to request patient remain in
full-code status.

Joseph Cramer

9/2 01015—At Dr. J. Cramer's request, I have seen this
84-year-old man whose x-ray shows a leaking aortic
aneurysm. In light of the age and unstable condition of
the patient, surgery is not a realistic possibility at this
time. Thank you for asking me to see this gentleman.

R. G. Bell

The last note was from Dr. Purdy. In blue fountain pen
he'd written in a shaky scrawl:

9/2 1300 hrs.—Pt. much deteriorated. A sad case.

David Purdy

Disgusted, I slammed the chart shut, picked up a pad and
pencil, and went in to Turk. When he saw me, he pulled at
his restraints and tapped the side rail angrily with his ring. I
fought with him briefly to hold his hand.

"Turk, will you please listen to me?" I said, a few inches
away from his face. "I know how angry you are, and I am
sorry. I told them you didn't want this. Dr. Cramer tried, too.
It's hard for them; it's hard on everybody." Turk pulled at
his restraints and started to tear.

"I brought you a pad of paper and a pencil. I want you to
write to me, but I'm counting on you not to touch your
tubes."

Turk nodded toward the pad and nodded excitedly. I untied
his hands, holding on to the ties; my experience with Scotch
Moore still lingered vividly in my memory.

Writing slowly, one wobbly letter at a time, Turk took several minutes to complete his message. The results closely
resembled Simon's first efforts at printing: "Please. Stop
this."

I read the note with a sense of helplessness. "I'll talk to

Dr. Cramer again, Turk. Do you understand that's all I can do? I wish you didn't have all this crap to deal with either."

In response Turk grabbed the pad again and wrote so hard the point of the pencil cracked and broke. Not pausing for a second, he blindly pressed the wooden point into the paper. In his rage he was laboriously breathing faster than the respirator, setting off the alarms continuously.

He handed me the pad. "Not right . . . want to die without all this. Torture."

I cleared a place among the wires and tubes and sat down next to him. "Turk, Louis and John don't want to let you go. You must be able to understand that."

Turk made writing motions, and I handed him back the pad and my pen.

"It is *my* death . . . not theirs! Stupid system."

Reading the message upside down, I laughed bitterly and took the pad back again. "You have no argument from me about that, Turk," I said, getting up.

Weak from the exertion of writing, Turk closed his eyes and lay back on the pillow. Feeling the need to stay close by him, I suctioned him, did a physical assessment, calibrated all the machines, printed out strips, took down numbers, and emptied containers of body waste.

At five-thirty Joe came in and sat down behind the monitor screens. "Well, Miss Heron, it's nice to see you could manage to be here with us today—" Joe stopped and took in my expression; Jan called it my "premenopausal intimidation" look.

"What's wrong? What did I do?" he asked, not very seriously.

"I'm upset and angry, I guess."

Joe pointed to himself. "With me?"

"With all of you, and don't pretend you don't know why all the nurses are angry. How could you let this happen to the old guy, Joe?"

Before Joe had a chance to speak, I pulled out the pad with Turk's messages and shoved it over to him. "Here, look at this; he wrote that."

Joe glanced at the pad without picking it up. "Look, Echo, I tried. I met with the family and had a big powwow this morning, but the older son is adamant. He feels very strongly that—"

I threw up my hands. "For Christ's sake, Joe! Who's in charge here? Don't Turk's wishes mean anything? I mean, it's his life—"

Joe raised his eyebrows at the phrasing.

"Okay, okay, so it's his death, but everybody is just ignoring him like he's not there. And then here's this jerko, stubborn son of his who says, 'No, Pop, you gotta stay around and go through all this crap because I can't handle the discomfort of grieving.' It makes me wonder if the guy has some subconscious grudge against his father or some incredible guilt or something."

Joe waited patiently until I'd quieted and put my hands in my lap. "Are you done?" he asked.

I nodded.

"Turk is eighty-four and in what is legally known as a 'compromised' position. He's intubated and frequently sedated. The family could argue he isn't mentally competent to make his own decisions. If I signed off the case now, the son would just go out and hire someone else who'd continue what we're doing and probably be even more aggressive.

"Listen, I regret this, but I look at it differently from you, which is why I don't get all worked up. Sure, I wasn't crazy about inserting those lines either, but since I didn't really have a choice, I ignored looking at the moral issues. I saw it more as an opportunity to keep in practice for the fifty-year-olds who come in and *do* have a chance for living twenty more years."

Joe picked up the chart and continued. "Listen, just to relieve myself of a little guilt here, Dr. Morrison thinks we should go to the limit."

Dr. Morrison, one of Joe's partners, was one of those physicians who liked the finer things in life. He more often than not thought of his bill first, the patient second.

"What's his problem?" I asked. "A little repressed sadism coming to the surface, or does he have a balloon payment due on that mansion he lives in?"

Joe shrugged and began leafing through the lab slips. "In the words of the infamous Shadow, 'Who knows what evil lurks in the minds of men?' "

My stomach lurched. "God, that just makes me want to puke."

"Oh, come on, Echo, keeping this guy alive a few extra days isn't that bad, is it?"

"Yes, Joe, it really *is* that bad. You don't sit here watching him and worrying about what's going to happen next. You don't watch him suffer."

Joe took my hands, which again were flying about, emphasizing my frustration, and gently kept them captive under his own on the counter between us. "I just want you to see that things could be worse for the old guy. I'm actually going easy on him."

He let go of my hands finally and went back to looking through the chart. Presently he stood to go.

"Do you need any more orders from me? Are you all set?"

I nodded.

"I'm off call to Dr. Morrison, so if anything happens, call him. If I can remember my address, I'll be at home. My family has seen me so little this year my wife called the other day to say my daughter found a photo of me and wanted to know who it was."

I managed to crack a smile.

"What was really funny was my wife said she had to think a minute before she could give her an answer."

He looked through the glass at Turk. "If I can sneak into the den, I'll give you a call later to see how he's doing."

After dinner, I recalibrated Turk's machines and suctioned out his tube and the back of his throat. As I adjusted numbers and transducers, I found myself paying more attention to the machines and numbers than to Turk, a common, legitimate complaint of the acute patients and their families.

I turned to Turk and touched him to let him know I hadn't forgotten he was near. "I'm sorry if it seems like I'm ignoring you. It's this space age medicine, Turk; sometimes we spend more time taking care of the machines than we do the person they're attached to."

Turk kept his eyes closed, and at once I noticed he was dusky and sweating, his face set in pain.

"Turk? What's wrong? Are you having chest pain?"

In response, Turk grimaced.

His systolic blood pressure had shot up into the 200 range from 140 in less than a few seconds, and his heart rate was up to 120. Thinking the machines had erred, I took the pulse and the blood pressure manually and found the numbers to be the same.

In the space of a minute I gave him four milligrams of morphine, turned up the nitroprusside, and dialed in a higher level of oxygen concentration on the ventilator control board. On the monitor a run of three PVCs caught my eye; quickly I gave him another dose of lidocaine and ran to the phone to dial cardiology's number.

On the twelfth ring the exchange answered.

"This is Redwoods CCU and I need to speak to Dr. Cramer right away regarding his patient Alonso Turk."

"Is this an extreme emergency?" the woman asked in her nasal voice. Why, I wondered, did all doctors' exchange operators sound like Lily Tomlin doing her switchboard operator routine?

"Yes, it is an emergency. I need to talk to Dr. Cramer right away!"

"I'm sorry, but Dr. Morrison is on call, and he's in transit to San Francisco at the moment."

"What the hell is he doing over in the city when he's on call?"

"I'm sure I don't know, ma'am. I think maybe he had an emergency. Can the problem wait just another ten minutes or so, ma'am?"

I covered my eyes, trying hard to be civil. "No. No, it can't wait. What's the matter with his beeper? Can't you page him?"

"Yes, ma'am, I've already paged him for someone else a few moments before you called, but he hasn't answered. I'm sure he's on the freeway or halfway over the Golden Gate. He'll get to a phone as soon as he can."

"Okay, thank you and keep trying him. It's a stat call."

"Yes, ma'am. Will do."

I hung up and for a second thought of calling Dr. Purdy, but let the idea slide away, remembering the first time I'd called him on an emergency situation; not only did I have to repeat everything three times (Dr. Purdy was hard-of-hearing and on the edge of being senile), but he could not get the patient straight. He kept asking me if the woman moved her bowels regularly. I explained the problem had nothing to do with her bowels, and Purdy gave an order for a stat tap water and soapsuds enema.

I called Dr. Van Buren's exchange and had to put vocal stress on the word *emergency* a few times before the operator would put me through. I held for a full minute before Dr. Van Buren came on the line.

"Yes?" he answered, sounding irritated.

The man's rudeness didn't faze me; it fitted so well with the rest of his personality. Dark and handsome, with a body nearly as well developed as Arnold Schwarzenegger's, the brawny Dr. Van Buren had an ego that could have blacked out the sun. In my two years at Redwoods Memorial I'd heard enough bits and pieces of gossip to know by heart the intimate details of his private life; many of the incidents, I was sure, came right from the TV soaps.

So many of the nurses had been seduced and jilted by the iron-pumping physician, it was not unusual to hear them comparing notes on his slam-bam-thank-you-ma'am lovemaking and his methods of "easing out" of these affairs once the conquest had been made. One always had a pretty good idea where his latest "dumped" victim worked; there were certain wards he avoided like the plague.

Like all good rumors, news of his numerous amorous adventures made the rounds of the hospital staff from housekeeping to pathology like wildfire. When they finally reached administration's ears, several of the nurses involved were privately reprimanded by their head nurses while Dr. Van Buren was invited to become a member of the Professional Ethics Committee.

"Hi, Dr. Van Buren, this is Miss Heron in CCU. I'm taking care of Mr. Turk tonight, and he's going down the tubes. In fact, I think he's getting ready to code on us anytime now. His BP is up around two hundred, with a heart rate of one-twenty, plus a run of PVCs, but the main thing is, he's just got that code look."

After I'd run through the rest of the information, there was a long pause and then a sound as if the phone were being picked up from a table.

"Ahhh, let's see now, what's the patient's name again?" he asked. It was obvious he was trying not to laugh.

"Turk, Alonso Turk, the eighty-four-year-old in ACCU. You saw him this morning," I said dryly.

"Oh, yeah, Mr. Berk, nice old guy with the creepy son. What's the problem again?"

I heard the rustling of fabric (sheets?) and a muffled giggle; I wondered if it was anyone I knew. Holding down my anger, I repeated my spiel. When I finished, Dr. Van Buren sighed. "You know, this sounds like you should be calling Dr. Cramer, not me. It's obviously a problem for the cardiologists, not me."

"I'm aware of that, Dr. Van Buren, but Dr. Cramer's off call to Dr. Morrison, who is in transit to the city and unavailable for another ten minutes. The guy is going to code, and I don't want to be caught without a doc who knows him."

"Hold on a minute," said Van Buren. I could hear the muffling of the mouthpiece (a pillow?), the distant cooing of a female voice, and finally outright laughter.

Van Buren came back on the line. His holier-than-thou attitude could be cut with a knife.

"Okay, get stat blood gases, an H and H, a CBC, and a chest x-ray, and call me back with the results. Have the radiologist call me at home."

"Are we treating the number values or the patient, Dr. Van Buren?" I said, feeling huffy. "I am telling you for certain this man is going to try to go out on us very soon."

"Look, Miss Heron, if Morrison doesn't get back to you in ten minutes, call me again and I'll come in. If he goes out before that, you've got your standing orders and the ER doc's right downstairs."

I was silent.

"Hey! I don't know what else you want me to do here," Dr. Van Buren continued, in defense of himself. "The guy's eighty-four years old!"

There was another short pause until Dr. Van Buren spoke again, but in a lower, softer voice: "Ah, by the way, Miss Heron, are you the tall, pretty redhead that works up there every Tuesday?"

"No," I said. "No, I'm not . . . thank God!"

"What? What did you say?"

"Nothing. Good night, Dr. Van Buren." I hung up and went in to check on Turk. He was clammy and pale. I turned on the overhead light and studied his nose.

We all had our "special" weird warning signs of impending disaster. Annie, for instance, once told me hers was when the patient felt weak and then had a sudden, strong urge to move his bowels. Jan's telltale sign was a patient's complaining of feeling cold and sleepy with an accompanying "funny ache" right in the middle of the back. For me, it was a certain look of a patient's nose—when it started looking like gray putty.

Turk's nose was a blob of gray putty.

Alarmed, I ran to order the lab work and the x-ray, then darted to the intermediate side, where Jan was watching monitors and taking admitting orders off a new patient's chart.

The minute she saw my face, she stood up. "What is it?"

"Turk's going down the tubes, and I can't seem to get anybody to give a crap. I want to call Cramer at home."

"Where's Morrison? He's supposed to be on call."

"Morrison is halfway over the Golden Gate on his way to the city, if you can believe that!"

Jan put her hand on the side of her face the way an old woman might have done when she discovered the cat ate the canary. "What's he doing going into the city on an on-call night?" she asked.

"Jan, I don't know, and personally I don't care right now. I just want to call Cramer at home. Where's the number?"

"Ec, you know Annie's not going to like that."

"I don't care. Annie's been head nurse for a long time; my guess is she's probably done it once or twice herself. Listen, by the time the exchange reaches Morrison, it'll take him another half hour to get back here, and by that time this guy won't be alive. I'm willing to stick my neck out. I want Cramer in here; he likes the old guy, and I don't think he'd mind."

"The numbers are in Annie's desk in the right-hand drawer, and you won't remember how you got it, right?"

"I have Alzheimer's on and off. What was your name again?"

The phone rang twice when a timid little voice answered.

"This is the Cramer residence, Melissa speaking. How may I help you?" I could hear someone chuckle and applaud softly in the background.

I bit my lip. "Is your father at home, Melissa?"

"Yes, he is. And whom may I ask is calling?"

I swallowed hard. "Tell him it's Echo."

I heard the squeaky, mashed, and muffled phone sounds of small hands inadequately covering the mouthpiece.

"It's for you, Daddy . . . it's Ethel," she announced proudly.

I smiled.

Joe's voice came over the line, and I felt I'd touched land after swimming in a rough sea for hours. "Hello?"

"Oh, thank God, Joe. Please don't be angry with me for calling you at home, but the old man is going down the tubes real fast, and everybody is unavailable or unwilling to do anything concrete. I need somebody who knows him to get in here stat!"

"Goddammit! Where the hell is Morrison?"

Joe's reaction made me break out in a sweat. I'd never heard him swear before.

"Ah, believe it or not, your partner is supposedly on his way to San Francisco on some emergency and probably won't be able to get back here until it's too late. Dr. Purdy doesn't know what he's doing, and Dr. Van Buren wanted me to wait for Morrison or call the ER doc."

Joe sighed and was silent. In the background I could hear Mrs. Cramer and Melissa debating whether Winnie-the-Pooh was a girl or a boy bear.

"So, what's the problem?" Joe asked finally.

"Intuitively I can tell you he's going to code within thirty minutes; clinically, his BP is up in the sky, along with the rest of his pulmonary pressures, his color is poor, he's tachy, he's diaphoretic and clammy, his pain is severe and unrelieved by MS, he stopped putting out urine two hours ago, and—"

Joe interrupted. "You are trying to tell me he's sick."

"Please, Joe."

"All right. Give me the son's number. I'll call him to see if he might back off a little. Maybe we can make this old fella at least a modified code. I'll be there in ten—"

In the background I heard Mrs. Cramer's verbalized disappointment accentuated by the stamping of a foot. "OOOhhhh, nooooo, Joe! Where's Morrison?" Joe covered the mouthpiece, and from the mumbles I gathered being married to a doctor, especially a good one, had its drawbacks.

Joe came back on the line. "Ah, sorry about that. There's some dissension among the troops here."

"Tell Mrs. Cramer I'm really sorry, Joe. Tell her you'll take her to Bermuda next week or something nice. See you in ten."

Five minutes later Jan handed me the blood gas results: Turk's oxygen level was low. "Radiology called a second ago; his chest is a diffuse whiteout; he's blowing his aneurysm," she said. I turned to her to ask what I should do when she shot over me and hit the printout button.

"He's blocking down!" she screamed. Over my shoulder I saw the rhythm had dropped to a rate of 40. On instinct we both rushed into the room, dragging the crash cart with us.

Turk's blood pressure had dropped along with his rate and now hovered at 70 systolic. When I tipped the head of the bed down in Trendelenburg position, Turk wearily opened his eyes. From the vacant stare, I knew he no longer recognized me or anything else; he was stepping over the threshold into another world.

Jan was injecting atropine, a drug used to speed up the heart, into his IV. I turned off the nitroprusside and, moving on a pure adrenaline rush, prepared and hung a dopamine drip, hoping it might bring up his pressures.

I wiped the old man's mouth with a wet washcloth, untied his hands, and pulled his body over onto its side while I slipped an oval "back board" under him in case CPR had to be performed.

Taking advantage of the short lull, Jan slipped away to find someone to cover the intermediate monitors. Through the glass walls of the room, I saw the door open and Joe's tall, slim outline hurry in.

Entering the room, he looked at Turk and then at me. "You didn't lie."

I shook my head and lifted my eyebrows in silent question.

Joe looked away. "No. He wouldn't go for a code change," he said softly.

"Figures," I said, deeply disappointed, although I already knew Louis would have to play his stubbornness to the end.

Joe brought his face close to Turk's. "Turk? Turk, can you hear me?"

Turk was barely rousable but managed to turn his head a little toward the direction of Joe's voice.

"I just spoke to Louis; they're on their way."

Turk lifted his hands briefly to claw at the air; then he stiffened, and his eyes rolled back into his head. I looked at the monitor; the huge PVCs all close together, like a picket fence, went across the screen. It was a heart gone astray, dancing with undirected, pulsating energy.

I shook the old man and called to him; there was no response. Dropping him back onto the mattress, I yelled for Jan, who showed up instantly, out of breath and looking pale herself.

Lifting my fist, I slammed it into the middle of Turk's chest. I hoped it would stimulate the electrical system of his heart enough to get back on the right circuit; all it did was knock the wind out of him.

Jan started ripping open drawers in the crash cart while Joe prepped the defibrillator paddles by covering them with blue gelatin, which would act as a conductive medium. On his command we all jumped back from the bed, making sure no part of us was in contact with Turk's body. Joe bent over from the waist, placed the paddles on Turk's chest, and jolted him with four hundred-watt seconds of electricity. It was one of those certain sounds that stayed with me, never to be lost from recall. Among them were the calls of katydids on a hot summer day, the silence of fresh-fallen snow, voices I hated or loved, and the sound of the defibrillation of a human body: the hollow click, followed by a noise like a trap door falling open and then hundreds of synchronized fists hitting raw meat.

Turk's body lifted a couple of inches off the bed; his arms flew up crazily a foot or so, like a rag doll being shaken by a child.

Jan and Joe looked at the monitor, waiting to see the results of the shock. I glanced quickly at Turk's face. His mouth formed an exaggerated O, and his eyes were open in shocked horror, as if he'd seen the atrocities of hell. I closed out the vision and saw the gentle old man singing "Little Sir Echo."

The rhythm came back to the screen as a wide complex at a rate of 37. I pushed my fingers into Turk's groin. "No pulses."

"Start CPR," Joe said calmly.

Climbing onto the bed, I knelt next to Turk and started chest compressions, trying to produce enough pressure to circulate the blood, but not to break ribs. With an eerie slow motion, Turk wrapped his hands around my wrists and, with an amazing amount of strength, pushed me off his chest.

I looked down at his eyes. His eyelids fluttered, like two tiny wings, and briefly opened to reveal a soul completed.

Following my internal voice, I stopped doing CPR. "I'm sorry, Turk," I said, and glanced over at Joe. "I can't do this to him. This isn't right."

Joe turned to Jan. "Miss Tobin, take over CPR for Miss Heron, please."

Jan gently pulled me off the bed and restarted CPR. I looked at Joe watching the numbers on the monitor falling, despite Jan's efforts.

"I'll bet he's tamponaded," mumbled Joe. "Okay, stop CPR and let's check his pulses." Jan and I each tried to find a pulse; there was none.

Quickly Joe took the four-inch cardiac needle from the cart and inserted it very slowly just below the xyphoid until very little of the needle was showing. Aspirating gently, slowly, the syringe filled with fifty cc's of the dark blood that had filled the sac around the heart and kept it from being able to work.

Immediately I felt pulses. Turk's pressure numbers were changing rapidly from 38 to 46 to 62. I beamed at Joe, who kept a straight face.

He leaned over Turk again and yelled into his ear, "Hey, Turk! Can you hear me?"

Turk barely turned his head toward Joe's voice.

Forty seconds passed, and we all watched the numbers now plummeting in the opposite direction, 60, 43. . . . The crazy ventricular tachycardia had started again.

Joe grabbed for the paddles and squeezed out more gelatin. "Start CPR again!"

Jan climbed back up on the bed and began pumping.

I could see Joe hesitating before he shocked Turk again. "Give him five of MS push," he said quietly.

Both Jan and I glanced at Joe. "I don't think we should continue all this without giving him something," he explained.

I inserted the needle into the rubber stopper and pushed in the drug, instinctively knowing the MS would end his struggle forever. As I watched the drug swirling toward Turk's arm, my mind fled back to a beautiful mulatto boy named Richard Wilson.

I remembered how it felt when death was still new to me. Then I had not known about its two faces. I saw death only as the ultimate thief; I'd been too insecure to know him as the kind rescuer. Miss Telmack had been right: Freeing people of the pain from which there was no other release but death was another part of nursing.

Turk's BP plunged from 30 to 20.

"That's it," said Joe. "His pericardium is filling up again, and I think this man needs a rest. We've kept him up too long already."

Turk's body relaxed, and I pressed the alarm silencer on the monitor. Holding his hand, I thought of how somewhere it had been predetermined that I would be with this man when he died. Knowing how much Turk hated the endotracheal tube, I released the pressure valve on the internal cuff. Immediately from deep within Turk's throat came a strangled last cry, the strange gasping sound I'd come to recognize as life and death changing places.

From 20 his BP went to 0, and the slow, wide heartbeat stopped. Joe turned off the monitor.

When Joe opened the door to the waiting room, I could see Louis holding his hat with both hands, staring angrily out the window. John sat reading a black book I thought might have been a Bible.

Later Louis, who seemed amazingly stoic, came in alone and stood poised in his usual spot at the end of his father's bed for a long time, expectant, waiting . . . for what I didn't know. At length he walked to the side of the bed and slipped the gold eagle ring off Turk's finger and put it on his own. The rest of Turk's personal effects, which included a pair of urine-stained pants, a ripped T-shirt with the collar ribbing missing, a red wool plaid hunting jacket, an old pair of brown shoe boots, a pair of scratched bifocals, and several bouquets of flowers, he told us to throw away. He said nothing about John, and I didn't ask.

Surveying the room, I ignored the mess and walked to the bouquet of bachelor buttons and white mums which had arrived anonymously earlier in the day. I'd jokingly made the comment to Turk that they must have come from Ned, and he'd cried.

Taking one of the vibrant blue blooms, I pinned it in my hair.

"Okay, Turk," I said. "I'm going to clean you up and send you back to the earth." I bent over to pick up a bloodstained sheet off the floor, and from the corner of my eye I thought I saw Turk's chest move. I froze and stared at his chest, then relaxed. It was only an optical illusion, a figment of what I desired.

The process of removing all the tubes and wires from Turk's body gave me a great feeling of satisfaction, as if I were purifying him. I opened the morgue pack and took out the first of the three items in the bag, the tan toe tag. I wrote his name and hospital number on it and tied it securely to his left toe. The second item was a soft, absorbent pad. I rolled Turk's body to one side and placed it under his buttocks to catch any "leaks." The third article out was a thin piece of gauze about a yard long. Policy required me to bind the man's hands together tightly so they did not flop around during transport to the morgue and the mortician's.

Loosely I wrapped the gauze around one of Turk's wrists and left it at that. "There you go, Turk. Now when you find Ned, you'll be spiffy as an old polished shoe. Make sure you—"

"Echo?"

I whipped around and saw Milly, the house nursing supervisor, standing inside the doorway, staring at Turk.

"God, you scared me, Milly!" I said, irritated and embarrassed I'd been caught talking to a corpse.

"I need to speak with you if you have time," she said coldly.

"Right now, Milly? Does it really have to be right now? I'm not feeling very receptive tonight. We just lost this man and I—"

Milly didn't budge. That didn't surprise me. She was an older, rather regimented nurse whose life seemed fueled by rules, policies, and regulations.

"I think you need to hear this now, Echo." Without waiting for a reply she continued. "I've been informed that you are leaving the hospital on your dinner breaks dressed in sweat

clothes. I've also noticed"—her voice went up an octave—
"that you do not wear regulation nursing shoes.

"Both these actions are against policy. Would you care to
tell me anything about these matters before they're officially
entered in your personnel file?"

Without responding, I pulled a clean sheet out of the drawer
and covered Turk's body to protect him from Milly's stare.
She caught the edge of the drape midair and threw it back to
Turk's waist. Taking hold of the gauze tie on his wrist, she
jerked it. "You forgot to tie the hands."

I pulled the tie out of Milly's hand and laid Turk's arm
back on the bed. "I didn't forget. I hate tying people up like
that; it's barbaric."

Milly roughly pulled Turk's hand up again and without saying anything tied his hands together so tightly she broke some
of the paperlike skin around his wrists. Blood oozed over the
white gauze.

"The morticians don't like them untied," she said. Her
jowls jiggled with the force of her movements. "They say it
bruises their arms; it's all in the policy book. If you ever took
the time to read it, you'd know that."

"If all the nurses acted according to the policy book, we'd
never get anywhere. We'd be like little mice, afraid to open
our mouths or move." I stopped to look at Turk.

"And anyway, Milly," I said, trying to make my tone a
little less caustic, "since when have you seen a male corpse
laid out sleeveless?"

Milly ignored my comments and maintained her stone face.
"Do you have anything you want to say about the shoes or
the dinner break incidents?"

"You really won't give me a break, will you?" I shook my
head and faced her. "Okay. I have a comment about my
shoes: They're comfortable. I don't go home with backaches
anymore."

"Well, I'm sorry, but you can't wear them. All nurses must
wear regulation white nursing shoes." Milly's eyes roved to
the blue bachelor button in my hair, and she moved to pull it
out. I grabbed her arm and pulled back.

"It's also against dress code to wear hair ornaments."

"Come on, Milly, let's go for one broken rule at a time,
okay? The shoes are orthopedically correct for me. What's
more important? My back or dress code policy?"

Milly was getting angry; she sighed and shifted her feet. "The patients and visitors expect nurses to look like nurses, and nurses wear white shoes."

"Reasoning like that is exactly why I would never go into administrative nursing. You're so blind that you honestly think you can sit behind a desk and make up rules and policies about how nurses should conduct themselves.

"Here in front of you is a dead man who we tried very hard to save. I was his nurse, and I did my job the best way I knew how. I got to know him; he was a good man, and now he's dead. I wish you could ask him whether he gave a damn if I wore white shoes or purple shoes or green hair. I'm sure he would have had a great answer for you.

I stopped, and Milly dropped her eyes. "So are you saying you won't . . ."

"I'm saying I will continue to wear my running shoes to work, Milly, yes. You may write that down if you wish."

"And you are aware you will be disciplined for breaking dress code?"

"If I had to wear a dark brown lift shoe because one of my legs was five inches shorter than the other, would that be acceptable?"

"Yes," Milly answered a little uncertainly. "Just as long as it didn't interfere with your work."

"Good point! These shoes actually help me work more efficiently and longer, so why aren't they acceptable?"

"A lift shoe is ordered by the doctor."

"Okay, I'll get a doctor's order. Will that satisfy the policy book?"

Milly hesitated. "I don't know, but I don't think you can do that." She started checking her pockets as if the answer would be in one of them.

I interrupted her. "And I want to confirm the fact I do leave the hospital on my dinner break."

The admission surprised her. "Where do you go?"

"Even though it's none of your business what I do on my own free time, I'll tell you so rumors don't start flying that I'm meeting Dr. Van Buren in the parking lot—"

The corner of Milly's upper lip twitched; this was her look of shock.

"I started running a few months ago to keep in shape, and sometimes I can't run before I come to work, so I run a couple of miles on my dinner break, wash up, and change back into my uniform."

"In thirty minutes you do all this?" she asked.

"No," I said, "it usually takes me twenty-five."

Milly turned away. "You're going to have to stop that, too. The hospital can't take responsibility for you if you should be hurt while you're off premises."

"Are you telling me I can't leave hospital grounds on my dinner breaks?"

"It's really not a good idea, Echo. We'd prefer you didn't, especially since you work CCU; you never know when you'll be needed here."

I sighed. "Okay. I won't leave the hospital anymore."

Milly smiled.

"But—"

Milly frowned.

"I'll have to charge the hospital thirty minutes' overtime from now on.

"You can't do that," Milly said indignantly.

"Listen, Milly, when a nurse doesn't get a meal break because she's busy, she generally is allowed to ask for thirty minutes' overtime, right?"

"Well, technically, yes, but most of our nurses donate that time to the hospital, free of charge."

I laughed the most sarcastic laugh I could muster up. "This, my dear supervisor nurse, is one nurse you won't find smiling as she's bled." I covered Turk and pushed the crash cart past Milly. "How much do you figure a patient pays for each day spent in CCU?" I asked.

"Anywhere from six hundred to a thousand dollars a day."

"And how much do I make in a shift, gross?"

"About sixty dollars."

"Who's responsible for the patient every second he's in here?"

"The nurses, but you can't—"

"No, no, wait, Milly. Stop right there. You're right; it's the nurses. Therefore, I am not donating anything to the hospital when it's already got my time, my guts, my soul. All I want is thirty minutes out of eight and a half hours that I can call mine to relax. If I am confined to the hospital, listening for code or stat calls over the loudspeaker, then I'm still on duty."

"Okay," Milly said, "I'll talk this over with Mrs. Miller, but for now, at least punch out for the thirty minutes you aren't here, so if you do get hurt, there's a record of its not being on hospital time."

I turned my attention back to Turk and finished tucking the clean sheet around him. "Fine, Milly, whatever. Just let me finish taking care of my patient."

Two weeks after Turk's death I found a card in my mailbox. On the front was a close-up photograph of two sea gulls flying in the clouds. The caption under it read: "They can because they *think* they can."

When I opened it, I saw the handwriting was even and slanted forward.

Dear Echo Heron, RN,

It has been ten days since my father passed away, and each day still feels like something is missing. I suppose time heals all wounds and sorrows, but it goes so slowly.

Louis has kept to himself, locking up his feelings like always. I think he's falling apart inside, but I suppose we'll never know for sure.

Being so close to Dad, watching him for those two weeks were like watching my own death in a way. It would have been so frightening if it had not been for all of you who tended to him and cared so lovingly for him.

The small item attached to the back of this card is something my father carried with him for as long as I can remember. Because he liked you so much, and because you were there for him when he passed on, I think he would have been pleased to know it is in your keeping.

I hope it brings you much luck, and thank you again for all your kindness.

The card was signed "John Turk."

I turned the card over and pulled off the masking tape.

Stuck to the tape was a thin gold coin, the size of a quarter. On one side was an exact replica of the eagle's head on Turk's ring; on the other was the image of the bird in flight over a mountain.

Running a finger lightly over the smooth surface, I tried to imagine all the times over the years Turk must have rubbed it between his thumb and forefinger out of habit. Just before dropping it into the secret compartment of my purse, I set the coin on the back of my thumb and flicked it high into the air, giving it the illusion of a floating golden bubble. Plucking it out of the air, I slapped it on the back of my hand.

Carefully I lifted my hand away from the coin. The golden eye of an eagle stared right through me.

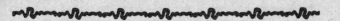

TWELVE

MR. LE FOIE'S FOOT in its pointed black shoe sprang back from my knee like a snake after an attack. The sharp, burning pain shot through my knee and traveled, like an electric shock, down my leg. Staggering to the bed, I got a stranglehold on the wild and dangerous foot and fought down the impulse to twist it off at the man's arthritic ankle.

Standing at the bedside, the rest of the CCU evening crew sucked in their breaths in sympathy with the pained look on my face. Then, as if they'd each taken the assault personally, they joined forces to overpower the confused man and led him back into the safety zone of his bed.

Jan and Linda each grabbed one of the old man's arms, while Catherine and Lucy struggled with his thrashing legs. On a count of three they hoisted him up onto the bed and locked the side rails.

"Help! Help me, someone, please," screamed Mr. Le Foie in a thick French accent. "I must get off this plane. I must find Maurice."

In spite of the situation, Linda giggled while struggling to keep Mr. Le Foie's hands away from her face. Infuriated by her joviality, he tried biting her; but Catherine had had the foresight to remove his dentures, and her arm went unharmed.

Lucy showed up with a Posey jacket and closed the door behind her so the man's screams would not disturb the other patients.

"You filthy hijackers, you. I will report you to the authorities. Maurice will put you in prison forever to rot, you whores, you Amazons, you terrible—''

"Okay Jean-Paul, that's enough," Jan said in her softest voice. "You're in the hospital, and we are the nurses taking care of you. We don't want to fight with you; we want to be your friends. We don't want you to—''

Mr. Le Foie swung at her. She successfully dodged the punch just as Dr. Cramer walked into the room.

"Mr. Le Foie's quite a handful, eh, girls?" Joe smiled.

At the sight of Joe, Mr. Le Foie rolled his eyes and put his hands together, begging. "Please, please, Captain, make these horrible women leave me alone. I must get off this plane, or there will be terrible consequences. Oh, Maurice will be so angry with them."

Joe put a hand on Jean-Paul's shoulder. "It's all right, Jean-Paul. You're not on a plane; you're in the hospital. These lovely girls are your nurses, and *I*''—Joe waggled his eyebrows and smiled mischievously—"am your captain."

"Joe!" I said harshly. "The guy's confused enough; don't make it worse!"

Joe turned around and glanced over his shoulder at me, rubbing my knee, which was now swollen to the size of a grapefruit. "Say, what did you do to this poor man anyway?"

I stopped rubbing and hobbled over to him. "All *I* did to *him* was put my unprotected knee a tad too close to his foot. Next time you send us an admission, it'd be nice if you'd warn us when he's a sundowner, and I'll make sure I wear a padded uniform."

Mr. Le Foie, the spry and kicking seventy-two-year-old Frenchman, had come to us directly from Dr. Cramer's office for overnight monitoring. He was pleasantly charming for most of the afternoon, flirting with us and showing off pictures of his grandchildren. At seven-thirty he awoke from his after-dinner nap and put on his call light.

When I entered the room, he saluted. Laughing, I saluted back and stood at attention. "Lieutenant, please tell Maurice to come in now. The poor man must be freezing out there."

I saluted again and innocently went traipsing off to the waiting room in search of a shivering Maurice, who I automatically assumed was Mr. Le Foie's son. Five minutes later I returned to Mr. Le Foie's room without the mysterious Maurice.

Sitting on the edge of his bed with his trousers on backward, wearing one shoe, and with a dinner roll stuffed into his shirt pocket, Mr. Le Foie waited patiently. He was ready, he informed me stiffly, to disembark from the plane without a fight. Only when he failed to laugh did I realize I had a sundowner on my hands.

Mr. Le Foie was among thousands of elderly people who, during the daylight hours, were pleasant, oriented, and cooperative but, as soon as the sun set, took on any one of a wide range of psychoses. At times they were hostile and combative, thinking they were hostages; sometimes they took on alter egos, and sometimes they were just themselves but had "invisible" company with whom they had lengthy and often lively conversations. Long-deceased spouses, parents, and friends rose from the dead evening after evening for these visits. More than once I'd been sharply reprimanded for stepping on their feet or sitting in their laps.

With the sunrise, ghosts and other disruptive personalities disappeared, and the sundowners returned to their normal states of being, having little or no recollection of the antics of the night before.

Joe scanned my knee and probed the sorest part with his finger. I jumped back in pain. "I think you'd better see a doctor about that knee," he cautioned.

"That's a good idea, Ec," said Jan, fitting Mr. Le Foie into the Posey jacket. "Put some ice on, and I'll have Lucy wheel you down to ER."

"I can't," I whined. "I've got two of my eight o'clock vitals to do and I still have to change two beds and make sure everybody's dentures get brushed."

Joe and Jan exchanged glances, and Jan put a hand on her bony hip. "What are you going to do?" she asked, exasperated. "Hobble around on that knee, making all the patients feel sorry for the poor crippled nurse? Forget it, sister, you're going downstairs. I'll divide up your patients between Cathy and Linda. Now go!"

Lucy wheeled me into ER ten minutes later with an ice pack sitting on my knee and turned me over to a young man wearing a paramedic uniform. He quickly moved the wheelchair out of the way, depositing me on bed five.

"It is just fucking nuts down here," the paramedic said, shaking his closely shaven head. "The nurses called the station to ask if we could help out. I've never seen this place so crazy.''

Without further comment, he took my vital signs, propped my leg up on a pillow, adjusted the ice bag, and hurried into the suture room to tend to the loud and high-pitched protestations of a young child.

The whole place seemed to be in a wild state of total confusion and noise. All the gurneys in both the main and suture rooms were filled. The trauma and pelvic room doors were closed, but from the number of nurses and lab techs hurrying in and out, I assumed they were occupied.

There was a short stack of charts of patients waiting to be triaged on one side of the clerk's desk and a larger stack of patients' charts with blue tags on the other—like in and out orders at a busy hamburger stand.

As far as I could tell, there were two ER docs on duty, both of whom I'd seen only briefly during codes in CCU. One was a tall, pleasant-looking black man, and the other was a small, swarthy man who seemed to be stressed, preoccupied, or both.

Both the evening float nurses were busy. One ran by my bed, recognized me, and said out of the corner of her mouth, "Now I know why I avoid this place." A candy striper was moving faster than almost anyone else, delivering medications, running off to the lab with specimens, and wheeling gurneys to x-ray.

Katy burst out of the trauma room and yelled for help. The black doctor quickly responded, and they both disappeared back into the room. Katy, I noticed, was about seven months pregnant.

The other doctor came over to the Asian woman in bed four. Dressed in a hospital gown but still wearing stockings and shoes, she was holding her stomach, grimacing. In a businesslike manner, he began asking her questions, speaking in a language I didn't recognize. She answered in a subdued tone, occasionally using sign language and pointing to different places on her abdomen. With obvious distaste the doctor touched her belly in the places she'd pointed to in a cursory way and nodded his head after each palpation.

A few minutes passed, and two cops walked in with a young light-skinned black woman who was handcuffed. Her hair was wild, and her clothes were ripped or cut, I couldn't tell which. She was crying and babbling incoherently; blood streamed from a deep laceration down the right side of her face and dripped onto her Windbreaker. From what I could catch of the conversation between the paramedic and the cops, there'd been a knife fight over a man, and the other woman was dead; our patient was under arrest for murder.

Katy came out of the trauma room again, her movements much slower and more relaxed this time, and turned to the man at the clerk's desk. "Tyrone, call the techs and ask them to bring up the M cart. The trauma room needs transfer to the basement."

Noticing the woman in handcuffs, she examined the wound, hastily wrapped a pressure dressing over it, and directed the policemen to keep her in the lobby until a place could be made for her. Turning around, she caught sight of me.

"Oh, my God, look what the cat dragged in," she said, coming over to hug me. I returned the affectionate greeting feeling as if I'd been drawn from the cold chaos of being a patient into the warm circle of recognition.

"God, I haven't seen you for ages." Katy drew the curtain just enough to be hidden from view.

"I know, and I'm sorry," I said, embarrassed. "I should have stopped in to say hello, but I usually arrive with two minutes to spare and waste no time getting out."

"I know what you mean. It's the same with me. Like to-night—I haven't had a chance to think straight." She sank appreciatively onto the gurney and put one of her feet up. It was slightly swollen around the ankle. "Since they closed Brand X's ER for remodeling, we've been insanity city every night; it never lets up. They asked me to work evenings for a few weeks because the shift is so short-staffed. I couldn't turn down the shift differential, plus—" Katy tenderly rubbed her belly—"I get to sleep in with Bruno here."

"When did all this happen?" I asked, giving her balloon-like abdomen a pat.

"Steve and I were married a year ago, and he suddenly got this bug to do everything all at once: buy a house; get a dog; have a baby; then go to the poorhouse. What about you? Any special men? How's that blond doll of yours?"

"Simon's great. He just left two days ago to spend the summer being spoiled by his grandparents in Texas. As far as men go, it's not easy meeting someone when the statistics

tell us there are three single women for every one single man.
Oh, occasionally I meet someone who asks me out, or my
well-meaning friends arrange a blind date, but it never turns
into anything. I mean, no one's swept me off my feet. Besides, I'm too busy spending most of my time here or with
Simon and my friends.''

Katy peeked under the ice bag.

''What happened to your knee?''

''Oh, nothing much. I got nailed by a sundowner with
shoes on.''

''Gotta watch out for those sundowners; if they catch you
off guard, they can make your life miserable.''

Straining to see through the loose weave of the curtain, I
was distracted for a moment by a sudden surge in the mad-
house activity of the room.

''So, who are all these people?'' I asked.

Pulling back the curtain a little, Katy surveyed the room.
''Assuming you mean the staff, the black doc is Dr. Judd—
sweet guy, very sharp. The other man is Dr. Kin. He's okay,
too, but gets a little weirded out with the craziness. They've
been here about a year now.

''Of course, Dr. Mahoney and Dr. Menowitz are still with
us, although I think Dr. Mahoney's starting to burn out a
little. With the exception of a short reprieve, Menowitz's been
burned-out for years, so there isn't much difference there.
Gus quit to take a job over in the East Bay in an even busier
ER, if you can imagine that, but she got tired of the pace and
is coming back next month as an on-call person.'' Katy did
a quick spot check of the room. ''I was surprised how much
I like working with the evening staff; they're mostly young,
independent, and strong-willed, yet so much friendlier than
a lot of the day shift people. They pull together more or
something. It's hard to explain.''

''It's the same upstairs,'' I said. ''We're like this close-knit
family unit of crazy women.''

Over the noise a particularly shrill scream came from the
child in the suture room, reviving my curiosity in the commotion.

''What's wrong with the kid in the suture room?'' I asked,
straining to see what was going on.

''He's commenting on Dr. Judd's sewing techniques.'' Katy

laughed. "His father smashed him across the head with a beer bottle when he walked in front of the TV by accident."

I winced. Katy caught the look and snorted. "Are you kidding? That's mild compared to the rest of the assortment that's been in here so far tonight. We started this afternoon with a gay guy from the Castro district who came in sniveling and babbling on about all this weird stuff. We thought he was just one of the garden variety weirdos until we examined him. It turned out he'd been drugged and then gang-raped by a bunch of his 'friends' last night, and then, for fun, they pinned his penis to his belly with thirty-three safety pins. He was still in surgery last time I checked."

The scene in the main room seemed wild, and I could feel the old crises addiction stir within me and rear its curious head. "What else you got down here?"

Katy thought for a moment, leaned back on her elbows, and put her other foot up on the gurney. "Let's see . . . the lady in the pelvic room is an ectopic pregnancy waiting for her GYN to come in. There's a dead man in the trauma room who arrested at home. The lady on bed two is a severe asthmatic we can't control with breathing treatments or an aminophylline drip; she's getting ready to poop out on us. The twin babies on bed one have croup; bed three is a chest pain, rule out MI, waiting for a bed in your acute unit; bed four is an abdominal pain; and the well-dressed lady in suture room two is very strange: She won't take off her clothes so she can be examined but has a temp of a hundred and two."

She leaned close to my ear. "The woman next door, we think, is bleeding into her gut. She's been waiting for a medical bed to open up for two hours."

"Jesus!" I said. "I forgot how different the ER is from the CCU."

Katy stood and lazily stretched her heavy body, like a pregnant cat tired of carrying her litter.

"There's going to be another on-call position available," she said, watching me out the corner of her eye. "It's supposed to be posted in the next few days."

My stomach contracted with a shot of excitement. "Do you think they'd hire me for on-call in ER and still let me work CCU?" I asked, trying not to get my hopes up, although I was already figuring how I could split my time. "I don't think anybody works two units in the house, do they?"

Katy shrugged. "So? What does that matter? Go ahead and apply. C'mon, Ec. I know you love it down here. We can use somebody with all that CCU experience, plus you're already familiar with the department. All you have to do is take the next MICN class."

"MICN?"

"Mobile intensive care nurse—you have to take it before you can work in ER. It's a certification class on trauma medicine and radio protocols for the county, so you'll be licensed to take paramedic calls over the radio and give them instructions on what to do for someone who's hurt in the field. You know, ten-four, over and out . . . all that stuff."

A nurse with red hair ran by us toward the lobby, yelling, "Quick! There's a seizure in the first-floor ladies' room!"

Katy squeezed my arm. "Gotta go, sport! Think about it." She disappeared, waddling after the red-haired nurse.

Dr. Judd ordered x-rays of my knee and, when it was determined nothing had been fractured, wrote out the standard prescription for pain pills and gave me the standard advice about using ice packs and keeping my leg elevated for two days.

Equipped with a pair of hospital crutches, I hobbled down to the nursing office to fill out the required employee accident form and apply for the ER job.

Milly was sitting at her desk sorting through a stack of files. She was smiling, and that threw me; it wasn't an expression I was used to seeing her wear.

"Hello?"

The woman started and looked up. The smile stayed for a moment, then faded when she saw the crutches. "What happened to you?"

"I got kicked in the knee by one of our more active patients. I need to fill out an employee accident report." I answered defensively, expecting a lecture about safety on the job and what an inconvenience it was going to be to find someone to replace me.

Instead, Milly turned to the gray file cabinet behind her. "I sympathize," she said, sounding like she really meant it. "I know how those knee kicks can hurt." Opening the second drawer, she pulled a yellow accident form from one of the folders and gave it to me. "Make sure you keep ice on it, and stay off your feet if you can. Do you need a ride home? If you want to wait for a few minutes, I can drive you."

I glanced briefly at the woman's pupils, looking for signs of drug use. Milly's personality change seemed as drastic as that of Ebenezer Scrooge on Christmas morning, and just as hard to believe.

"Ah, no, I can drive . . . I don't have far to go, but thanks anyway." Suddenly I looked away, speaking rapidly, the way I did as a child when asking for something I really wanted but was certain I wouldn't get. "I also want to fill out an application form for the on-call position in ER. I want to work in both units."

A hint of sour crossed her face. "I don't know if you can do that," she said slowly.

"Is there a policy against it?" I asked. Thoughts of new battles over more ancient policies were making my stomach tighten.

Milly got up and walked around the desk. "You know, there actually isn't," she said carefully. "It's never come up before. I don't know anybody masochistic enough to want to work in two different critical care units . . . especially those two. Of course, you'd have to be certified as an MICN." Milly thought for a moment and leaned toward me smiling a little. "Aw, why don't you go ahead and fill out an application anyway and see if it goes through? I don't know why there should be any rule that says a person can't . . ."

Milly stopped when she realized I was staring hard at her feet and smiling. She was wearing a pair of dark gray running shoes with magenta stripes.

Blushing, she stuttered, "Oh, those . . . well, I've had sore feet and a bad back most of my life . . . well, I mean, since I started nursing . . . then when you told me that you . . . when I tried a pair . . . I mean, they're really awful looking things, not really professional at all, but . . ." Milly stopped stuttering and laughed. "To put it plainly, they're the most comfortable shoes I've ever worn in my life, and I'm retiring in four days and three hours anyway, so what the heck?"

I almost laughed. Of course that was the reason for the Dr. Jekyll—Mr. Hyde change. Milly wasn't schizophrenic, she was simply getting out.

"Congratulations," I said, meaning it. "By the way, what

ever happened with that policy about leaving the hospital on meal breaks?''

"That one was in the rule book all right, but dust had covered the fine print at the bottom of the page where it said it was okay to leave the hospital grounds as long as you clock out and in. It isn't something the hospital likes to advertise to its employees. They like to keep you on the premises in case they need you.''

"And the dress policy on white shoes?'' I asked, pointing to her feet.

Milly smiled and shrugged. "Oh yeah, well . . . that's the part I rewrote.''

I was sitting in the window seat watching my ice pack melt, preparing to crutch it into the kitchen for a replacement from the freezer, when the phone rang.

"How're you doing?'' Jan asked as soon as I answered.

"I'm able to sit up and take nourishment, how're you?''

There was an almost imperceptible pause, like the guilty hesitation before a lie.

"Okay. Want to see the new movie playing at the Sequoia, or would sitting for that long bother your knee?''

"Have ice pack and crutches, will travel. I need to get out of the house before I go nuts. Since Simon's been gone, it's like a tomb around here. I've already read every book in the library and I've sunk as low as darning socks to keep busy. Can you come and pick me up?''

"Will do! See you at seven.''

An hour later Jan pulled up to the front of the cottage. From the window I watched her as she walked to the door. She was different; her gait was slower, and her head not held quite so high. I opened the door and reached out to pull her hair; it was our way of saying hello.

"Hey, fatty, how're you?''

There was the same pause as before, and her abstraction and inability to look at me sent a silent, dull ache through my guts.

"Okay,'' she said flatly. She held the door, and as I passed, she gave my braid a tug.

At the theater the familiar popcorn smell blasted my nose while my eyes were drawn immediately to the colorful posters of men with straining, sweat-covered muscles and pleading, large-cleavaged women hanging among the standard black-and-whites of W. C. Fields, Mae West, and Clark Gable.

I bought my popcorn; Jan purchased her usual corn chips and soda. We were heading up the ramp into the dark inner sanctum when Jan stopped and leaned against the wall, right under the poster of Clark Gable. His gaze seemed to land on the top of her head.

She turned to me. "Hey!" she said.

I'd just deposited a handful of popcorn into my mouth.

"Yeff?" A kernel of partially popped corn flew out and landed on her blouse. I picked it off and looked at her, waiting for her to speak.

"I'm out of remission; start chemo next Tuesday."

I didn't flinch but stopped chewing, then chewed like a maniac and swallowed the mouthful with difficulty. The corn kernels felt like lead pellets scraping down my esophagus.

It was beginning, I thought, *it was beginning, and I had to let it come.*

"Okay," I said slowly. "When do we go shopping for wigs? I know of this great place down on Market Street where we can buy a wig and get a fake mustache at no extra cost. Guaranteed, no fleas, no moths, or your money back on the whole deal."

Jan laughed out loud. "Brother," she said, turning and walking into the theater, "I should know better than to try and get a little sympathy from the infamous Nurse Wretched."

After the movie Jan drove halfway up Mount Tamalpais, to a place known among the locals as "Four Corners." From the car we were able to see the entire bay. Jan was calm and quiet and, I sensed, satisfied just to be alive for that moment. The deep bass beat of Marvin Gaye's "I Heard It Through the Grapevine" made the dashboard vibrate.

"So, when did you find out?" I asked, facing the subject head-on.

"Three days ago," answered Jan casually. "I didn't want to tell you right away, because I had to sort out my own feelings first. For all my philosophizing, it still threw me, believe it or not.''

"I believe it," I said.

"I wasn't aware of it really, but I'd built up a little stockpile of hope in a small corner of myself, and as soon as I was told, it was like having everything ripped away all over again, like I'd been betrayed or something.''

She rolled down the window, and a cool breeze from the bay filled the car. After taking in a deep breath, Jan let it out slowly and rested her head against the frame of the door.

"I had to go to work that afternoon, and I didn't know what to do except get angry with everyone who's alive and well.''

"Why didn't you tell me before?''

"I had to get back to base by myself, to reaffirm the acceptance I'd worked so hard for. I had to get rid of that stockpile.''

"But, Jan . . .'' I protested.

"Don't worry, I'm not quitting. I'll continue to wage my war with the chemo, but I'm resolved to live every second as it happens. If I go before I've done everything I want to do . . . well, I guess I just go.''

We were quiet for a while, listening to the golden oldies station. "Blue Moon,'' then "Teen Angel'' played while I tried to ignore the pressure in my throat by concentrating on who I'd been when those songs were popular. It didn't work; I kept losing the memories and thinking about Jan.

"What about during the chemo? Do you get sick?''

"If it's anything like the last chemo I got, yes.''

"Can I be there to help you? Hold your head, rub your back?''

"No," said Jan quickly, as if the idea were totally unacceptable. I looked away, trying not to feel hurt. Jan put her hand on my shoulder.

"I know you want to help, but I don't like to have anyone around while I'm sick; I don't want anybody to have to deal with that part except me. I need to know I can handle this by myself.''

"Okay for you," I said jokingly, "but you're gonna miss out on some great nursing care.'' I resumed looking out the window, knowing better than to argue with Jan. Besides myself, she was the most stubborn woman I'd ever run across.

"Let's change the subject for right now," Jan suggested.

I thought for a minute. "Okay, here's a tidbit for you: I applied for an on-call position in ER."

"That's great," Jan said, and then changed her expression to one of concern. "Wait a minute, that's terrible! What about CCU? Have you told Annie yet?"

"No problem, boss. I want to work both places, divide my time. CCU is beginning to get to me. We see so much of the same thing every day: heart and lungs, and always the same age group, fifty and up. I'm starved for variety. ER wants me, and I don't think Annie will mind the idea of having a good will ambassador from CCU working down there."

Jan tilted her head to the side and spoke to me in the same tone as that which a mother might take with a headstrong child who was demanding to swim in shark-invested waters. "It's up to you, of course, but I think you'll get more than variety down there . . . in the pit."

As her last administrative act Milly fought the system of unwritten policies to make sure I got the on-call ER job. Somehow she managed to get around the Catch-22 that stated I had to have my MICN before I could begin work in any emergency room but that in order to take the MICN course, I had to be presently employed in an emergency room.

Arranging it so I could do both at the same time, I worked evening shifts in ER and CCU and drove in to San Francisco each day to take the MICN course.

By July I was definitely getting my fill of variety. Just as Katy had said, the department was always chaotically busy. The summer was particularly hot, the mercury frequently staying above the seventy mark until long into the early-morning hours. I learned very quickly that heat, coupled with a full moon, created an emergency room nightmare.

Heat seemed to melt the holds on tightly guarded violence and insanity. The hotter it was, the more people were out and about, drinking, then driving to the beaches for some relief or up the narrow mountain roads to watch the fog roll in under the Golden Gate Bridge. It all guaranteed bad accidents, drownings, and overdoses.

Even worse than the heat, however, was the time of the full moon. People simply went a little nuts, and not necessarily just the high-risk groups but the so-called normal people as well. The first night of the new moon was a signal to all that the free-for-all was on. Emergency room personnel generally put great faith in the popular saying "A full moon fills the emergency room."

One steamy Friday night I stepped out of my car and looked into the sky. The sun glinted brilliantly on one side, and the moon glowed faintly on the other. I pulled my purse over my shoulder and headed for the ER doors, thinking of Dr. Mahoney's comment when I had shown up in the department my first scheduled shift; I repeated it to myself all the way to the end of the parking lot: "Oh, you fool . . . you fool . . . you fool . . ."

The doors swung open, and I walked expectantly into the pit.

The commotion was unbelievable. There was a patient on every bed and two in the hallway on gurneys borrowed from surgery. Three chairs, placed by the side door, were filled.

Two guards from San Quentin, a San Rafael policeman and a highway patrolman were doing their best to stay out of the way of the paramedics, doctors, and nurses, who ran from bed to bed. A large blond woman of about thirty was weaving unsteadily toward the bathroom door when she walked into the wall, excused herself, then fell to her knees, laughing. Carol, one of the day shift nurses, picked her up, quickly helped her into the bathroom, then rushed off to the suture room.

The tense atmosphere propelled me to run to the back room to put away my purse. In my mad rush, I tripped over a half-folded wheelchair which had been left in the middle of the tiny walkway. Angrily I maneuvered it out of the space and unfolded it completely. "EMERGENCY ROOM—PLEASE RETURN" was printed in bold black letters across the orange vinyl back; *Halloween chariots*, I thought, and wheeled it toward the others stacked against the wall.

At the clerk's desk Irene was busy stacking the charts to be triaged, while people threw questions and demands at her. Two of the phones were ringing, but she ignored them. Feeling sorry for her and to help lower the noise level, I picked up one of the lines.

"Hello, this is emergency."

"Oh, uh, hi," a girl responded, sounding surprised. I could

barely hear the timid voice over the noise, most of which was due to the big blonde, who was now out of the bathroom, waddling around with her panty hose around her knees and screaming at no one in particular that we'd stolen her purse. The CHP officer came over and escorted her out the side entrance.

"My boyfriend just told me he has gona . . . gonher . . . gon . . . you know, the clap, and I think I have it. I just looked down there, and there's this little red—"

Feeling a little like a calloused ogre, I cut her off mid-sentence and gave the standard answer the nurses were instructed to give to people who called in and wanted to tell all about their medical complaints.

"I'm sorry; but we're really busy right now, and we aren't supposed to give out advice over the phone. If you want to come in, we'd be glad to help you."

"But I don't have any money," the young voice complained, "and my boyfriend said—"

"If you have no means, go to the county clinic; it charges only what you can afford." I glanced up and saw Joy, the day charge nurse, drumming her fingers impatiently, waiting to give report. The girl began to cry, and I felt the squeeze of the famous rock and hard place. For the hundredth time since I'd started working in ER, I vowed never to answer the phones again.

I tried softening my voice as much as I could yet speak quickly at the same time.

"Look, sweets, pull yourself together and go over to the county clinic before it closes. Do you know where it is?"

"Yes." The voice faded away even more, adding to my guilt.

"Then go over right now and have them check you out, okay?"

"I'm fifteen, and I don't have a car."

Joy touched my arm and motioned for me to get off the phone—immediately.

"Take the bus."

"Do you think it could wait till tomorrow?" the girl asked, sounding just a little less mournful.

"Yeah, sure." Exasperation broke through and entered my voice. "You won't die if you wait one more day."

"Thank you," the girl said breathlessly, "You've saved my life."

"That's wonderful," I said without enthusiasm, and hung up.

As soon as I put the phone on the hook, Joy started in giving report. I turned around to see who else I'd be working with and saw Gus and Beth, both good ER nurses, both hard workers. I felt safe.

"We are nuts down here if you haven't noticed." Joy started, "We've got people stacked up like pancakes waiting for admission to the floors . . . plus one coming in for CCU and there're no beds left in the house. Dr. Judd and Dr. Mahoney have both been working nonstop. Dr. Judd just went down to administration to see if a few inpatients can be transferred out or discharged. I told the supervisor that if they didn't do something, we were going to have to close to paramedic and ambulance traffic and start directing people elsewhere. I figured a kick in the cash register might give them some incentive to find us beds."

The blond woman burst into the department, screaming, and the CHP officer tackled her and pulled her back out. Joy didn't even look up; she just raised her voice, speaking over the commotion.

"The waiting room is full. Most of these new charts haven't even been triaged yet, and we've got a couple of people out there who should be seen pretty soon. A lot of those people have been waiting as long as two hours. I'm afraid to go out there anymore; people are starting to get really angry.

"None of us got to eat lunch, and there hasn't been time to check the crash carts or restock the cabinets, plus we're running low on linen, narcotics, and suture supplies. Irene has called housekeeping and central supply three times to come up and restock, but I have yet to see them."

Joy scanned the room as a whole and squared her shoulders.

"Okay, now. On to the serious business: The lady in the pelvic room is an incomplete abortion, waiting to go to surgery. In bed one is a man brought in by the San Rafael police to be cleared for crisis. He's claiming he hasn't killed enough Vietcong, and he wants to 'slit some yellow throats.' Interestingly enough, they sent an Oriental guy from the crisis unit to talk to him."

Gus burst out with a Cousin Ralph, and Joy stopped long enough to giggle.

"We hope, when crisis goes, they'll take him with them. Bed two is another admission: an eighty-year-old total body failure, supposedly going to west ward. Notes are done, and the floor has been given report; we're just waiting for the bed to be cleaned. Bed three is a kid with a possible broken clavicle who's waiting for his pediatrician to come in. Bed four is a deep second-degree burn to the leg that needs to be dressed, and then he can be discharged. Bed five is another crazy who's also here to be cleared for crisis. He says voices keep telling him to masturbate in front of old women."

Joy stepped away from Irene's desk and in a low voice said, "He tried it in front of Irene twice, and she's still upset. We had security in here with him until a worker from crisis could get here, and you'll never guess who was sent."

"Oh, my God," Beth said, chuckling, "an older woman?"

"With white hair, no less," said Joy, then continued.

"Suture room, bed one is a stab wound to the chest from San Quentin who has chest tubes in already and is also waiting for surgery. Bed two is a bad laceration of the buttocks from a motorcycle versus plate glass window accident; he's being sewn up now, and the trauma room is a bad status asthmaticus who's intubated and waiting for an ICU bed; respiratory is in with her. We've also got someone in the scanner that we've been keeping in the hall: a woman window cleaner who fell off some scaffolding and down two stories. Apparently she has two bad fractures, so we've got her on strict spine stabilization precautions."

Joy turned around, and we followed suit. "Moving on to the blue chairs: The young boy with the yellow skateboard has a possible broken shoulder and is waiting to go to x-ray. The older Japanese man with the cap is a sprained finger waiting for a splint. The guy without any shirt or shoes has a broken nose and has been to x-ray but is waiting for the films to come back. He also has a blood alcohol level of point-two and is waiting for jail clearance to San Rafael PD."

Gus held up a hand and started for the door. "That's enough for me. I think I'm going home now."

Laughing, Joy grabbed her by the sleeve and pulled her back to the desk.

"The other hallway gurney is a sixteen-year-old-aspirin OD

who was ipecaced and watered. She vomited up enough pill fragments to fill two bottles. We're waiting for a salicylate level on her before crisis evaluates her. Her mother refused to come in, and the father is on his honeymoon with his new twenty-one-year-old bride.

"The crib is a two-year-old with a high fever who was seizing when he got here . . . also waiting for the same pediatrician as the other kid. His lab work has already been drawn. I noticed the mom has a PID shuffle, and she looks like she's running a fever. I haven't had time to suggest she sign herself in to be seen."

With that Joy put down her pen and rubbed her lower back.

"I'll stay over for an hour or so until you guys are cleared out a little," she said, stretching. "I conned my sister into picking up my kids and feeding them, so I'm free for a while . . . until my husband gets home anyway."

Gus appointed herself charge nurse and was to take radio calls and help out generally. To Beth she assigned the suture and trauma rooms, plus the crib. Beds one through five and the pelvic room were my areas.

When Joy finally left at 7:00 P.M., we had cleared out the first group and gone through most of the stacked charts. No one had been to dinner or even had time to go to the bathroom.

Dr. Mahoney and Dr. Judd both were short-tempered, and although we tried to make light of the confusion, nothing could dissipate their foul moods.

Lori, the new evening supervisor, showed up around eight with a tray loaded with sandwiches, fresh fruit, and soft drinks. We ate as we worked, gulping down mouthfuls of tuna fish and bananas between seeing patients.

By nine there was enough of a lull to switch off the automatic pilot and think about what to do next. The three of us restocked as many carts and cabinets as we could, until at nine-thirty we got the prize of the evening in the form of a white male in his late twenties who'd attempted to shoot himself through the head. Most of his face was blown off, and he'd lost an incredible amount of blood; but he was still alive.

Gus and Beth disappeared into the trauma room, while I finished discharging or admitting the patients left in the main room.

By ten, four of the five gurneys in the main room were

empty, and I wanted to weep with joy at seeing the clean, unoccupied sheets. I sat down for a minute, and the acrid smell of my own sweat hit me. I rolled my eyes and pretended to be knocked out from the stench. Then, for no reason other than the fact I was exhausted, I started to laugh. I stopped only when I heard the pneumatic hiss of the door opening and the sorrowful sound of a woman weeping.

Flanked by a man and woman police officer, an attractive woman I judged to be in her early twenties was helped into the main room. She wore a pair of baggy white cotton pants and a sleeveless white blouse that was ripped open at the right shoulder and over the left breast.

The male police officer walked over, turned his back to the sobbing young woman, and whispered, "She's been raped."

Immediately I got up and led her into the pelvic room, requesting the policewoman to stay with her for a moment. Then I asked the male officer to step outside with me.

As we came out, two more police appeared in the main room, roughly dragging a man in handcuffs. I noticed the policemen both were quite tall, while the man was short and slightly built; their difference in size caused the man to stumble every few steps as the police pulled him along. From where I stood twenty feet away, I saw he was covered with dirt and was bleeding profusely from his scalp and face. On his arms were several open wounds.

"That's the asshole who did it," said the policeman.

Motioning to the officers to bring the man into the suture room, I went in ahead of them and got down a box of gauze pads, which I soaked in germicide. The handcuffs had cut off the circulation to the man's hands, and I requested they be removed, mostly so I could more easily apply the pads to the wounds on his arms.

Sheepishly, softly the man said, "Thank you." Immediately the bigger of the two cops flushed red, grabbed the man by his head, and forcefully smashed him down into the pillow. The action was so unexpected and violent I jumped out of the way.

"Hey, scum, don't you talk to this nurse," he shouted. "Don't you even dare look at her."

The policeman who'd come in with the girl touched my arm and motioned me out of the room. At the clerk's desk he gave me the essentials of what had happened.

"The girl's name is Kirsten Searles, lives in Mill Valley. She was out walking on Stinson Beach when this asshole jumps out of nowhere and holds a rifle on her. He tells her he's going to kill her if she doesn't do as he says and proceeds to rape her."

"What happened to him?" I asked.

The man smiled wryly, the same way Joe Friday used to on "Dragnet." "The girl did that." He snickered. "And didn't do a bad job on the bastard either. We've been looking for this guy for a week. In five days he's raped two other young women that we know of; one was a thirteen-year-old girl. Besides that, he's wanted for armed robbery in Salinas and a hit-and-run in Monterey." The policeman shook his head. "What can I say? The guy is a bad dude."

The evening clerk interrupted by handing me the two rape forms and several stickers stamped with the girl's name and birthdate. Reading my mind, he informed me that the only float nurse available had been assigned to pediatrics but that a woman from rape crisis was on her way.

A minute later I entered the pelvic room. The small seven-by-ten closet held one pelvic exam table, a blanket warmer, and several small cupboards. The girl was sitting on the rollaway stool with her head in her hands, trembling. Her short light brown hair was wet and caked with sand. I nodded to the policewoman, indicating she could leave.

"Kirsten?"

Without looking up, she nodded.

I knelt in front of her and put my hand on her knee. "I'm Echo. I want you to know you don't have to be afraid now, and you can cry as much as you want and say anything you'd like."

Kirsten put her hand on mine and squeezed. The action was small yet so tender that it broke through the thin layer of hardness I'd built around myself and awakened my compassion.

"Let me tell you everything that's going to happen now, okay?"

Kirsten nodded and covered her eyes with her hand.

"You've been brought here because we want to make sure

you're okay and because we need to collect evidence from you for the police.

"After I take your vital signs and ask you some questions, Dr. Mahoney will do a complete physical and pelvic exam; she'll draw some blood and take some samples from your vagina. Someone from rape crisis is coming in to bring you a change of clothes and to help you out in any way she can. The women they send have been through this, so they're pretty understanding."

Kirsten raised her head to look at me for the first time. The attractive face was like a child's in its innocence, but the eyes reflected such sadness I immediately choked up.

She took my hands. "Do you know what he did to me?" she asked with a kind of desperation.

I nodded.

"Do you know that he killed my dog? He killed Lady, just like it was nothing. I've had her since I was seven years old, and he killed her."

I found my voice, though my throat was tight. "I'm sorry, Kirsten. Please tell me what I can do."

Kirsten bowed her head and started to cry again. Standing, I held her head gently to my stomach and rocked her.

Finally, she threw her head back and shook it; sand flew in every direction.

"I'll get undressed now. I'm sorry for being such a baby."

"Kirsten, you have no reason to be sorry. You have every right to feel the way you do. You deserve some tender care."

Kirsten stood, and I handed her a gown, then opened the rectangular brown box marked "RAPE KIT," took out two brown paper bags marked "CLOTHES" and placed them both on the floor next to her. "Put everything in those," I instructed.

Kirsten laughed through a sob, and I looked at her questioningly.

"My mother always told me to wear clean underwear every time I went out in case I ever had to go to the hospital—I should have listened."

I smiled. "That's okay. Nobody in the history of the world has ever listened to their mother's advice about clean underwear. I have yet to see a clean pair on anybody who's come in here."

While she undressed, I went into the main room, where

Dr. Mahoney had brought back two patients and was doing vitals on them herself. Gus, Beth, and Dr. Judd were still in the trauma room with the gunshot wound.

Dr. Mahoney looked up from a chart briefly. "Get him in a gown," she yelled across the room, jerking her thumb in the direction of the suture room. "And wash out those wounds so I can see what we're dealing with."

Once in the suture room, I found I could not look directly into the man's face, and when I spoke to him, I directed my eyes to the policemen instead.

"You need to remove your clothes and get into a gown," I said, looking at the bald-headed policeman. "Then I need to clean your cuts with germicide soap and get them ready for suturing."

"Yes, ma'am," said the man. His voice was soft, with a midwestern twang. "Would you like me to take off my socks, too, ma'am?"

Looking at him for the first time, I saw two dark eyes, a thin, acne-scarred face, and a mustache. His teeth were badly stained, and one of the front teeth was half-gone. He was wearing a gold earring on his left ear and a gaudy turquoise and silver cross around his neck.

The evil-looking face threw me. I wasn't sure why, except the voice didn't match up with it. "Ah, yeah, the socks, too," I said.

I left and glanced in the window of the trauma room door. There were several doctors, including one of the neurosurgeons, all standing around the patient. The man was intubated and seizing violently. Gus and Beth were so busy I did an about-face and left without opening the door.

I took a peek through the one-way window in the pelvic room door and saw Kirsten on the table, lying on her side in the fetal position. I went in. "Are you okay?" I asked.

Kirsten nodded, though I could see she was ready to cry. After I took her vital signs, I wrote them on her chart, picked up the two bags of clothes, and sealed them. I pulled a blanket from the warmer and wrapped the girl in it, covering her toes. When I tucked the upper edge around her chin, she started to sob again and hid her face. I rubbed the back of her neck for a minute until she turned her face to the wall and seemed to doze off.

Letting her rest, I went back to the suture room. Without looking at any of the three men, I drew a basin of warm water, mixed in the red germicide soap, and carried it carefully to the gurney. Reaching over my head, I switched on the surgical lamp.

"Lie down please," I said, looking into the basin.

The man did as I asked, and one of the police officers left the room. The other one leaned against the sink and began filling in a report form.

I dipped a washcloth in the orange suds, wrung it out, and then started wiping through the clumps of hair matted with blood, attempting to get to the loose flaps of scalp. As soon as I cleaned out most of the sand from the wound, more would fall in. Within a few seconds the area under the other flap began to spurt.

I stood back and studied the man's arms and hands. There was one deep wound about three inches in diameter on his left arm and two smaller ones on his right forearm. On his hands I saw the tattoos common among street people; on the webbing between the fingers of each hand were spelled the words *evil* and *hate.*

"This isn't working," I said. "I think it would be a lot easier to wash your whole head and both arms under the sink faucet."

The officer snapped to attention, watching every movement of the man's body as he sat up, slipped off the gurney, and shuffled to the sink. About two feet from the sink, his knees sagged, and he extended his hand and gripped the edge of the basin for support. Without thinking, I started to go for the man to support him, but the cop pushed me out of the way and grabbed his belt from the back to hold him up.

"What's the matter, Donatini?" the cop asked gruffly.

"Nothin', man, just felt like passin' out for a minute. That's all. There a law against that, too?"

The cop jerked the man's belt and growled, "Shut that fuckin' mouth, asshole."

Gingerly I stepped in between the two and pressed the foot controls. The water came out warm, and I indicated to the man to put his arms under the running water. After soaping the wounds and rinsing the sand and blood off, I wrapped both his arms in towels, and he dipped his head under the water.

I watched the rose-colored water flow from his head and into the sink for a moment, then soaped his scalp, rinsed it, and gave the man a towel.

He dried his head and then lay back down. Methodically I shaved the hair away from the lacerations on his scalp and covered them with a sterile towel.

"When was your last tetanus shot?" I asked, studying the man's chart. I did not want to look into that face again.

"I got one back in high school when some asshole tried to take off my head with a beer bottle. I don't remember the year, but it was just before they throwed me out. That was in Minnesota. You can look it up."

I checked the birthdate: October 25, 1943. "Was your tetanus more than five years ago is really all I need to know."

"Pssssh, sure—that was a long time ago." The man laughed, and the sound was unpleasant.

Without saying anything more, I prepared a tetanus booster and injected him. Standing close to him, I saw the man's eyes bore into my face, then travel down to my breasts. Feeling repulsed and a little frightened, I hurried out to the medicine cabinet and checked my name tag. Thank God, I'd remembered to wear my emergency room tag—the one that gave only my first name.

When I opened the door to the pelvic room, Kirsten sat up, hugging the blanket to herself, and I noticed she'd stopped crying.

"Are you up for this, or do you want some more time?" I asked, setting the rape forms in front of me.

"I'm okay," she said. "I want to get this over with."

I went down the list of questions and checked off the ones that had to do with the description of the assailant.

"Ready?"

Kirsten nodded.

"Okay. Where did this happen?"

"Stinson Beach, a little ways from the rest rooms."

"What time?"

"About nine-thirty, I think. I drove out to the beach about seven-thirty with Lady to take a walk. It had gotten dark, and I was heading back to the parking lot. There was this noise, and I saw this guy walking toward me; but I wasn't afraid because I had Lady with me.'' Kirsten started to tear again.

"He passed me, and I saw that he was carrying something under a jacket or a shirt. He said something like 'Hey, baby,' and I just kept walking, but a little faster. Then Lady started growling, and I didn't turn around because I could feel him behind me. I started running, but he grabbed me by the back of my blouse and threw me down. Then he stuck the rifle in my neck and told me to get up.

"Lady was barking and jumping on him, and all of a sudden he took the end of the rifle and swung it around and hit Lady in the head. She yelped and fell; then he hit her again, and her head went to the side, and she didn't move.

"I didn't know what to do.'' Kirsten's voice was rising, and she'd started to tremble again.

"I tried to run away, but he caught me and told me if I did that again, he was going to kill me. He said that it made no difference to him whether he killed me or not and that he'd killed a lot of people. I begged him not to hurt me. I told him everything I could think of: that I was pregnant and I had syphilis. He just laughed, grabbed my feet, and dragged me off to the edge of the beach, where there were some big rocks.''

I put down the forms, reached over, and held her hands.

"I really got scared then because I knew I didn't have any control over what was going to happen. I kept trying to think of a way to get away, but he had that rifle on me.''

Kirsten wiped her face with her shoulder.

"I blacked out, I think, 'cause I remember only pieces, like when you try to remember a movie you saw a long time ago?

"I was hating him so much I got sick and threw up, but even that didn't stop him. He just kept pulling on my pants, I screamed and kicked, but he shoved the rifle into my throat so I could barely breathe.''

Pushing herself back, the young woman looked almost apologetic.

"I was afraid to die. I knew if I kept fighting, he'd kill me. All I saw was this turquoise and silver cross on a chain around his neck swinging back and forth, and he was saying, 'Like it, baby? Huh? Like it, baby?' ''

Kirsten leaned her forehead against my arm and pressed her hands over her mouth to muffle a scream. She was trembling, her eyes were shut tight, and the long wail ended in a whimper.

I stroked her head. "It will fade, Kirsten. You can't know that now, but someday it will fade."

About five minutes passed until the young woman sat up straight. In with the sadness was now mixed anger and defiance.

"At the end he'd put the rifle down, so I grabbed it and bit his arm. I don't remember how, but I managed to get up; that's when I kicked him in the balls, and then I hit him in the head with the end of the rifle. I thought I knocked him out, but he stood up right away. He wasn't standing too good, but he tried to punch me in the face. I hit him in the head even harder and really knocked him out that time.

"I thought about killing him. I wanted to, but I couldn't; I don't know why. Now I wish I had.

"When he woke up, I made him crawl in front of me to a house, and the people called the police and they took him to the jail, and the other police brought me here."

Kirsten stared at her lap and looked very tired. "The police said they'd find Lady and take care of her." She sighed and shook her head. "I should have killed him."

We both were sitting silently when the woman from rape crisis arrived a few minutes later. I met Dr. Mahoney at the door as she was ready to come in, and motioned her back outside. Off to the side of the main room, I related Kirsten's story as she'd told it.

At the end Dr. Mahoney shook her head, took the forms, and started back into the room without saying a word.

"Dr. Mahoney?"

Dr. Mahoney sighed and slumped. "I don't want to talk about anything right now, Echo. I'll take care of the forms; you take care of the suture room. The creep has been sewn up and is in x-ray for skull and chest films. When he comes back, give the slug a dressing, bring me the x-rays, and get him the hell out of here. I want housekeeping down here to clean everywhere he's been." She opened the door. "I'll buzz when I need you for the pelvic."

All the beds were empty, except bed four, which held the enormous weight of the asthmatic black woman. She was being given a breathing treatment, inhaling the medicated vapor greedily.

I found Gus and Beth restocking the trauma room and generally cleaning up. The man with the gunshot wound had been considered a "save"; he was in surgery, having what was left of his brain glued back into place.

I had watched Gus work for a minute when she looked up and stopped long enough to put her hands on her hips. "Do you believe this shit?" she said. I assumed she meant the whole evening.

"Yeah," I answered. "Please remind me to be off call on the next full moon, okay?"

"Sure, Ec. We say that every month, and every month we always get duped into working."

"Not this cookie," I said, pointing at myself. "I'm getting myself a lunar calendar and referring to it every time I take call."

Dr. Judd walked up behind me, smiling. "Sheeeit, girls, quit your complaining. You should work a hot full-moon night in Atlanta sometime. This is downright sophistication compared to that."

The pelvic room buzzer went off, and I'd started in that direction when the rapist, surrounded by the two policemen and x-ray tech, walked into the main room. We crossed paths, and he smiled at me in a way that made me feel sick.

Taking the x-rays from the tech, I turned back into the trauma room and spoke to Beth from the door. "Could you do me a favor and dress the suture room's lacerations and get him ready for discharge? He makes my skin crawl."

Reluctantly she agreed, and I brought the man's films to Dr. Mahoney. She looked at them quickly and shrugged.

"Normal," she said, and turned her attention back to Kirsten, who was holding the rape crisis lady's hand.

Explaining everything she was doing, Dr. Mahoney gently conducted the pelvic exam, collecting the samples required by the county, while I labeled and sealed them in the appropriate containers and envelopes. When the exam was over, Dr. Mahoney gave Kirsten a prescription for a round of antibiotics in case the man had infected her with some form of VD. Then Kirsten was free to dress and go with the woman from rape crisis.

"The first thing I want to do is take a long, hot shower," Kirsten said. "I feel filthy."

Helping her on with the jeans and sweat shirt the rape crisis woman had brought, I wanted to tell her it was going to take more than a shower for her to feel clean again; it was going to take years before she no longer felt soiled by what had happened.

I found her a pair of paper slippers and went with her to the door, where she gave me a hug. "Thank you. You were so nice to me. Thank you for not making me feel I'd done something wrong." I hugged her back, and the three of us exited the small room.

As Kirsten walked out into the main room, so did the man who'd raped her. They faced each other moving with jerky, halting steps in the first horrible moment of recognition. In a split second, everybody slowed down and stopped like film jammed in a projector.

With wild, proud anger Kirsten screamed and lunged in the man's direction, her hands clawing. When I threw myself in front of her, she knocked me back, but I managed to push her away.

Upon seeing her, the man changed: His eyes glazed and turned hard, then leering. "What'sa matter, baby?" he sneered in a taunting tone. "Couldn't get enough?"

Instantly both cops hoisted the man up, then threw him to the floor. The bigger cop put his foot on the back of the man's neck and held it to the ground.

"That was a real dumb move!" the cop shouted at me; his face was red, and the veins in his neck were bulging. "Get her out of here . . . *now!*" Grabbing Kirsten's arms, the rape crisis woman and I half dragged, half carried her out of the main room and into the lobby.

Painfully I had begun stuttering explanations and apologies when Kirsten stopped me short.

"It doesn't matter anymore," she said, starting to cry. "Nothing can hurt me anymore."

When I got back to the main room, the man and the cops were gone. On the floor where the cop had held the man's head with his foot was a small pool of blood.

I pulled up in front of the darkened cottage and switched

off the Chevy's lights. The unlighted driveway looked sinister, and the three feet to my front porch seemed a long and dangerous distance to travel. Gathering my purse and sweater, I opened the car door, changed my mind, and slowly closed it without getting out.

Straining to hear over the pings of the engine cooling down, I tried to discern any unusual noises.

Five minutes passed, and without so much as breathing, I left the car, looked in all directions, and crept noiselessly to the front door.

Aware of my heart pounding in my throat, I touched the doorknob but couldn't turn it, terrified there would be a man with hard eyes waiting on the other side.

At once my fear turned to anger. For a lifetime I'd been taught that limitation by *that* particular fear was the normal order of things for women. How many times had I been robbed of the simple pleasure of taking a walk alone after dark because I was a woman and "men like that" roamed the streets, waiting?

Behind me came the sharp sound of gravel as someone stepped onto the porch.

Unable to scream, I doubled over and backed into the corner. My eyes refused to focus, but I heard a familiar voice. "I'm sorry. It's—it's me, Joan. Are you all right?"

My eyes cleared, and I saw my next-door neighbor step backward with her hands up. "I didn't mean to frighten you. I heard you come in, but I didn't see your lights go on, so I thought I'd come over to see if everything was okay."

In pure relief I let out the breath I'd been holding and tried to laugh. "I'm okay. I was scared. I should leave a light on, but tonight I forgot, and—" I stopped and hurried to unlock the door. "Please, won't you come in for a beer or a glass of wine?" I asked, opening the front door boldly.

"Sure!" She smiled. "A nice glass of wine sounds great."

I poured us two healthy glasses of Chablis and told her the story of the evening. As I talked, I noticed she looked at me as if I were telling her something hideous. At length she shuddered. "How can you do what you do?" she asked.

"I don't know," I said. "I used to think it was all just wanting to help people, and now . . . ." I had to think of how I could put into words what I was feeling without sounding callous. "Now I just feel removed at certain times, as if I were an actress in some awful, exciting, gory movie."

Joan shook her head and finished her wine without saying much. I felt alienated from her, as I did whenever I talked about hospital business to my "normal" friends, people who had nothing to do with the field of medicine.

"I respect you a lot," she said finally, then added, "but I know I could never do what you do. I'd either go nuts or become an alcoholic."

The statement made me laugh as I thought of the number of "closet" alcoholic nurses I knew who were just barely hanging on to their sanity.

When Joan left, I went through the house and locked all the windows and doors and prepared for my long-awaited shower.

The hot water relaxed me, and I laughed at myself for being so foolish about coming into the house. I was soaping my hair when my mind took a cruel path, and the shower scene from *Psycho* flashed on loud and clear. I stopped, then shook off the vision, humming a lively tune, out of breath from the sudden jolt of self-induced fear.

In a minute I felt better and was singing outright when, through the shower curtain, I saw the bathroom door slowly open, four, five, six inches.

Screaming at the top of my lungs, I grabbed the back brush, jumped out of the shower, and slammed the door open the rest of the way.

Emelio, who had mistakenly thought the bathroom door might be a good scratching post, arched, hissed, and flew down the narrow hallway into Simon's room.

By 1:00 A.M. I lay exhausted in my bed, unable to sleep. The thought of taking one more glass of wine as a tranquilizer came up, but my ulcer balked at the very notion. Five relaxation techniques later, I was still hearing noises and seeing the man's rat eyes, hearing him say, "What'sa matter, baby? Couldn't get enough?" Strangely, I couldn't remember what Kirsten looked like, but I could picture her hands holding my arm.

I wished Simon were with me, asleep next door. After a few more minutes I tiptoed down the hall to his room, stepped over the wall-to-wall toys, and climbed into his bed. The smell of him lingered on his sheets and dispelled some of my anxiety.

Emelio came out from his hiding place under the empty toy chest and cautiously crept up my leg. Reaching my stomach, he hesitated, sniffed the air, and, satisfied that I wouldn't have another frenzied attack, curled around to sleep on my chest.

Good, I thought. *If there's anything in the house, the cat will warn me.* In the moonlight I watched his ears carefully for any signs of twitching.

Eventually my body relaxed enough to allow the gold and purple presleep swirls to appear on the back of my eyelids. My Man's Inhumanity to Man scale made a brief appearance in my thoughts, and I wondered why some things failed to infuriate me the way they used to. Sometimes I felt so removed from all the insanity.

Drifting, I found myself watching a Jimmy Durante type character and a chorus line of women dressed in nursing uniforms, doing a soft-shoe routine to a tune called "How Do You Do What You Do?"

The act wasn't going at all well when suddenly everybody disappeared and the bare stage metamorphosed into the usual setting for my dove dream.

While I dreamed, another part of me watched the visions of this recurring unconscious phenomenon with keen interest, making note of every detail.

The dream was exactly the same as it was the first time I'd had it one year before. It begins in the house where I grew up, at the top of the concrete basement steps. Standing alone, I am in a state of absolute panic and dread, for I have just remembered the dove.

Who entrusted the bird to my care, or the reasons why this precious creature of the sky must be kept caged in the basement, are hazy. What *is* clear is that I have once again neglected to feed or otherwise tend to her needs for too long a time.

Rushing down the stairs, I entered the cold dampness only to find what I fear most: At the bottom of the cage the bird lies on her side, barely alive. Gently holding the delicate body, I feed the dove by hand and resolve not to forget again my responsibility to her. After a moment she raises her head, blinks, then weakly flutters to her perch unassisted, while I cry with relief.

As I climb the stairs to the upper levels of the house, the truth of the dream reveals itself to me again: This white bird, the symbol of peace and love, is somehow part of my soul.

THIRTEEN

IT WAS A USUAL MONDAY swing shift in CCU, and the basic story lines were more than familiar: the same diagnoses and prognoses, life and death, pain and release.

Jan and I sat talking at the intermediate station while keeping our eyes glued to the monitors. The ten continuous geometric patterns moved smoothly from one side of the green phosphorescent screens to the other, shapes and lines translating into life.

"It's going to be a nice, slow night," I said, taking my eyes off the monitors to look at Jan.

"Could be," she said. "I don't like making those kind of predictions. The minute you open your mouth, it always turns out to be just the opposite. Enjoy the calm now; it could be the one before the storm."

Smiling peacefully, Jan adjusted the clasp holding her long hair in a ponytail at the back of her neck. Her hair had thinned badly, but by wearing ice packs on her scalp before and during each chemotherapy, she had not as yet had to resort to wearing a wig; this small victory was her secret pride and joy.

From skin and bones she'd gone mostly to bones but wore loose, bulky clothing to hide the fact. Only a handful of people in the unit noticed that her coloring was changing to a yellowish hue and that she was plagued by a constant cough. Old rumors sprang up from the grave but somehow didn't spread beyond CCU. When the gossipmongers approached me to ask for the real scoop, I simply directed them to ask Jan themselves, certain no one ever would; no one ever did.

Jan, Simon, and I spent as much time together as we could now. It was at this time Simon began to ask the questions his intuition formed. I found I could no longer hedge with vague, broad answers—and to lie to a nine-year-old was, in my opinion, unthinkable. I finally told him the truth, more to prepare him for the inevitable than to satisfy his curiosity.

He took the news wide-eyed but quietly, asking only when she would die. I answered that no one knew for sure, months, maybe years, but not too many.

Later I overheard him on the back stoop, making bargains. Holding Mooshie on his lap as a witness to his good intentions, he prayed. "Don't let her," he pleaded in a whisper. "I'll give her some of my blood to kill the bad cells, but just don't let her . . . not for a long time."

"I'm starving," Jan said, glancing up at the clock. "Would you relieve me for dinner?"

I nodded and turned my attention back to the monitors. "Go ahead, my patients are settled, and I've given my six o'clock meds. Take your time, but try not to stuff yourself. You've been packing on the weight lately; pretty soon they're going to start calling you Tub o' Lard Tobin."

Jan tried not to laugh but did.

"What're you up to, anyway, seventy, eighty pounds?"

Jan's attempt to look offended failed. "I want you to know, twerp face, that I am ninety-six pounds and gaining."

Before I knew what she was doing, she stamped me with a rubber stamper she'd concealed in her pocket. In red ink my arm read; "RETURN TO MEDICAL FLOOR" "Take that!" She laughed.

Lucy and Catherine happened to be passing the desk and joined in on the act. After a five-minute "stamper" fight Jan walked off to dinner with "DISCHARGED" smeared across her cheek, while Lucy and Catherine each had a copy of the standing medication orders imprinted in various places on their uniforms.

As I leaned back in my chair, the tranquillity of the unit was almost disturbing. In front of me, the cardiac monitors beeped out ten different rhythms, each representing its unique, troubled human heart. Reaching over, I turned several of the auditory control knobs to "loud."

Like a complex musical composition, the slow waltz beat from room 17 provided a basic rhythm, while room 5 sounded out a consistent pacemaker rhythm in four-four time. Finally, room 8's atrial fibrillation enlivened the melodic ode to life with its erratic syncopation.

I closed my eyes and listened; reminiscent of crickets on a lazy summer evening, the sound was just on the edge of being soothing when the ringing of the phone interrupted my auditory fantasy.

"Heart unit. May I help you?"

"This is the emergency room," said Gus, not recognizing my voice. "We're sending you a patient of Dr. Peters's for admission to the acute side of your unit. Her name is Sondra Nelson. How soon can you be ready to take her?"

I sighed; Jan may have been right about the calm before the storm.

"Hi, Gussie. It's me, Echo."

Gus's voice relaxed, and she dropped the stiff formalities. "Hey, reverb, how're you guys doing up there? We're scattered down here, and boy, have I got a weird one for you."

Chucking calm out the window, I heaved a rather dramatic sigh just as Jan walked in the main doors, carrying a dinner tray. I motioned for her to pick up the other line and covered the mouthpiece. "Listen in; it's ER with an acute admission for us."

Jan set down her tray and picked up the phone.

"Okay, Gussie, I got the boss on the line with me, so fire away."

"Like I said, this one is stranger than fiction," Gus said, "and to be honest, it's not really clear just what the story is on this lady. Her husband brought her into us, saying she was having trouble breathing. Dr. Judd saw her briefly, then called Dr. Peters in on the case. Both of them are being pretty closemouthed about whatever the problem really is. They've kept the curtain closed around the bed since she got here. My guess is mum's the word because of who she is; you'll recognize her for sure."

A longtime student of melodrama, Gus paused for effect, then continued.

"She's the wife of Gavin Nelson, Nelson Enterprises . . . San Francisco, New York, and London."

Without straining, my memory produced a vivid photograph from a recent society page which pictured the petite, impeccably dressed socialite and her successful husband posing in the winners' circle at Bay Meadows Racetrack.

Holding a bouquet of roses, her gloved hand raised to wave at the crowd, Mrs. Nelson was classically beautiful in a homecoming queen sort of way. She was smiling an exquisite cover girl smile that revealed perfect teeth.

With his arm slipped about her small waist, the debonair and handsome Gavin Nelson looked admiringly into her face. The Nelsons were the very picture of health, happiness, and storybook romance.

"Dr. Peters's present diagnosis is . . ." Gus cleared her throat and said sheepishly, "Uh, shortness of breath?"

Jan and I glanced at each other. "Shortness of breath?" I repeated, wondering if I'd heard correctly. "I get short of breath, too, just thinking about how short-staffed this is going to make us tonight. That's not enough to warrant an admission to CCU, let alone the acute side, Gus. This is starting to sound a little like a bogus admission."

The reasons behind bogus admissions were many. Sometimes they simply involved an innocent misdiagnosis by the doc: a patient who came in appearing sicker than he actually was. More often, though, they involved a "difficult" situation for the doctor, usually political in nature.

Nurses hated bogus admissions; not only did they take up needed beds and make poor use of nursing time and skills, but nine times out of ten, the patients were demanding and disruptive.

In the case of Mrs. Nelson, I suspected the politically based, fluff-my-pillow variety of bogus. This situation often involved a member of the wealthy elite who came into the hospital with minor problems. They, or their families, insisted on one-to-one nursing care, private rooms, and special diets. The doctor, usually considering such a client a valuable financial asset, admitted them to a critical care unit, where most of their whims would be catered to.

"I know, I know; I *told* Dr. Peters you guys would have a fit," Gus piped up "but he assures me there's more to the story. Says he'll fill you in on details later. For now he wants her brought up to your unit as soon as possible.

"All I know about her is she's forty-two years old and looks healthier than I do. She keeps insisting she's perfectly well and is allowing herself to be admitted only to appease Dr. Peters. She 'allowed' me to take her blood pressure and temperature, but that's where she drew the line. Her temp is up to one hundred point seven, and I noticed she did have some shortness of breath with exertion, but nothing spectacular.''

In the background, I could hear the frantic sounds of the usual emergency room chaos.

''Sorry I can't give you more information, guys, but I simply don't have it. By the way,'' Gus said, ''I'm sending her up fully dressed; she flat out refused to put on one of our lovely Yves Saint Laurent hospital gowns. When can you take her?''

Jan put down the phone and walked to the assignment board; she was the only charge nurse I knew who was meticulous about matching staff personalities with the patients'. Making up her mind quickly, she assigned Ella, the no-nonsense, let's-get-down-to-business nurse, my type A chest pain patient; to Catherine, the always happy chatterbox, she gave my withdrawn congestive heart failure, and to Lucy, the kind, quiet one of the bunch, she assigned the woman who was grieving over the recent loss of her leg. To me, she gave Sondra Nelson.

''How about fifteen minutes?'' I asked.

Gus hesitated, and I could almost hear her wince. ''I guess that's okay. We're a little tight on beds, but I suppose we can swing fifteen minutes.''

Jan brought her dinner to the monitors and sat down. ''It's okay, I'll eat at the desk; you go ahead and get the room ready.''

I hurried to the kitchen to grab an apple from the refrigerator, knowing it would be the only dinner I'd get. Munching, I walked over to the acute side, speculating on the unusual circumstances surrounding the socialite's admission and flicked on the lights in room 3.

I turned down the bed, found an extra pillow, and pressed the bedside monitor power button.

Towels, electrodes, water pitcher, oxygen bottle, wall suction—all present and accounted for.

Elias Peters, one of the county's handful of oncologists, was a really fine doctor in every sense of the word. I'd never seen him make a bogus admission before; why would he start now? What political pressures had he succumbed to and why?

I set up the IV: five percent dextrose and water, a tourniquet, and a medium-gauge needle. I called for a standby IV pump and took a quick look around the room. Right on cue, the doors flew open and the tanned, attractive Nelsons were ushered in by a distraught transport attendant pushing an empty wheelchair.

Seeing me, the attendant hurried over to explain. "She refused to come up in a wheelchair!" he said in loud disbelief. "I have never had a patient just walk up to critical care on her own before! It's—it's against policy!"

I laughed and patted him on the arm. "Everything's okay. Don't worry about it. You got her here safely anyway. Thank you."

Red-faced, the attendant stared at me as if I'd betrayed him by not reprimanding the patient, shrugged, and wheeled the chair away, holding his head rigidly to one side.

I introduced myself to the couple, seeing immediately the newspaper photograph had told only half the story. Set in a delicate oval face, the woman's large hazel eyes drew my attention right away. Although her tan did not hide the dark circles under them, they were brilliantly clear and seemed to penetrate everything they saw. Her frame was quite small, but she carried herself with a physical dignity that made her appear larger and taller than she actually was.

There was no question the woman was impressive, but something about her disturbed me. Studying her more closely, I was startled to detect a hint of terror in the unique eyes, something like a small animal caught in a trap.

"Mrs. Nelson, I'll be taking care of you this evening until midnight, when the night shift relieves me." Mrs. Nelson glared at me. "I'd like to have you come into your room and get—"

Mrs. Nelson's face took on a wild look, and she tossed back a shock of shining, carefully tended blond hair from her face. "I should *not* be here!" she finally exploded in a heavy, loud whisper. "This is absurd, all this fuss! There is nothing wrong with me, and you should know I fully intend to be home by Thursday no matter what happens. I'm sorry, but you—we're wasting hospital time."

Mrs. Nelson's breathing had become rapid and shallow, and after her outburst she was almost at the point of gasping.

I fought down my urge to reason with her and instead reached for her hand, which was small and cold to the touch. A childhood memory of holding a dying bird flashed through my mind.

"I don't think I'll be wasting my time," I said as calmly as possible.

Mrs. Nelson tried desperately to avoid looking at me by staring at the antiseptically clean, white-tiled floor.

"I'm here to help you get better and get you home as soon as possible. I'd like—"

"I've already told you, there is nothing wrong!" she snapped. "I am perfectly healthy. Why, I'm as healthy as—as healthy as . . . ." Mrs. Nelson was trembling.

Gavin Nelson put his arm protectively around his wife's shoulders.

Abruptly the woman jerked her hand out of mine and brought it awkwardly toward her chest as if she didn't know quite what to do with it. She finally let it rest on her collarbone, where her trembling fingers pinched at the skin of her neck.

My smile faded into an expression of concern. Mrs. Nelson was obviously the kind of patient who needed to be in control, and if she weren't, my instincts told me, she would simply walk out and I'd be blamed. Doctors took a dim view of nurses who scared their patients away.

The distinct feeling that there was more here than met the eye caused me to stretch my patience, and I softened to the point of being syrupy. "I'm sorry about this, Mrs. Nelson, but why don't you let me help you get settled in your room before Dr. Peters arrives? It won't take but a minute, and your husband can stay in the waiting room until you're ready."

Mr. Nelson put his head close to hers and spoke to her as one would to a stubborn, spoiled child. "Yes, sweetheart, do what the nurse says. I'll be close by. Don't worry, everything will get straightened out, and then we'll go home. Everything will be fine. I promise."

Sondra Nelson looked up at him. "Do you really promise, Gavin?"

"I promise. You'll be home by Thursday." He looked over

at me and winked as if that would give his promise more validity.

Resisting the urge to wink back, I pulled a chair up to the nurse's station for Mrs. Nelson, who stared at me blankly.

"I prefer to stand," she said dryly.

I decided "intimidating" would be a good adjective to use when I described Mrs. Nelson to the night nurse.

I led Mr. Nelson to the waiting room. As the door closed behind us, he turned to me and with urgency said, "You must be very careful with my wife. She has definite ideas about the way things are."

"Definite ideas?" I repeated, wondering if that meant Mrs. Nelson was going to be even more difficult than I already anticipated.

"She doesn't always see things the way other people do. You might say she's a bit eccentric that way. When Sondra gets an idea into her mind—well, that's the way it is. Simple as that. She thinks she's perfectly healthy.

"I practically had to force her into coming to the emergency room, never dreaming they'd insist on admitting her." Mr. Nelson faltered. "She's very angry with me."

"I'll be as gentle as I can with her," I said, and dropped the subject. I sensed the man was walking on eggshells; it was as if he wanted to say more but was too embarrassed.

When I returned to the nurse's station, Mrs. Nelson was leaning against the counter, impatiently tapping her foot.

"Took you long enough," she complained. "What did my husband tell you—that I wouldn't face reality or something equally ridiculous?" She tossed her head, then, without waiting for my reply, tucked her purse under her arm and started walking toward the glass rooms. "Let's play this farce out, shall we?"

Taking the lead, I ushered Mrs. Nelson into her room. I couldn't help being amused at the scene. Here was a patient, fully dressed, in no apparent distress, walking into an acute care room as if she were being shown a hotel suite.

It was so different from the usual manner of bringing a patient to this room: gurneys wheeled in at breakneck speed, IV lines, and monitors bumping around, while nurses and doctors, their adrenaline flowing, ran alongside, shouting orders.

I handed Mrs. Nelson one of the blue patient gowns. "I'd

like you to put this on, leaving it untied and open to the back."

She scrutinized the shapeless garment with distaste. For a moment she said nothing and played with the buttons on the front of her dress.

"Do I really have to wear this? Can't I send for something from home?" Mrs. Nelson pleaded.

Taking the gown from her, I held it up and laughed. "Well, it's not exactly Dior, but while you're being examined, you'll find it easier to wear this."

What I didn't tell her was that the simple cotton gown was designed to provide easy access to a patient's veins and arteries, and in the event of having to resuscitate a patient, we could quickly rip or cut it off altogether.

Resigned, she began to undress in exaggerated slow motion, stalling for time. Sensing her extreme discomfort with my presence, I excused myself and left. Such a display of modesty was unusual in a woman as young as she, but I'd grown accustomed to the fact that few people were what they appeared to be or, at least, what I expected them to be.

When I returned, Mrs. Nelson was in bed, clutching the covers to her chin. Dominating the room was a strong, musty odor, one I knew I had smelled before, but I couldn't put my finger on what it was or where I had encountered it.

"Okay," I said as casually as possible, "what I want to do now is hook you up to the monitor, then take your blood pressure and listen to your lungs and heart before the doctor gets here."

With a terrified expression Mrs. Nelson looked about the room, as if searching for the fastest escape route. The look went straight to my heart, and without really thinking about it, I, too, found myself speaking to her as if she were a child.

"It's all right, nothing I'm going to do now will hurt you in any way. I'll explain what I'm doing in detail, and if I think something might be painful, I'll let you know in advance, okay?"

Mrs. Nelson nodded, and I grabbed a handful of the white electrode pads and continued my explanation in the same nursery schoolteacher voice.

"I'm going to put these sticky white pads on your chest, and then I'll snap a lead onto the outside of each one. That will help me see the pattern your heart makes on this screen right here next to your bed.''

Smiling, I draped the three monitor leads over her knees and pulled away the bed covers.

Left unfastened, the blue gown fell down, away from her chest, and immediately both of us froze in position. For a moment neither one of us breathed.

My heart beat wildly as I stared at what used to be the woman's left breast. The area was nothing more than an eroding mound of hardened black and gray tissue riddled with small spots of what appeared to be green mold. In the center, where the nipple should have been, was a two-inch hole from which brown pus oozed. It was a volcano of putrid flesh.

Mrs. Nelson inhaled sharply, and for an instant I thought I saw the muscles of her chest wall. The strong, musty smell rose to my nostrils, and my stomach churned. Automatically I cupped my own breast in my hand, as if to protect it from what I saw.

This was the source of the smell which lingered in the room: the odor of human flesh decomposing, one of the smells of death. I remembered where I had encountered it before; it had been the subtle odor which permeated the cancer ward of the hospital in Oakland where I'd trained with Miss Telmack and Tessie.

Glassy-eyed, Mrs. Nelson stared at me vacantly, until I saw a small flicker of realization that I had discovered her secret. She pulled the gown up over her chest.

A rush of emotions hit me all at once: pity, sadness, but mostly disbelief. Any shred of inward tranquillity I may have had was broken.

Scrambling to find some kind of emotional hold, I remembered the conversation between my father and me just after my graduation. With bravado, I'd been relating some of the horror stories I'd run into in the ER, hoping to shock him. Unmoved, he wisely assured me that as long as I worked in the medical field, even after I was sure I'd seen it all, I would still run into situations that would jolt me anew. His advice was first to have compassion, not only for the person but for myself, and, second, to use that compassion to guide any strength I could find within.

Not knowing what else to do, I listened to my father's voice and pulled to the surface all my strength.

"Mrs. Nelson, look at me please," I whispered.

As if being called from a trance, she turned her face toward me, looking tired and stubborn, like a child who doesn't want to stop playing at bedtime.

"Yes?" she answered vaguely.

"Mrs. Nelson, how long has your breast been like this?"

Mrs. Nelson looked down at the grossly disfigured breast as if she were seeing it for the first time. "Oh, that? That's just a bruise I got from working in the garden a few months ago."

My mind reeled. Incredulous, I repeated the word. "Bruise?"

Mrs. Nelson read my look and stuttered. "What I mean is that—that I—I bumped myself with a pair of long-handled shears last year while pruning roses, and the bruise kept getting bigger. I don't know why it hasn't gone away."

In all those months had she really not seen the horror in front of her eyes: her own body?

I remembered the large quantities of morphine given to the patients who carried the musty smell. "Do you mean to tell me you've had no pain?"

"No," Mrs. Nelson replied calmly, believing in her own answer. "No pain."

There was a long silence; then, abruptly, she spoke in a rapid, high-pitched voice. "It's so silly, really. I, well, I've been so . . . I mean, it's been hard for me to catch my breath lately, but it's just allergies. I'm quite allergic to summer grasses, you know, it's just that, it's just . . ."

Her voice trailed off as I caught her gaze and held it.

"Mrs. Nelson," I said quietly, "the tissue of your left breast is badly damaged. It's not just a bruise. It's much more serious."

Mrs. Nelson looked like a child being told some fantastic fairy tale. "It is?" she asked, her eyes full of wonder. Then, as if she'd caught herself in a foolish position, she stiffened.

"Well, whatever it is," she said, regaining composure, "I'd better be home by Thursday. I'm giving a dinner party for twenty people that evening, and I can't be bothered with this nonsense."

In emphasis, she patted her chest just once. A few seconds passed; then she started to cry without making a sound, coughed, and tried to catch her breath.

"Oh, please, can't they just give me some antibiotics and send me home if I promise to rest for a few days?"

She was pleading, and the pitifulness of the situation made me think of how many times I'd heard the same bargaining before, people desperately begging for health if they just did this or that or *anything*. The worst part of it was, it was almost always too late by the time they reached us.

"No," I answered finally. "You won't be home by Thursday. You may have to have some special intravenous drugs and some x-rays; you might be here for a while."

She looked lost and frightened, and a terrible sadness rushed into my chest. How much could I tell this woman? How much would be heard? Not much, I thought, at least not now.

I placed the electrodes and leads on Mrs. Nelson's chest, carefully avoiding the discolored tissue. Sitting her forward, I listened to her lungs. The air exchange was minimal.

In my mind I pictured the chest x-ray. It would be nothing but large white spots that translated as a tumor growing out of control.

I placed the drinking water next to the bed and saw her eyes fixed on the bedside monitor. The slightly irregular pattern moved across the screen.

"I will be out of here soon, though, won't I?" she asked, never taking her eyes off the monitor.

I was bound by policy not to say anything regarding what I thought the diagnosis would be until Dr. Peters talked with her. I'd already broken one rule by telling her the situation looked serious.

I turned my face away. "I don't know," I lied, "I'll get your husband now, before the doctor comes."

Mrs. Nelson reluctantly stopped staring at the monitor and asked, "Do you think you could bring me a pen and some paper? I want to make a list of things I have to do for the party on Thursday."

She caught my look and quickly added, "Just in case."

Just in case of what? I thought. *A miracle?*

In the waiting room Mr. Nelson looked relaxed as he perused the newspaper. His manner conveyed a feeling that life had been easy for him, as if no tragedy or sadness had ever touched him.

Smiling, he greeted me warmly.

As I sat on the edge of the chair opposite him, my immediate reaction surprised me; I felt a surge of resentment toward the man.

"Do you have any idea what is going on here?" I asked in a quiet but deliberate voice.

For a moment he said nothing, looking confused. Then: "Well, she seems a little short of breath, and—"

I cut him off sharply. "When did you last see your wife's breast?" I demanded. My voice wobbled, and I felt my face flush from the effort of keeping my temper in check.

"Oh, you mean that bruise? I saw that about eight months ago and told her I thought she should see a doctor about it, but like I said earlier, Sondra has a mind of her own. I guess we just let it slip by.

"We're pretty busy people. She's very active in community functions, you know." Mr. Nelson smiled broadly and added, "She'll be fine. You won't keep that girl down for long."

My anger swirled beyond the fringes of my control. *This was insane*, I thought; *no one could be that blind. . . .*

"Didn't you see that your wife's breast tissue was badly damaged, couldn't you smell that odor? I don't understand how you could just let something like that 'slip by' for so long."

I didn't realize I'd raised my voice to a shouting level until I noticed two people in the hallway had stopped to stare at me. I shut my mouth and touched my face. It was burning.

Mr. Nelson moved to the edge of his seat. His smile was gone, and he rubbed his forehead with the tip of his fingers.

"I—I don't know what to say. I just didn't think it was so bad. She's been so active. It's not as though she's been sick or anything. I haven't really seen the bruise since, uh—" He stopped speaking and looked at the floor, embarrassed. "You see, quite a few months ago," he said uncertainly, "she, uh, began having some problems sleeping at night and"—he shifted uncomfortably in his seat and lowered his voice—"uh, she moved out of our bedroom and into the guest room so she wouldn't keep me awake. She said it was her allergies.

"I just didn't think about it until she started looking so wornout all the time, and she was having more trouble breathing during the day.

"Once every so often I thought there might be more to it,

but we've been married for almost twenty years; phases like that come and go.''

Mr. Nelson acted as though that were the long and short of it.

"I'm planning a surprise second honeymoon trip as soon as she's out of here, an extended stay on the Mediterranean. I think that may snap her out of it.''

So that was how she managed to keep the truth successfully hidden from him. The last time he'd seen her breast, the tissue had probably just begun to discolor.

My anger slid into compassion, and a familiar internal tug of war commenced. It wasn't right to vent anger at this man; I had to be professional, but on the other hand, wasn't he an intelligent, educated person? Even if he had no idea of what was happening to his wife's breast, how could he have ignored the problem of her obviously failing health and let it "slip by" as if it were as bothersome an errand as returning overdue books to the library?

Mr. Nelson still seemed reluctant to face what I told him. "Come now, is this really that serious?" he asked.

The policy regarding giving out information again loomed before my eyes, but the rules had ceased to bother me at this point. What I'd seen gnawed at me, and I was furious with Mr. Nelson's denial.

"Serious?" I repeated, shaking. "The bruise you saw a few months ago has grown into something very serious. It could mean her life.''

From the way Mr. Nelson looked at me, I knew my medical opinion had little validity. In his mind I was only the nurse, the person who did the dirty work of emptying bedpans and dispensing medications. No matter how brilliantly I explained it, he would never hear the word *cancer*, not for her.

We both stood at the same time. It was an awkward moment; there was nothing more to say. Now there was only the matter of the woman's survival.

"Why don't you go in and stay with her now? I have things I have to do at the nurse's station. Dr. Peters will be here any minute.''

I cocked my head. "This might be a good time to talk honestly with each other, maybe pull together more than you have recently.''

In the room Mr. Nelson shyly smiled at his wife, but she averted her eyes and did not return the smile. There was a long silence while he fidgeted with the newspaper and she rolled the bed sheet between her fingers.

Perhaps left along, they would face the reality of the situation and talk to each other. Surely, they couldn't stay silent forever.

I went back to the desk, feeling exhausted, and glanced at the clock. It was 7:00 P.M. Only an hour had passed since the woman's admission. Glassy-eyed, I watched the monitor without really seeing it. I was surprised at myself; it wasn't like me to go so upset. A moment later the squeak of the back door roused me. Listening to the footsteps, I recognized the soft shuffle of Elias Peters.

The bearded young physician sat down heavily beside me, took off his glasses, and rested his head on his hand. For several minutes we both stared at the monitor bank in silence without moving. That made me a nervous; Elias was not the kind of man to stay still for more than a second.

Finally, I looked over at him. His face was pensive, tinged with discouragement.

"Elias, I don't get it," I said. "How could this happen?"

"I don't know, kid," he answered. "Never in my career . . . I mean, I've seen cancer in some of its ugliest forms, and I've also seen people try very hard not to believe they were ill, but never have I encountered denial like this before: the patient; the husband; everybody. She must have had friends who knew *something* was wrong." He sighed and leaned back in his chair, making it creak.

"From the look of her breast, my guess is the disease had been spreading for about two years, maybe longer. We can only guess at the dynamics that went on in her mind. I doubt we'll ever know the full story, but all in all, it's pretty amazing."

"What's her prognosis?" I asked.

Elias looked at me as if I were crazy, then ran a hand through his shaggy black hair. "*What* prognosis? The disease had probably metastasized everywhere.

"If she had come in even two months ago, we could initiated some agressive therapy, and she might have had a year or two left." Elias stood up. "Now it's just too late."

He went into Mrs. Nelson's room and pulled the curtain.

Trying to listen and not to listen at the same time, I caught a few words of his low, muffled voice. "When? . . . Too long . . . doesn't look good . . . why? . . ."

He returned to the desk, looking even more discouraged, and opened the chart. "Well, I told them," Elias whispered, slowly flipping through the various papers. "They didn't say a word. No questions. Nothing. They just sat there and looked at me like I was some kind of murderer."

"They'll have questions later, Elias. It takes awhile for news like that to sink in."

He looked up from the admission notes. "The problem is, Ec, even if they do want to talk with me later, what can I tell them?"

"You can tell them to prepare for death," I answered.

Over the remainder of the evening I saw an incredible change take place in Mrs. Nelson. For months she had managed to appear fairly healthy, fooling everyone around her. But now, after only a few hours of hospitalization, she deteriorated before my very eyes.

Her cardiac rhythm became erratic, and her shortness of breath was more pronounced. But the most incredible change was her overall appearance; she seemed to have aged twenty years. Her face sagged, and she paled to the point of grayness.

I'd seen the phenomenon before, though I had no explanation for it, at least none that would be acceptable in the very logical and scientific world of medicine. I believed it had something to do with the final defeat of the spirit.

Every comfort measure I tried to enforce, Mrs. Nelson resisted. She flatly refused the pain medication Elias had ordered and could be persuaded to use oxygen only with the condition she have full control of the green plastic nasal tubing it flowed through.

Denial continued to protect Mrs. Nelson while she was engrossed in watching television or making lists of things she had to do for Thursday. Whenever I tried to engage her in conversation, she would hedge my questions with monosyllabic answers and act perturbed until I reluctantly decided the best thing to do was just to leave her alone.

The frustration of not being able to help or comfort this

woman ate at me, and at midnight I clocked out, feeling as if I'd failed in some major way.

The following evening I refused to give in to my desire to check on Mrs. Nelson. I was afraid of finding she'd signed out against medical advice and gone home to prepare for her dinner party. Secretly I hoped working in ER might give me some excuse in the form of a chest pain or a congestive heart failure to visit CCU, but it just wasn't a coronary kind of night; instead we were having a run on abdominal pains and migraines.

The department was moderately hectic, although no one could pinpoint exactly why; it was Tuesday, the weather was neither hot nor rainy, the moon was not full, it wasn't near any holiday, and Brand X's ER was fully functional. By nine we'd seen twelve abdominal pains and seven migraines; that, we were sure, had to be a record of some kind.

At nine-thirty a stocky red-haired woman wearing a Burberry raincoat showed up at the registry desk and demanded a doctor come to her car to examine her ninety-year-old mother, who, she claimed, was too ill to walk.

Informed our doctors didn't see patients in the parking lot, the woman reluctantly registered her mother while Beth and I wheeled a gurney out to the car. Curled up in the back seat of a vintage Mercedes-Benz, the shriveled old woman was blind and extremely hard-of-hearing, unaware of any world outside her own. Her legs were so atrophied and contractured in a severe bent-at-the-knee position that nothing, save an act of God, or a stick of dynamite, could have moved them. Here, I thought, using Turk's phrase, was a real live bed potato.

As soon as we parked the old lady in the space of bed two, the daughter, pacing like a military man, flew into a rage.

"Where is the doctor?" she yelled. "No one is to touch my mother without the proper certificates."

Confused as to the woman's meaning, Beth and I gave her a blank look. "Everyone is seen in order here, ma'am," I said, "and anyone who touches your mother is properly licensed to perform whatever it is she's doing." I took the BP cuff from the wall and started wrapping it around the old lady's arm. "For instance, I'm the nurse, and I'm going to take your mother's blood pressure and pulse—"

The woman grabbed the back of my uniform and pulled me away from the gurney. "You are not a nurse; you are a liar. I want the doctor, or I shall call the newspapers and tell them about this slaughterhouse."

A hush was spreading over the room as several of the patients noticed a disturbance brewing and were straining to see who was doing all the yelling and why.

Dr. Mahoney came from the suture room, removing a pair of bloody gloves. "I'm Dr. Mahoney. Is there a problem here?" From the way she barely moved her lips, I knew her temper was brewing.

"My mother is ill. I want her seen by a doctor," the woman repeated.

"I *am* a doctor." Dr. Mahoney flushed. "What is the emergency that can't wait?"

Without warning the daughter roughly shoved Dr. Mahoney. "You're no doctor; you're a woman," she screamed shrilly. "I want a real doctor. No one goes near Mrs. Caballero without showing me credentials first. I have personally been given the names of all the qualified doctors by the CIA, so you can't fool me." She shook her fist close to Dr. Mahoney's face. "Let's see who has the power, you or the government."

Complete silence fell over the room.

Backing away, Dr. Mahoney stared at the woman in shocked understanding. Calmly she requested Mrs. Caballero's old records and told the clerk to call the security guard. As an afterthought, she instructed the candy striper to take the other patients out of the room.

Slowly, so as not to incite mass panic, all patients who could walk were taken to the lobby; the ones who couldn't were herded into the trauma and suture rooms, and the doors closed tightly behind them.

In what I felt was a daring display of bravery, Dr. Mahoney and I turned our backs on the daughter and skimmed the admission sheet from Mrs. Caballero's last admit, dated two years before. The note read like a feature article from the *National Enquirer*.

When Mrs. Caballero's only daughter, Evelyn, had called an electrical repairman to find the faulty wiring in the attic of her home, she hadn't bargained he'd also discover her aged mother locked in the hallway broom closet. For almost two years Evelyn had been secretly "guarding" her mother from the FBI, Russian spies, various viruses and bacteria, and nuclear fallout by keeping her in the small room, opening the door only to feed her and change her soiled linens.

Once removed from her daughter's home, Mrs. Caballero was placed in a convalescent center, and Evelyn, by order of the court, was enrolled in a psychiatric treatment program in lieu of being charged with elder abuse.

The head nurse at the convalescent home almost cried with relief as she filled in the rest of the story for us over the phone. Earlier in the day Evelyn had been allowed to take her mother for a stroll in a wheelchair to a neighborhood ice cream parlor. When she failed to return by noon, the police had been called and were presently in search of the abducted nonagenarian.

Beth picked up the red phone marked "Hot line," connecting her directly to the sheriff's office, while Dr. Mahoney and I again approached Evelyn, who was now making ferocious faces at us.

"I'm sorry, Evelyn," Dr. Mahoney said, "but your mother has to stay here with us for observation."

Evelyn laughed and snapped her fingers under Dr. Mahoney's nose. "Ha, like hell she does. I'm getting out of this two-bit dump and taking my mother with me. We'll see what the president of the United States has to say about this."

Unsuccessfully she fumbled with the lock on the side rails. As her frustration gained momentum, she tore at the metal bars, trying to get them down. "You can't take Mother away again," she shrieked. "She's mine."

Dr. Mahoney inched closer. "We've called the sheriff, Evelyn. Your mother needs to stay here with us, and you need to calm down."

"You can't do that. I'm a citizen; I have the freedom to report you to the newspapers. I'll have you arrested for impersonating a doctor; I'll report you to the radio stations—"

Mrs. Caballero, who had been quietly rocking herself, stopped and cocked an ear toward the commotion. "Eh, what's that you say, dear?"

I stepped in from the other side of the gurney to pat Mrs. Caballero's arm. "It's okay, nothing for you to worry about."

"Eh? What's that? Who're you?" Mrs. Caballero leaned in my direction.

"I'm the nurse, you're in the hospital, and—" I broke off as Evelyn's fist flew over the gurney and grazed the side of my head.

"If you don't get away from her, I'll kill you. I've got a gun in my purse that the president gave me, and he taught me how to use it." Evelyn fussed with her purse clasp, and from the corner of my eye I saw the clerk rapidly slide off his chair and crawl under his desk. Beth slipped into the trauma room, and one of the candy stripers crouched down and crawled into the suture room. I backed away toward the pelvic room, but Dr. Mahoney stood perfectly still, staring over the woman's shoulder.

Behind Evelyn, two sheriff's deputies appeared, and behind them, two men from crisis; trailing was the security guard. Fanning out, they came slowly toward her. Following Dr. Mahoney's gaze, Evelyn turned.

Instead of trying to run away, Evelyn laughed and ran toward the group, swinging her fists. She landed her first punch on the jaw of a surprised deputy, then kicked him square in the groin.

The ensuing scuffle lasted a good two minutes before the four remaining men were able to wrestle the woman to the floor, flip her onto her stomach, and handcuff her wrists to her ankles.

Beth, who'd been watching from the trauma room window, ran out to help Dr. Mahoney tend to the deputy, still doubled up in front of the clerk's desk.

Now aware of some major disruption, Mrs. Caballero called out, "What's going on over there?"

"It's okay, it's over now," I said.

Leaning over the edge of the side rails, the elderly woman clucked her tongue against her loose dentures. "Is it Evelyn? Is she fighting *again*?"

The three men, Dr. Mahoney, and I lifted the hysterical woman onto a gurney and covered her with a sheet. Rolling toward crisis, she assured us the president would not be pleased with the way things had turned out.

I picked up the purse, which had been kicked under the laundry cart, and out of curiosity opened it. Inside, under multitudes of pink Kleenex and packages of breath mints was a shiny black Saturday Night Special.

"Evelyn?" the old lady called. "Is that you, Evelyn?"

"Evelyn's all right, Mrs. Caballero," I said or, rather, yelled. "She's being taken care of down the hall, and we'll take care of you, too. Then you'll be able to go home."

The old woman pulled away from me and spit in my general direction. "Aw, fuck you!" she screamed. "I'm not staying in no goddamned hospital!"

Dr. Mahoney and I glanced at each other. "Like mother, like daughter," we said in unison.

Throwing back her head, Dr. Mahoney roared an infectious laugh that had a slightly insane ring to it. The clerk, Beth, the deputy, and I followed suit, adding the perfect, final touch of hysteria.

Wednesday was a day off, and although the incident from the night before provided a momentary distraction, Mrs. Nelson stayed in my mind, always hovering on the edge of my thoughts. I rarely thought about patients outside the hospital anymore, except when Simon begged for a gruesome bedtime story, but when I prepared for bed, I still carried Mrs. Nelson inside me.

At 4:00 A.M., during my usual rendezvous with nightmares and truths, my mysterious obsession with Mrs. Nelson was solved. I dreamed I was walking through a gallery of fine paintings and stopped before a Salvador Dali I'd never seen before. On closer inspection I saw a likeness of myself floating above an ethereal desert, my eyes lifted toward one of the artist's famous melted clocks. My breasts had been replaced by a window through which could be seen a grapefruit.

The dream jarred a memory I had long since buried out of shame. In my early twenties, during the time I was a secretary by day and a patchouli-reeking frequenter of City Lights bookstore by night, my well-ordered double life was threatened by the appearance of a small lump in my left breast. Like Mrs. Nelson, my fears grew and solidified into an impenetrable wall of denial. The obvious physical changes were invisible to me for some eighteen months until, during a routine exam, my doctor discovered what my mind had hidden;

the innocuous pea-size bump had grown into a mass the size of a tangerine.

I hadn't even been allowed to go home to get my toothbrush. Two hours later, as I lay between sanitized hospital sheets, a nursing student came to my room to shave a portion of my thigh, explaining it was routine; in case of a mastectomy, the skin from my thigh would provide the graft for my chest.

That afternoon, as I slowly crawled out from under the death-heavy blanket of anesthesia, I listened to someone retching close by as my gingerly exploring fingers informed me my whole chest was one large bandage. My pain receptors hinted at a burning sensation in my armpit.

Terror-struck, I found my voice and asked the recovery nurse if I still had my breast; she told me she didn't know and to go back to sleep.

Back in my room, three more nurses came to check on me at regular intervals and went away, each one unwilling to disclose what mystery lay underneath the dressings. At the sink next to my bed the broad-hipped cleaning lady wrung out her sponge over the acrid-smelling pail of suds and, with meticulous care, wiped away the day's buildup of hospital germs. She looked over at my mournful face and found the kindness to smile and say hello.

I clung to the smile and the low, gentle voice as if they were a life raft. In a torrent of stuttered sentences I explained my internal torture and begged for help. Wordlessly the kind woman put down her sponge and lifted the covers away from my legs. She laughed at my puzzled look and pointed to my leg; from her own study of common-sense medical wisdom, the woman knew if there was a bandage on the thigh, there was only one breast.

"It's okay, lady." She reassured me with a wide grin. "You gots em' both."

Thursday morning my first conscious thought was of Mrs. Nelson; I was resolved to reach out to her while there was still time. I'd tell her about my experience, trying to let her know she didn't have to feel alone or ashamed. I wanted to apologize to Mr. Nelson for my anger, tell him that it had all been projected.

At 2:45 P.M. I drove into the hospital parking lot with my speeches memorized and bounded up the stairs two at a time. Swinging open the acute side door, I sensed something was wrong immediately. The tension in the air was so high it felt like the inside of a circus tent while a performer balanced on a tightrope with no net below.

The bright red crash cart sat in the doorway of Mrs. Nelson's room. The overhead lights were turned up full, and at least six pairs of legs were visible from under the curtain surrounding the bed. From the monitor bank the continuous EKG strip rolled off the counter and onto the floor. I knelt and, through countless yards of paper, searched for the beginning.

The strip read like a story. At first, Mrs. Nelson's normal pattern slowed, then became slower still, then wider. Suddenly there was a change, and the slow, wide complexes melted into a wavy, crazy line resembling a child's scribble: ventricular fibrillation. Next came the large dark vertical line denoting the stylus jumping off the paper with the first defibrillation.

That was enough. I didn't need to see the rest. I left the paper on the floor and walked into Mrs. Nelson's room.

In the bright fluorescent light she looked ghastly, like one of the figures I'd seen in the House of Wax. Blood trickled from her mouth, and I noticed one of her arms hung loosely off the bed.

Although the hands of the nurse doing the chest massage were in the way, I caught a fleeting glimpse of the disfigurement. No miracle had happened; it hadn't disappeared.

The IV line coming from her left arm jiggled with every chest compression, causing the IV bottle to hit the metal pole it hung on in a steady, clanking rhythm. Unconsciously I began tapping my toe to the beat, realized what I was doing, and stopped.

Elias stood by the head of the bed, looking sad and tired. I watched him for a moment, then studied the face of every person in the room.

The respiratory therapist was pumping extra oxygen into the patient's lungs with the green plastic balloon while the laboratory technician concentrated on palpating the femoral artery with her fingers, trying to find the spot that would yield the most blood.

The pharmacist stood by the crash cart, drawing up syringes of various medications, then lining them up on the bedside table, each one carefully labeled so no mistakes could be made.

CCU nurses ran in and out of the room, bringing in supplies as they were needed. Lori, the supervising nurse, stood in the corner with pen and paper, recording every action, while Luce, with her back to the rest of the room, concentrated on the monitor, calling out the rhythms as they came over the screen.

No one was looking at Mrs. Nelson, the scared, dying woman.

I wondered if as healers we had forgotten that every body has a soul and a brain, that each patient is a person with a past, a lifetime lived?

The laboratory saw the patient in terms of how good the veins were, and the pharmacy saw a body as a certain number of kilograms for proper drug dosage calculation. Even the nurses saw the patient as a unit of work: acute, intermediate, or self-care. Who saw the patient as someone's mother or a loved husband or simply a valuable human being?

I looked at Sondra Nelson and imagined her laughing as she ran down a sunny beach. She was a woman who'd loved, laughed, hated, and cried; she had walked in the rain, eaten chocolate ice cream cones, comforted a friend in need, and ridden bicycles. She had done all those things. Didn't that make her kin to all of us standing over her?

From the corner of my eye I saw the intubation instruments on a small surgical stand. On the end of the tray was the long, straight steel blade which would force her tongue aside so her vocal cords could be visualized. Next to the blade lay the twelve-inch opaque white endotracheal tube. During the procedure the tube would be pushed to a point beyond her throat, just at the top of her lungs, and finally be connected to the respirator through an endless series of blue and clear plastic tubes.

The resuscitation stopped as a normal heart pattern smoothly slid across the monitor screen, and Mrs. Nelson again began to breathe spontaneously.

A desire to comfort her engulfed me, and I gently pushed my way to her side. Recognizing me, she started to cry and groped for my hand. The strength of her grip surprised me.

I bent down close to her face. "I've thought about you a lot the last two days," I said. "There was so much I wanted to tell you. I know how terrifying all this is, and I wish I could change it."

Her eyes widened and filled with tears. She shook her head back and forth several times as if to make everything disappear. Her breath was coming in gasps.

She gripped my hand as if she were holding on to life itself, weakly mouthing words I couldn't hear.

I leaned closer, my ear almost touching the woman's lips. The smell of old blood and vomit made my stomach turn, but I held my breath.

At first all I heard was the word *Thursday*. Then, listening with every bit of concentration I had, I heard the entire phrase she repeated over and over like a litany. "Home Thursday, home Thursday, home Thursday . . ."

Time stopped for us. The confusion in the room slid far away, and there was only silence. We saw no one except each other. Our hands gripped tighter, and our eyes steadfastly held each other's stare.

My brain seared with the thought that except for sheer luck, this living nightmare could, at one time, have been mine.

Two inches from her face I said simply, "It's okay now. You will be home today, Sondra Nelson. Today is Thursday, and you are going home, I promise."

The woman's grip relaxed, and her eyes closed. Tears began to roll down her pale cheeks. Transfixed, I watched one tear stop when it hit a small crust of blood, mix with it, then continue on until it dropped off her chin to the pillow. It created a small pink smear.

My speeches were no longer important. All of us had fears that we locked away from ourselves. For Sondra Nelson, her fear had gone out of control and clouded her mind from the reality of the cancer which would consume and eventually destroy her.

I leaned closer to her. "Sondra, I have to go to the nurse's station for a few minutes, but I'll be back. I am going to help you. Don't worry, I won't leave you alone for very long."

The beautiful hazel eyes stared into my face. In a cracked whisper she asked, "Promise?"

I gave her hand a squeeze. "Promise."

Elias followed me out of the room and motioned me over

to him. I could tell by the look on his face he was miserable.
He shook his head. "What do you think, should I intubate
her? If I do, she won't live but a day or two more. The cancer
has metastasized everywhere." Elias put his head against the
wall. "I just don't feel we've done anything for her, you
know, like if we don't do something, we've failed."

In the battle of dying there was often the divided dilemma
of how much pain was worth the struggle of keeping someone
alive for just one more day or one moment longer.

We could put death off for possibly two more days, keeping
her drugged just to the point of a semicoma. She would still
feel the respirator pushing air into her through the endotracheal tube, her hands would be restrained, and she would be
unable to speak, a mute prisoner of the fears locked inside
her. Eventually she would die during the chaotic ordeal of
the resuscitation procedures, just as Turk had.

On the other hand, we could make her comfortable; there
would be no invading tubes, no probing needles.

The facts made the choice clear. "It's time to let her go,
Elias," I said. "Don't put her through this anymore. It's the
best we can do."

After a moment Elias nodded in agreement. "Guess I'd
better talk to Mr. Nelson. He's the one who has to make the
final choice. It's not going to be so easy for him. The poor
guy is really coming apart at the seams. They both were so
totally unprepared for this."

Elias went to the waiting room, and I methodically cleaned
the nurse's station, pasting the various EKG strips on Mrs.
Nelson's chart, and filing away the laboratory result slips.

On the progress sheet Elias's scribbled note from the day
before caught my eye: "Patient and husband told of prognosis. Both beginning to relinquish their denial of the situation . . ."

I put down the chart and looked up. Mr. Nelson stood over
me. He looked years older, and when he spoke, I heard a
voice that was much lower than it had been only two days
ago.

"The doctor says she's going to die. I don't understand.
She said it was only a bruise. That's what she told me. Then,
somehow, there was—there was this . . . cancer."

He struggled not to be too loud. His shoulders hunched
forward, and one hand went to his face. "Why didn't she tell

me? Why wouldn't she let me help her? If only I had paid more attention, I—How could this happen? How could—"

The man started to cry with the full realization of the truth. He wiped the tears from each eye with his thumbs but kept his eyes downcast.

"I don't know what to do." Mr. Nelson's voice softly wavered. "I don't want her to suffer. I don't want her to die." He cleared his throat and looked at me with reddened eyes. "Isn't there anything else we can do?"

"No," I answered, feeling as if I were twisting the knife in his heart. "Not without causing unnecessary pain for her, and nothing that will stop death for very long."

I stood and put my arms around the man and held him until he stopped crying. He didn't fully realize it yet, but he was doing all there was left to be done; he was grieving.

Mr. Nelson and I walked to the entrance of his wife's cluttered room. In the center Mrs. Nelson lay moaning, rhythmically turning her head from side to side.

The day shift nurse was finishing up by medicating her with a small amount of morphine. I made a note of the time. It was 3:42 P.M.

Mr. Nelson stared at his wife, and his face was tired and pale. To no one he said softly, "God help me."

Elias quietly came up behind us and put his hand on Mr. Nelson's shoulder.

Without turning, Mr. Nelson whispered, "Okay. That's enough. No more pain. No more suffering. Just let me be alone with her now."

He had made his decision. It was a decision made from the deepest love one person could feel for another.

Immediately Elias cleared Mrs. Nelson's room. The crash cart was removed, and the harsh overhead lights were turned off. Only the intravenous medicine which kept the woman's rhythm stable was left hanging. The emergency was over; Mrs. Nelson could die without interference.

Mr. Nelson and I entered his wife's softly lit room. I went to the bedside monitor and turned it toward the wall, away from their view.

When I turned around, I was startled to see Mr. Nelson lying on the bed next to his wife, holding her. As her head rested on his shoulder, he spoke to her quietly, every so often kissing her hair or the tip of her ear. Too weak to speak, Mrs.

Nelson squeezed his hand now and then, as if it were some secret silent code.

I watched for a moment. From the well of emotional overload tears came to my eyes. Cancer, the master thief, had won again.

I found Elias sitting in the doctor's conference room, completing his notes on Mrs. Nelson.

Seeing my red eyes, he stood up and put his arms around my shoulders. Glad for the warmth of another who'd known the same lonely place, I let my head rest against his chest.

"Ah, kid, sometimes I think we're all in the wrong business," he whispered.

I sniffled in reply.

Elias slipped into his jacket and put away the chart. "It's so hard to be looking fate right in the eye and struggle to change something that just won't be changed," he said.

We gave each other small, sad smiles.

Elias opened the door to the unit. "Well, kid, I'm off to try again. Hang in there."

Right. Try again. That was all any one of us could do.

Three hours later, still in the arms of her husband, Mrs. Nelson ceased breathing. The sound of her husband's crying escaped from behind the glass door and etched itself in my memory.

On the monitor the heartbeat slowed, widened, and then melted into a single, straight line.

It was Thursday, and Mrs. Nelson was home.

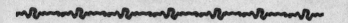

FOURTEEN

THAT SEPTEMBER was a month to remember in CCU. It was the month Jan achieved one of her life's goals and went to Italy. On top of that four more CCU senior staff nurses decided to take their vacations at the same time; everyone knew September was *always* the slowest month.

For twenty-five straight days not one CCU bed on either side of the unit was empty for more than an hour. The order of the day was to take just one more patient, one more admission, get everything done, but do it quickly and without appearing rushed or impatient in front of the patients.

We were pushed to the limit, working double shifts and extra weekends and coming in on our days off. Tempers ran high, but most of us quickly learned to take it all with good grace.

We survived by reminding ourselves and each other that it was okay to have only one pair of hands and legs per nurse. We did what we could, scrambling to cover the essentials of patient care. The pampering details, like back rubs, long talks, and hourly offerings of snacks, we saved for another time—another month perhaps.

In the midst of all the confusion Mrs. Mather repeatedly sighed and said she just didn't understand modern nurses.

Mrs. Mather was the wife of one of our patients, Charles Mather. Right from the first day of Mr. Mather's large posterior wall infarction to two days before his discharge, Mrs.

305

Mather went down in CCU history as setting more precedents than any family member to date.

I wasn't sure how much her having been a retired RN had to do with it, since it was a fact that medical professionals usually went an extra mile for their own kind; but Mrs. Mather got what she wanted, and what she wanted was to run Charles's show.

Mrs. Mather unofficially moved into CCU as a kind of honored permanent visitor. She was allowed to be present at any and all of Mr. Mather's procedures and examinations and was given license to read his chart at will. In the course of two days she took over most of his secondary nursing duties, while making it difficult for us to tend to the primary ones.

Mrs. Mather ate all her meals with her husband, slept next to his bed in a lounge chair, and used the staff shower and bathroom; nobody said anything about her hand laundry hung neatly in the conference room closet.

But try as we might, Mrs. Mather made it difficult for us to ignore her. Not to be bettered by the younger set, she never let go by any opportunity in which she could voice her opinion on our new techniques. When we gave Mr. Mather his medications, she had to check each pill or injection to make sure it was the right dose. In order to do a physical assessment on the man, we practically had to climb over her to get to him, and the lab was forced to listen to her lecture on exogenous infections every time he was stuck for blood.

Mrs. Mather wasn't really rude—she never raised her voice or used abusive language—but she had a way of watching every small move, clearing her throat loudly, and raising her eyebrows when she didn't agree with something we were doing. Our clever explanations made no difference, her counter explanations (often lengthy and tedious) clearly proved the old way was best.

Many of the nurses resented her interference and her untrusting attitude, but most of us shrugged it off, realizing the woman had a driving need (some thought of it as tenacity; others saw it as a deep-seated psychological problem) to be near her husband, proving her worth as wife and nurse.

My brief time with the Mathers came on the afternoon Charles was "bumped" from the acute side to make room for a twenty-eight-year-old code waiting in ER. After receiving a skeleton report from the charge nurse, I was assigned to pack Mr. Mather up, wheel him to bed nine, and add him to my flock of three other patients, it was hoped, all within ten minutes.

When I entered the acute room, Mrs. Mather was sitting on the side of Mr. Mather's bed, taking his pulse. Noticing my bright colored smock with its marsupial-like pockets, she stopped counting and stared.

"Hi, Mr. Mather, I've come with good news: You've been promoted to the intermediate side effective immediately."

Mr. Mather smiled, proud of the progress his body had made. "Well, it's about time I got some new walls to stare at. I hope to hell there's a bathroom in this new room; I'm tired of using that damned bedpan."

"Not only is there a bathroom you can use, but you also have privileges to be up in a chair for meals."

The creases between Mrs. Mather's eyes puckered. "Why weren't we told about this earlier? Whose orders are these?"

"Sorry, Mrs. Mather, but we need the bed quickly. There's a code in ER, and Dr. Cramer feels Mr. Mather is more than ready for the intermediate side."

The answer wasn't enough. "Don't you think he's being a little too hasty with this transfer?" Mrs. Mather asked. "It hasn't been a full week yet."

I noted a look of doubt veiling Mr. Mather's prideful expression and spoke quickly to restore the man's confidence.

"Oh, no, nowadays we move people right along . . . get them up and about as soon as possible. Your husband has done very well. As a matter of fact, he could have been transferred over yesterday."

"See Mother?" Mr. Mather chided. "Stop your worry." He glanced in my direction. "Will you please tell my wife to stop her worrying?"

I looked directly into Mrs. Mather's eyes. "Stop your worrying."

After a cursory two-minute physical exam in which Mrs. Mather behaved like a hard-to-move piece of furniture that was always in the way, I prepared Mr. Mather for transfer. Heaping the end of his bed with clothes, oxygen bottle, magazines, books, the portable monitor, his flow sheets, and the conspicuous blue urinal, I jockeyed it into position. An ache in the small of my back reminded me my spine was no longer made of indestructible rubber, my Gumby days having been over since the eighth grade.

Pulling back the curtains of the glass wall, I observed the rest of the unit. The overabundance of chaos in the other three rooms was obvious. Each of the patients was on a respirator, Dr. Morrison was inserting lines in the patient in bed two, and the other nurses, including the nurse who'd previously been assigned to Mr. Mather, had their hands full. I looked through the double doors to the intermediate side; call lights buzzed, phones rang, while nurses, float nurses, and the clerk ran in every direction.

I paged the orderly, only to find he was booked solid for the next two hours, not an uncommon state of affairs these days, since the administration had cut back on "unnecessary" expenditures by doing away with one of our two evening orderlies. The administrators insisted the position was a waste of good money; the nurses who depended on these men to help move heavy patients or keep dangerous ones under control had a different opinion. Our petitions asking for the reinstatement of the second orderly had been ignored to date.

Administration versus nurses was the name of the game, and in every hospital, big or small, it was always the same political hoopla. Administrators knew or cared little about the needs of the nurses, although they ultimately knew we were the backbone of the hospital.

I was still a rookie when I made the discovery that if all the nurses got together and walked out of the hospital, there wouldn't be a hospital anymore; it would simply be a flophouse for sick people and nothing more. Yet, year after year administrators came to the bargaining table, ready to argue our worth, pushing for pay cuts, decreases in benefits, fighting to ignore the cost of living while they enjoyed yearly salaries most of us couldn't even dream of. The fact that our salaries and benefits were less than grocery checkers' meant nothing; nurses were replaceable.

I looked back at the heavy bed, felt the ache in my back, and sighed, disgusted. Against my better judgment, I finally asked Mrs. Mather to help me steer.

We had got all the way to the door of Mr. Mather's new

room without a problem when Mrs. Mather stopped in her tracks.

"What's wrong?"

"There's another patient in this room," she whispered.

I glanced over my shoulder at Mr. Mastro, who was waving happily. "Charles and Vivian Mather, meet Arthur Mastro, your roommate."

Mr. Mather waved back, delighted. "Hiya, Art. Do you play gin rummy perchance . . . penny a point?"

Mr. Mastro nodded. "Forget the pennies, Charlie. I'll play you for shots of good bourbon, though."

Mr. Mastro and Mr. Mather laughed, recognizing they were kindred spirits; here was someone else in the same boat, someone with whom each could commiserate over the same tasteless hospital food and the same rules and regulations. They could support each other when they had minor setbacks, and more important, they could make each other laugh.

I was pleased; when two roommates got along well, it could turn a depressing, dismal time to a close sharing experience which often launched lifelong friendships. These patients healed faster and were less likely to have recurrent bouts of pain.

Mrs. Mather's scowling face came back into my frame of vision. "I want a private room," she said. "Charles needs peace and quiet to recuperate."

I opened my mouth to protest, but Mr. Mather spoke up for himself. "Don't be silly, Viv, this is fine," he said, then winked at Art. "Besides, Art and I need a night out with the boys."

I smiled reassuringly. "He's right, you know. It's really better for him to be a little distracted."

In silent retaliation Mrs. Mather would have nothing to do with helping me move the bed the rest of the way into the room.

Mr. Mather regained the rest of his health quickly, and by his third intermediate day he was walking the halls, anxiously looking forward to discharge. Despite looking a bit worse for wear, Mrs. Mather walked proudly at his side as living testament to the fact she had carried her husband through the valley of death.

* * *

Before I even pulled into the driveway that night, I could see all the cottage lights blazing through the cool September evening. Simon was spending the night at Patrick's, and the cats weren't clever enough to have figured out how to work the light switches. I'd been increasingly forgetful, but I was certain *I* hadn't left them on, at least not to the extent they were lighting up the creek.

I tiptoed onto the porch and softly knocked on my own front door. The smell of cooking garlic and basil came from inside, making my mouth water. It was a friendly smell, and besides, how many robbers or rapists cooked while they waited for their victims?

I opened the door and quietly went inside the warm, steamy hallway. Mooshie and Emelio greeted me by wrapping their tiny Burmese bodies in and around my feet, making it difficult for me to sneak into the living room.

I heard the clamor of dishes and pans being washed, then my wooden spoon hitting the edge of my largest cooking pot, the one I used for spaghetti sauce.

Peeking around the kitchen door, I sucked in my breath and let out a scream. "Janeeeeeeeeeey!"

Throwing the spoon in the air over her head, Janey screamed along with me. Through the laughter and hard hugs, fragments of our conversation were half-cried, half-squealed out.

"What are you doing here? Oh, my God . . . you look great. . . ."

"Wanted to surprise you. Oh, you look so good . . . oh . . ."

"Oh, God, you don't know how I've missed you. . . ."

"Yes! Yes, I do . . . me, too . . . letters aren't—"

"Aren't enough. I know. . . . How . . . when—"

"That nice landlady let me in. I just had to see you. Flew up on a moment's notice . . . got to go back tomorrow . . . made spaghetti . . . bought a bottle of sake for later. . . . Oh, God, it's so good to see you."

"Damn, Janey, I swear, I'm so happy I think I'm in my right mind!"

"Then thank God I'm here!"

"Oh, God, me, too!"

* * *

The night was lost and gone. Everything we wanted to tell each other about our lives was suddenly urgent; nothing could wait till morning. After the dishes had been washed and put away, we took a walk through the light rain toward the library, a good four-mile round trip.

Janey owned the first two miles with her funny running commentary on the joys and tribulations of being madly in love with and married to a doctor. "My life is everything I always wanted it to be now. Not only do I have a nice, healthy son and a great relationship with a wonderful man who loves me dearly, but I'm ready to embark on a new challenge: I've been accepted into law school!"

My jaw dropped. "Law school? Are you crazy? The law is so"—I tried to find a nice way to describe my experience with the law—"so bleeech! Since when did you want to be an attorney?"

"Ever since I was a kid and fell in love with Perry Mason. You know how I always liked to diagnose patients by putting together clues? That's where it came from. The mysterious nooks and crannies of law have always fascinated me." Janey got that faraway look. "It's—it's in my blood: Scotland Yard, Agatha Christie—"

"Inspector Clouseau?"

By the time we reached the library, the wind had come up. Taking momentary shelter in the doorway, Janey pulled two small cups and a corked serving bottle of warm sake from her jacket pocket. The powerful rice wine was enough to make the cold wind inconsequential.

I took the two miles back as mine. Tear- and laughter-studded stories of Jan and Simon and some of my more disastrous blind dates took up the first mile and a half. The last half mile I saved to give her bits of news I had heard about some of our instructors and classmates. Tessie had written and published a book about keeping oneself within a certain budget. The book was doing well enough that she was no longer teaching. Miss Telmack had moved to St. Paul or some such city to live with her sister, Mavis, and Mrs. Z. and Burl were still at Buchanan. Pearson, I'd heard tell, had blended into the woodwork and disappeared.

When I mentioned that P.J. had started beautician's school

less than a month after graduating and that she had worked ever since as a manicurist in Novato, we laughed until we had to sit down on a curb and wait while we steadied ourselves. The police stopped to make sure we weren't vagrants or escapees from some home for the mentally incompetent. I wasn't so sure we convinced them otherwise.

At the cottage we shed our wet shoes and socks, placing them close enough to the fire to steam. Pouring the last of the sake, we made ourselves comfortable and waited for dawn to arrive.

Spread out on the futon, Janey lay still as Emelio made a home under her chin. As if halfway through a thought, out of the blue, she said, "Ah, yes, that horrible profession that sucked us in like flies." She pulled herself up on her elbows.

"You know what really gets me? I keep remembering Tessie's speech about what an honorable and special profession nursing was. Then I remember all the shit we had to go through to get there, and I can't believe how much I hated being a nurse. It's a profession of malcontents; one or two years after you're in, you'll do anything to get out. I swear, everybody I meet is an ex-nurse: car washers, lawyers, bums, business execs—"

I roused and sat up, facing her. "Wait a second. Back up. Did you say 'hated' . . . as in past tense?"

Janey smiled. "Two glorious months ago. No more nursing, never again . . . never! Hubby is doing well in his new practice; there wasn't any reason for me to stay at something that was making me so crazy and miserable."

There was quiet while I took in the news and tried to figure out what I felt. "I envy you in a way, and I'm a little jealous. But mostly, I'm just glad to see you happy."

Janey came over to the window seat and put her arm around me briefly. "Oh, Ec, it's so great to be out in the world and feel almost normal. I couldn't take nursing anymore. It drained me of every ounce of self-respect and energy. I honestly don't know how you stay in it. Aren't you burned out yet?"

I threw another log in the fire and rearranged the embers. "I don't know. I'm not a quitter by nature. It's hard for me to let go of something I fought so hard for. I envy you, but I guess I'm also disappointed that you gave up, like you didn't try hard enough or something."

"Yeah, but, Ec, there's a difference between sticking with something you struggled for and getting rid of it when it's rotten and starts to make you sick."

I shrugged and turned my eyes to the fire. "I'm still getting too many rewards to quit. I try to ignore all the shit like the rules and regulations and the nursing administration and the doctors' power games. When it's just between me and the patient, it's still great, and I'm fine. I still get a lot of mileage out of touching people who need that kind of caring."

"But don't you ever get fed up? I mean, let's face it, there ain't a whole lot of respect or recognition that goes along with the job. You spent five years in college so you can be treated like a bedpan-wielding handmaiden with an I.Q. of 70? Not me!"

Janey's face was flushed with anger as she headed in the direction of the kitchen with our empty sake cups.

"I don't know, Janey. I see a patient walk out of the hospital when I know if it weren't for something a nurse did, that same patient would be carried out in an undertaker's truck. Right now that still means enough."

Janey came back from the kitchen, carrying an apple and an orange. "Okay, I won't mess with your ideals, but just don't go around thinking nurses who stick with it go out in five-star glory. Believe me, I've seen them: They quietly drop in their tracks when they're sixty-five, are given one-liners in the hospital newspapers, and that's the last you ever hear of them."

I smiled. "But I bet the people they took care of remember them."

Janey rolled her eyes. "Incurable optimist at heart . . . God help you!"

Touching base with Janey had infused me with enough new energy and inner smiles so that I got through the next few days of filling in on the day shift without feeling tired or cranky.

The only reason I was late for work on Friday was not a faulty alarm clock but that finding a sitter at six in the morning for a child who has just awakened with a runny nose and sore throat was close to impossible. After fifteen calls I finally deposited an uncharacteristically lethargic Simon on the next-door neighbor's couch with a gallon of orange juice and a two-quart saucepan full of chicken soup.

The unit was quiet, not the normal day shift level of noise and confusion. The night nurses weren't talking much to each other, rushing to finish up charting and get out. Morning report moved slowly, with a depressed feeling.

Between report on beds eight and nine I prodded Annie in the ribs. "What the hell's up?" I whispered. "Somebody die or something?"

She drew me close. "Mrs. Mather."

I smiled uncertainly, not quite sure how to decode her cryptic answer. "You mean, Mrs. Mather finally went home?"

Annie shook her head sadly. "No, she was found dead in the lounge chair next to Mr. Mather on five A.M. rounds."

"Oh, my God! How's Charles taking it?" I asked.

"Feeling responsible; he admitted that she had a long history of cardiac problems and that she'd been complaining of chest pain for two days but wouldn't do anything about it—swore him to secrecy. The poor guy's been having chest pain since it happened."

Posthumously Mrs. Mather had created yet another precedent.

I'd just finished having another one of my dove dreams and was beginning a dream that had something to do with a dog barking at Mrs. Mather in her lounge chair. At least, that's what I remembered as I drifted lazily back through the dark to sudden, complete wakefulness. A sharp sense of danger crowded out the hazy blue spots on the periphery of my vision, and my heart pumped hard enough to make the cat move off my chest.

The dog barked again and then again in a rhythm faster than my breathing. I listened harder. A bark? No.

Bolting out of bed, I covered the hallway to Simon's room in three strides and turned on the overhead light. On his knees next to his bed Simon stared with glassy eyes out the window. "Can't"—he coughed, making the barking sound—"can't . . . breathe, Mama." With every inspiration he lifted his shoulders to assist his diaphragm. The hollow whistling of his wheezing made him sound as if he had a squeak toy in his chest. I lifted him easily and carried him into the bathroom. Against my arms, his skin was hot, and his pajamas were soaked through with sweat.

With the shower going full blast, we sat on the edge of the toilet, waiting until steam billowed down from the ceiling, like falling clouds. Familiar with the procedure, Simon eagerly stuck his head through the opening of the curtains and tried to breathe in the warm mist. Breathe and pull . . . one . . . two . . . three . . . breathe and pull . . . one . . . two . . . three; it was the rhythm of an asthmatic's nightmare.

The steam did its job, and Simon coughed until he practically vomited. In a moment of pride he showed me the results—a greenish mucus plug, uglier than sin. I stared at it and made a face. "Yeeechhh!" Simon tried to laugh, but he was breathing too fast and couldn't even manage a smile.

I acted calm, patted my son on the back, and left him in the bathroom. Like a madwoman, I frantically searched his room for the magic inhaler and found it under a pile of laundry in the corner. Regaining composure, I sauntered back into the bathroom, smiling.

Simon had his head inside the shower and was trying to cry without making any noise. He gave it up when he realized it took too much energy. He grabbed the inhaler out of my hand and desperately sucked in the medicated vapor. Two puffs, I reminded him gently, only two puffs. Not paying attention, he continued to pull on the inhaler until I had to pry it away from him. He looked at me with the pleading expression of a starving child. My heart wrenched, and I considered letting him have as much as he wanted but knew it could hurt him more than help.

Instant relief did not come, as it had so many times before. Both of us were surprised, then disappointed, then frightened. There was something different about this attack that was truly ominous; it made both the mother and the nurse in me uncertain and hesitant.

The hot water turned warm, then cool, and the steam clouds turned to water drops, which ran down our faces and the walls. I watched Simon's intercostal muscles suck in and out, working hard to keep him breathing.

"Can't . . . can't . . . oh, my God . . . please."

Shocked by his words, I looked into my son's face and saw the essence of a child's fear.

Trembling, I drew up a small dose of epinephrine and injected him. Ten minutes passed, then twenty, and there was no response. I injected another small dose and waited, certain it would begin to open the airways. Trying to rush the minutes, I dressed myself and put a light cotton robe over Simon. Passing the hall mirror, I saw our images: he with his head on my shoulder, pale and shaking from the adrenaline; me pale and worried. Simon was patting my back as if to comfort us both.

Ten minutes later my nurse side slapped me to my senses, and I called the doctors' exchange. It was 5:15. At 5:21 I pulled into the empty parking lot of the pediatrician's office. After getting out of the car, I lifted Simon into my arms and discovered he did not have the strength to hold on. I pulled back to look at him in the new morning light. His color was dusky, and his nostrils were chalk white and flared. I hesitated, then, holding him to me, walked around the front of the car, headed for the street; if I saw a police car, I would flag it down.

I stepped off the sidewalk, and I heard Simon gasp once and sob, "Mama, please help me. I'm going to die."

I was running for the car when Dr. De Laney pulled into the lot next to us. Seeing Simon's color, she rolled down her window.

"Oh, my God! Go straight for the hospital; it'll be faster than paramedics; don't stop for signs."

Strapping us both in and jamming the horn, I watched between Simon and the road: *chest moving . . . watch out for the yellow VW . . . vacant stare . . . second red light . . . run it . . . my son is blue . . . where the hell are the cops when you need them? . . .* Simon's eyes closed, and I had driven nine miles in less than seven minutes.

In an extremely irregular move Dr. De Laney and I ran with Simon directly to pediatric ICU and put him in the first unoccupied bed we saw. After tearing off his robe, I held his head, counting the number of breaths, trying to hear if there was any movement of air. Both night nurses entered the room and looked questioningly at Dr. De Laney. "Status asthmaticus," she said.

Within fifteen seconds the page system belched. "Respiratory, PICU, STAT. Dr. Branzburg, PICU STAT!"

My mind whirred, and I felt as if I were in a nightmare.

This was my child here . . . right now. This was happening to Simon, not to some stranger in ER. Look, look closely.

A nurse who seemed familiar tried to take me away from the bed, away from Simon, and I screamed at her. "This is my *son*, goddammit. Don't you dare try to move me out of here."

Dr. De Laney pulled me away and sat me in a chair twenty feet away from the bed. "There isn't enough room in there," she said sternly. "Give us space. Don't try to be a nurse now; it won't work." And she was gone.

A girl from registry shyly approached me and adjusted her clipboard. "Name of the patient?"

"Simon Heron . . . one *r*."

"Middle name?"

"Day . . . d-a-y."

"Address?"

"Address?" I couldn't remember my address. I knew it was Mill Valley, California, but I couldn't remember the street, let alone the number. I knew the cottage was pink.

"That's okay; we'll get to that later. How about your phone number?"

I bit my lip and tried to envision the numbers written in runny blue ink on the front of my phone. "Ah, let's see . . . three, three, eight . . . no, wait, uh, three, eight—unh-unh, that's not it either . . . I can't seem to remember right now . . . I don't know what's wrong with me."

The girl was looking at me sadly, yet I detected a small strain of impatience.

"How about a birth date?"

I knew it was December. Simon had been a December baby. I could even see the doctor who had delivered him and the wonderful nurse with the English accent who had helped; I could remember that but, for the life of me, not the date.

The girl smiled apologetically and casually took my purse. "It's okay. I know you're upset. No problem." She went directly for the small leather case at the bottom and pulled out my insurance card. I watched her, thinking of all the people I'd seen come into ER rattled to the point of not remembering anything beyond their own names. I'd never believed before that they couldn't really remember.

I recognized the respirator tech who was so good with the patients in CCU run in to join the crowd forming around

Simon. In a brief moment I saw a mottled hand with the dirty fingernails of a typical ten-year-old. I flashed to Amy's hand and shook my head to get rid of the thought.

Inching my chair along the wall, I stopped when I was about ten feet from the bed; if I stayed in my seat and didn't yell again, they wouldn't make me go back. I bit the back of my hand to remind myself and tried to see as much as I could.

One of the nurses tied off Simon's arm and palpated the back of his wrist for a vein. Taking the angiocath, she stuck him, swore, pulled out the needle, opened a new one, repeated the process, and failed again. I'd just started to get out of my chair when Dr. De Laney took over and probed for Simon's antecubital. Backing into the chair, I bit my hand harder, still watching as the lab tech did a deep arterial stick, searching for a gusher. The blood came back so dark that someone questioned whether it was really arterial. Simon had not flinched at any of the needle sticks, and I wondered if he was unconscious or just too weak to react.

Hands and arms stretched over Simon again, and the monitor screen flickered then from a faint shadow, came up brighter to show a heart rate of 170. How long could a child's heart beat at that rate without problems? I couldn't remember, and didn't want to.

Dr. Branzburg, the only pediatric pulmonary specialist in the house, walked through the room. Half rising out of my chair again, I almost screamed at him. What the hell was he doing walking as if this were a Sunday stroll? *Run, you son of a bitch, run! This is my child that's in trouble—mine!*

I could see the man recognized me as a CCU nurse, was puzzled for a split second as to why I was in PICU in my street clothes, but didn't make the connection. He walked right by me and into Simon's room.

Dr. De Laney didn't even look up. "Hi, Vince. This is a ten-year-old with a history of asthma. Had a cold for a day or two, last night became febrile and coughed up a couple of mucus plugs. Steam, metaproterenol inhaler, two doses of epi—nothing. Trying to get a line here for some aminophylline. If I can't, I may have to do a cutdown, he's constricted as hell."

Dr. Branzburg hastily listened to Simon's lungs and stood just as the nurse came in and handed him a slip with the blood gases. "His oxygen level is forty-eight, and his carbon dioxide level is sixty on room air," he said, scowling. He rubbed his eyes, took a deep breath, and let it out in a stream of orders. "Okay, let's get this kid a nebulizer with Alupent stat, and when the line gets established, have an aminophylline drip ready and some Solu-Medrol."

The man from respiratory started the nebulizer, the respiratory treatment which forced medicated mist deep into the lungs and dilated the constricted air passages. More people seemed to be in the room now, although I wasn't quite sure who they were. One of the nurses moved away from the bed to pick up a roll of tape, and for a second I had a clear line of vision of the right half of Simon's body. He wasn't moving or responding to the confusion around him. His lungs looked as if they were expanding more than before, but I couldn't trust my judgment; he still looked dusky.

Dr. De Laney whooped. "I got it! I'm in! I'm in! Give me that aminophylline line, quick!"

There were a few stray laughs and sighs of relief. Then the monitor went out of rhythm for a second, and all eyes went to the screen: PVCs . . .

I caught the glances between the people in the room and the fleeting, subtle panic that crossed their faces.

"Okay, folks, let's get going here," said Dr. Branzburg, sailing on his adrenaline rush. "This kid's pooping out. If we don't get him going here pretty soon, we're going to have to intubate—if we can. Somebody get the crash cart and have it ready. Why the hell did the parents wait so goddamned long to get him—"

One of the nurses elbowed him in the ribs and said something in a low tone. Shocked, he turned around to look at me, then turned his back. I heard him growl under his breath, "Why the hell didn't somebody tell me, for Christ's sake?"

My mind's whirring now wobbled, and I felt myself losing control. Intubation, like all those other people with the suctioning and the ugly tube all the way down and the spasms . . . Simon? No, unh-unh. Somebody has this all wrong. Not my kid—not my—

A hot knife of panic and guilt stabbed through my brain. Did he say I'd waited too long? I'd done something to hurt Simon? Was I the cause of this?

I started to stand up and move toward the room and stumbled over my feet. One of the nurses whipped around and pointed at me with a look that could have felled trees. "Get back on that chair!"

Numbed with pain, I kept walking toward Simon. Why couldn't I see my own child? I wanted to see him for a second just to touch him once, only once. . . .

"Get her out of here!" I heard somebody say. I thought it was Dr. Branzburg's voice, but it could have been anyone.

An arm slipped securely, tightly, around my shoulders, and I let myself be guided out of the room. I wasn't sure how my feet were because I no longer felt anything physical. At the door I looked back once and saw Simon, the most special little person, my child, my friend, engulfed by a horde of distantly familiar people in lab coats and blue scrubs.

I was sitting on a couch and someone was holding both my hands. Out of the corner of my eye I saw a Buchanan College insignia patch on the sleeve of the someone, a nursing student, a young girl.

"It's all right, Mrs. Heron. They'll do everything they can."

How do you know that? I've used that line, too, but nobody really knows if it's going to be okay. It's something we say to make the relatives feel better. I promise, if you let Simon live, I will never use it again; it's not right to set people up.

The girl was silent, and I wondered for a second if I'd spoken aloud; then my mind wandered back to the place of pain.

Could there be brain damage from lack of oxygen? . . . Could there? Of course, Nurse, you know that.

But—but—the mother side speaks—not to my son . . .

Yes, to your son. Why do you think your child is immune? Because you are a nurse?

I cleared my mind and tried to think. Had she said his blood gas was only 48? How long could a child—

From around the corner I heard someone shout for another line, and the feeling of confusion swelled. I headed back toward the main room on two stilts made of flesh and bone, but the nursing student blocked my way.

"Let me go! I want to know what's happening to my son." I frantically tried to go around her but saw her worriedly look over her shoulder for help and felt sorry for her. I let her pull me back to the waiting room.

"Mrs. Heron, it's okay. Please let's go sit down. Your son will be okay."

I know better than to believe you. Do you think I don't know what's going on in there?

"Concentrate on something else," she said. "There's nothing you can do in there."

I know that. I know there is nothing I can do, and that is the worst of the pain.

I turned and focused on the girl. She was blond, not very pretty, and nervous. There was a sleep wrinkle still on her left cheek; it looked like a scar. "You're second year?" My voice sounded like a warped record playing far away. I felt like throwing up. Bending over, I put my head in my hands and rocked back and forth.

Please, please make him well. Please, please . . .

The girl rocked with me. "Yes, I'm just starting second year."

Poor thing, she can't think of anything else to say, but did you when you were with Amy's mother?

"What's your name?"

"Penny."

"Talk to me, Penny, tell me about nursing school."

Take my mind away from this awful place. Make my son be well. Don't let him die.

"Oh, it's hard. Our instructors are nice, though—really fair."

She said something about the instructors? Tessie met Simon once, said he looked like a happy and whole child, said he— Oh please, God, I'll do anything, I'll do everything.

"So next rotation I go to Oakland and do my surgical intensive care rotation. . . ."

Oakland? I knew a boy in Oakland who died. His name was Richard Wilson. I failed him, too; I waited too long then, too.

"I want to work in a pediatric clinic, somewhere near the ocean. . . ."

I continued to rock back and forth, hoping for some relief from the pain.

Simon and I share a love of the ocean, of music, of . . . so many things. We are so alike, but that shouldn't surprise me.

We've raised each other, haven't we? We are more like friends than mother and son—always have been. Oh, Jesus, Buddha, Muhammad . . . hello? Anybody listening? Please help my son, my friend.

I tried again to concentrate on the girl's voice, which faded in and out like an old car radio when you're traveling over the mountains.

". . . so the field is wide open. There's so many nurses who can't deal with children who . . ."

Die? Did she mean to say die? Death. I am always surrounded by death, and now it has come to pay me back for all I have stolen from it. Not my child—do you hear me, you fucking son of a bitch! Get away from my child.

A hot panic-pain choked me, and I remembered how the Eastern religions preached about embracing a moment until it exhausted itself. I threw myself into the pain, then backed away instantly, allowing myself to be distracted by a voice.

". . . it's the best stethoscope I've ever had . . ."

I turned my head. The stethoscope was red. I remembered being as old as Simon and coming out of anesthesia. The nurse's hands were tipped with red nail polish. In my confusion I thought they were drops of my blood and got hysterical. But Simon was so much braver than I. Did he know? Was he aware of what was happening to him?

I was still rocking when the body next to mine rose and another, heavier body took its place. The strong smell of a man's perspiration filled my nose. I heard a man's voice and felt a hand on the small of my back. Someone had come to tell me the truth.

"Echo?"

I stopped rocking.

Is the voice a yes or a no?

"Echo?"

I couldn't move, not even to nod.

Concentrate. It's only a dream, you'll see. . . .

But why am I so afraid? Please, God. Please, God . . .

"Echo, your son is okay. We broke through. He's a lucky boy . . . getting ready to intubate when he started responding to . . . bronchitis with asthma . . . went too far . . . status asthmaticus . . . PVCs resolved with the correction of acidosis . . . intravenous aminophylline, Solu-Medrol, erythromycin, Alupent nebulizer treatment . . ."

What is he saying? Speak to me like I'm a normal person. I don't understand all this medical lingo stuff. Aminophylline? Solu-Medrol? Those are drugs, but what are they for? Wait—drugs are for the living. Simon is alive? Is he saying Simon is okay?

I opened my eyes and saw the pediatric ICU waiting room. The rug was mauve, and I saw feet dressed in a pair of brown men's shoes, the kind with the little holes in a swirl design— wing tips?

My neck and back felt stiff, but I sat up and looked into the man's eyes. Dr. Branzburg had brown eyes and very bushy eyebrows. The fuzzy, faraway feeling started to fade. This had to be reality: eyebrows like that happened only in reality.

"What did you say?" My voice stuck to the sides of my tongue, like peanut butter.

"Simon is going to be okay. Of course, we'll need you to stay with him. He needs a good CCU nurse to keep an eye on his monitor for overnight." Dr. Branzburg smiled and patted me on the shoulder. "You shouldn't have waited so long. Next time, if he doesn't improve right away with the epi, call me or Dr. De Laney, or just bring him to ER."

I nodded, feeling horrified and ashamed of myself. What had I been thinking of? Simon could have died because of my inability to act.

Dr. Branzburg stood up. I followed suit; but my knees gave out, and I fell back onto the couch. I tried again, and the man reached out to support me. On an impulse I put my arms around him and hugged. "Thank you" was all I could manage to say. Dr. Branzburg was embarrassed, laughed, and patted my back nervously.

Suddenly Pat was there, pale and speechless, out of breath. He was wearing pajama tops over a pair of sweat pants. His white socks were inside out, and there were little threads sticking out everywhere. His rubber thongs were barely staying on his feet.

I smiled. "He's okay now." I was aware it sounded as if I were referring to a skinned knee.

Pat sank to the couch and started to cry. "The nurse called . . . she said he was serious . . . I thought he was—"

His tears and the sound of his sobs pushed the fuzzy curtains back from my brain, and I relived everything from the barking dog dream to this moment. I sat down next to my son's father and in compassion for him, for myself, wept.

Moments later we went into the room where Simon lay sleeping, exhausted from his battle. There was a green oxygen mask covering most of his face except his eyes, and I touched his arm for a final reality check. He was warm.

His coloring was good, and his heart rate was still in the 150 range.

Probably from the aminophylline drip and/or the Alupent nebulizer. I'll have to check with Joe to see how long his little heart can handle this. Not that I don't trust Branzburg, but—

He was covered with sweat. Patrick knelt next to the bed and stared at Simon's arm where an IV was running into one of the veins in the back of his wrist.

Erythromycin? I'd better look that up in the PDR or ask George, the pharmacist; he'll know if there's something better on the market.

Patrick looked up to ask, "Can I touch his hand? Will it hurt anything?"

I shook my head. "You can even hold it if you want to. Just don't bend his wrist."

My nurse side was awake and smiling.

The next morning I left Simon's bedside long enough to call the nursing office to explain why I wouldn't be in to work evening shift.

"Are you ill?" The question was cold and unfeeling.

"No, *I'm* not, but my son, Simon, is in the PICU. See, yesterday, he—"

"Then we can't put you on sick call just because your son is ill, Mrs. Heron. We'll have to—"

The stinging vinegarlike bile came to my throat. "You don't seem to understand what I've told you. My son almost died yesterday. He is in intensive care. I need to be with him."

The icy voice cut me off. "That doesn't warrant a sick call, Mrs. Heron. We'll have to put you down as refusing to come in. Now I'll have to get someone from registry to replace you. I'll have to—"

I stopped listening and hung up.

* * *

Soon there wasn't enough space to keep all the gifts that were crowding Simon out of his bed; it was Christmas in September.

Hour to hour he improved, growing strong enough to demand a Coke, then to drink the whole thing down in a matter of seconds and burp loudly. When I told him he was the king of eructators, he laughed until he wheezed, in love with the sound of the word, saying it over and over, amusing himself by stressing various syllables.

When he was moved to the regular pediatric ward, I actually heard myself say, "Don't you think Dr. Branzburg is being just a little hasty? Simon hasn't been here for even a full forty-eight hours!" Silently I begged Mrs. Mather's forgiveness.

The pediatric nurses proceeded to spoil my son, and I was happily jealous. I kept my nurse side out of sight and under control as much as I could, knowing (Thank you, Mrs. Mather) how intimidating it could be to be scrutinized while you were trying to work.

Two nurses seemed to be assigned to Simon consistently. On the evening shift it was a middle-aged Filipino woman named Rosa who possessed a divine power and a kind spirit— the signs of a true master at working from the heart. Something about her drew people in; whether it was the easy smile or the genuine interest she generated, everyone wanted to be near her.

The woman touched naturally; her bed baths and back rubs were a ballet of the hands. Her clever methods of giving children their medications made them eager to receive whatever pills or liquids she held in the medicine tray.

At noon every day Simon began asking, "Where's Rosa? How long till she's here?" and I found I was as anxious for her calming, joyous presence as he, especially after a day shift with Ruth.

It was a fact of life that some nurses are better than others, but we all agreed that Ruth had missed her calling as a worker in a noodle factory. I knew by her angry sighs and impatient "Excuse me's" that she resented the way I watched her like a hawk whenever she was near Simon—but the woman *did* bear watching.

She never touched or spoke to her patients unless it was absolutely necessary, and when she did, she was abrasive.

She was sloppy about the care she gave; baths were neglected, meds were always given late, and when she changed
IV dressings, her aseptic techniques were so poor I couldn't
watch. On Simon's second day I broke from the ranks and
files of nurses long enough to insist the woman never set foot
in my son's room again.

   I returned to work on Simon's third hospital day, extremely
conscious of all I did and said around my patients. I imagined
them to be my father, or one of my brothers, or Janey or Jan.
The small things I never had had time for anymore, like using
a softer voice or listening for just a few more minutes, were
important again. I'd make the extra effort for as long as I
could remember what it had been like on the other side. I
hoped I could make it last.

FIFTEEN

HE WAS CLOSE BY, the indiscriminate gatherer of souls. Like other nurses who'd seen too much of him, I'd developed the special vision which enabled me to recognize him the very moment he appeared. He'd been held at bay for four years, since the night Jan and I sat on Four Corners, listening to golden oldies. Jan had managed to outsmart him, fighting valiantly, but this time he'd come in earnest to collect what was due him and left his calling card.

Gaunt and jaundiced, Jan's body had not kept in step with her spirit; physical limitations now began to surface and interfere with her life. A simple sore throat had turned into an ulceration which plagued her, not only because of the constant nagging pain but because now her normal diet was to be replaced with cold high-protein milk shakes and soft foods. Giving up her beloved corn chips was, as silly as it seemed, a crushing blow.

Frequent waves of nausea and increasing shortness of breath slowed her, but she would not stop until her sense of perfection was satisfied in every detail. Going with her desire to touch base one last time with all she believed in and lived for, she ignored her deteriorating health and constantly assigned herself to patient care, taking the sickest, most acute patients.

I'd watch her move about a patient's room, turning him, adjusting machines, running for drugs and supplies, and finding ingenious ways to hide her handicap from everyone. Graceful as a dancer, she would pivot and dip to check some nonexistent problem under the bed and, once out of sight, gasp noiselessly for air. On the way to the linen cart she'd step into the bathroom, quietly vomit, spray her throat, wipe the perspiration from her face, and emerge smiling, right as rain.

"I know I've functioned better," she said one night as we sorted through a mile-long EKG strip from a code, "but I just can't give up. This is my life line; the minute I stop, I'm dead."

To most of the nurses who worked with her, she seemed only quieter, sometimes short-tempered, but, all in all, more dedicated to the profession than ever. To those of us who loved her, her subtle withdrawal from us exactly coordinated and balanced with the approach of death; it was a dance to prepare us for her final absence. She was so set in her course that no one was more surprised than Jan when life gave her a final chance at the best it had and she fell in love.

The man involved was a childhood friend, who, on a whim, looked her up one day. Slowly the friendship was renewed, changed pitch, and exploded into a love affair of passion and joy.

Jan radiated with a new grace and a rich maturity which seemed to round her out and complete her. In the back of everyone's mind was the hope that her new strength would buy her time, keep the reaper at bay. But Jan, in her practical wisdom, surprised us again by ending the affair three months after it had begun.

"I let it go too far," she said. "I got so caught up in it I lost sight of what was fair to him. I couldn't let us both go on, dreaming dreams that won't happen. I don't trust myself. I want it too much."

"Come on, Jan," I argued, "every person who loves risks being hurt. It's the dance that matters, not the sore feet at midnight. Let yourself soar. Just once, let go of the safety bar."

Jan shook her head. "I couldn't do that to him. I love him too much to have him go through the ugliness at the end."

"Stop being so damned protective of everybody," I snapped angrily. "You rob him of being able to give you something valuable. It isn't like you've kept secrets from him, Jan. He knows what he's in for; for that matter, we all do, and it hasn't stopped any of us from hanging around."

Jan lowered her eyes and said nothing.

I took a deep breath and let it out slowly, envious of how simple she made it seem to act on what she felt was the right thing, but Jan was a woman of rare qualities. So many women, it seemed, were afflicted with mental blindness the minute it came to the men in their lives and the loving of them.

I sought Jan's gaze. "I'd understand why you're doing this if he's made you unhappy, but . . . ."

Jan looked at me fully. "Please," she said softly, "I may not be right, but try to respect me in this . . . it's the way I've chosen to go."

My head rested in the protective crook of my arm while I tried to block out the stabbing pain behind my right eye and concentrate on simple thoughts. ER had been moderately busy; but it was still early, and the rain promised more business in forms ranging from fender bender whiplash to indoor recreational mishaps.

The stress-related headache, which rarely left me these days, escalated to nausea-producing proportions after we'd failed to resuscitate an eighty-two-year-old man who'd intentionally rolled his wheelchair off a cliff. I'd hoped it might go away during the hour I got to rest in the quiet room while trying to help the wife through her guilt, but it didn't; it only became worse.

The onslaught of ingrown toenails and lacerations kept us busy but not crazy; each of us had been able to eat dinner sitting down.

It was about 7:00 P.M., and Dr. Menowitz had just come on duty to relieve Dr. Kin when his booming voice suddenly exploded in the main room. "For chrissake, why do I have to put up with this crap every single time I'm here?"

I smiled, hearing the familiar whine. It had been several months shy of a year since the last time I'd worked with the man, and I was pleased at the prospect of seeing him again.

My appreciation of Dr. Menowitz had been fully and irrevocably developed during the 3:00 to 6:00 A.M. stretch of an 11:00 P.M. to 7:00 A.M. shift I'd worked six months before. In an effort to stay awake or at least to remain aware enough to listen for the radio, I decided to do spring cleaning. Raiding the housekeeper's closet for a dust mop and a spray

bottle of cleaning fluid, I dusted ceilings and walls, then
wiped down cabinets and countertops. While rearranging one
overgrown pile of scrap paper, I found a pad of paper covered
with Dr. Menowitz's handwriting.

The first bit of writing which caught my eye read:

> When winter comes again,
> wrapped in pearl gray rain,
> the child I failed to save
> will run before me,
> splashing through puddles
> in a yellow slicker,
> and I will remember every detail
> of his small face.

Forsaking mop and dust rags, I unashamedly pried, devour-
ing pages of lines which gave black-inked invitation to consider the beauty of one physician's soul. I was sick to death
of the amount of backbiting that went on about him and kept
the discovery as one of my secrets, smug in the idea that I
knew an aspect of him few others would have believed existed.

In reply to Dr. Menowitz, Judy, the ER nurse trainee, in-
quired timidly, "What is it, Dr. Menowitz? Can I help you
find something?"

"The nose instruments—they're all mixed in with the eye
things, goddamm it to hell. Where's the nasopharyngeal mirror?"

"Here, is this what you're looking for, Dr. Menowitz?"
The nurse was almost whispering, afraid to disturb the lid
lightly covering the man's temper.

"Tell me," he said in the irritated, exasperated voice he
could do so well, "does this look like something I'd use to
look into a nose? If there's a brain in that thing sitting on
your shoulders, please, just for me, try to use it."

I smiled and, opening my left eye, peeked out in the direction of the clerk's desk. Judy, on the verge of tears, angrily
picked up a chart and ran off to the lobby. The clerk was busy
filing old lab reports, and Gus was hunched over, trying to
hear the paramedic call through the static on the radio. She
wrote down the report as it came through in bits and pieces.

Dr. Menowitz stalked past the partition, muttering under

his breath, unlocked the cabinet labeled with a piece of adhesive tape reading: "SACRED INSTRUMENTS—KEEP OUT UNDER PENALTY OF BEING TORTURED WITH A COLD SPECULUM," and searched for the nasopharyngeal mirror.

"So, how's the poetry-writing-in-a-one-room-log-cabin-in-the-woods-dream coming along, ranger?" I asked.

Dr. Menowitz turned around, smiling. "Hey there! I haven't seen you since the last time I saw you."

"Yeah, me either," I said dryly. I picked up my head, and the blue and white spots blocked out patches of my vision. "Seems every time I work either you're on vacation or you've just worked the opposite shift. However, I do know your reputation as the monster doctor who leaves a trail of dead or screaming nurse bodies behind him is still going strong."

Dr. Menowitz laughed, pulled out the long steel instrument, and stood up. "But can't you tell I'm more mellow? I haven't bitten anyone in a long time."

"What are you writing these days?" I asked.

Dr. Menowitz adopted a guilty look. "Not too much lately, lazy slug that I am. Every once in a while I get revved up and romance the typewriter for several days, then throw most of it out or have a big fire. Sometimes I actually submit what I consider my better things, get rejection slips, then proceed on to insecurity, depression, writer's block, and finally heavy suicidal threats—you know, the normal writer's sickness."

"And yourself? You look like you're studying to be an anorexia major."

I got up quickly, lost my balance, regained it, and walked to the sink, speaking rapidly. "Naw, I'm fine. This is my running weight; I've been doing a lot of hard runs; if I were any heavier, I'd be waddling up those trails." I forced a laugh and turned away. "You're seeing the headache I've had for two days, plus my ulcer's been yelling at me. A little Tylenol, a little Tagamet, and I'll call you in the morning, Doctor."

Dr. Menowitz looked doubtful. "Nope, that's not the look of a headache, not unless you're growing a brain tumor in there. You look really different from the last time I saw you. To be honest, you look like plague and famine warmed over. Why don't you go see Dr. Schupbach?"

I quickly declined his suggestion as Gus came back from the life line radio, waving the paramedic report slip.

"What's up, Gussie?" I asked, glad to get off the subject of my health.

"Thirty-six-year-old female was found semiconscious at home by the husband, who admits she's been doing lots of cocaine lately. He says she went through two grams by herself today and about an hour ago was so coked up she had a seizure, fell down, and hit her head. She was okay at first. Then she got pretty dopey, and he hasn't been able to wake her up.

"She has no past history of seizures, and the paramedic says she's not responding verbally but opens her eyes once in a while. She's tachy at one-ten, BP is one-thirty over ninety, and pupils are equal and reactive. There's some ecchymotic areas on her face and arms, and she's got a laceration to the forehead. Right now she's breathing okay, and they've established a line of five percent dextrose and water at a keep-open rate, given Narcan, dextrose, and drawn a red top for us. There was no response with the Narcan or dextrose, and ETA is less than five."

I noticed that as soon as Gus mentioned cocaine, both Judy's and Dr. Menowitz's attitudes changed from concern to disgust. Dr. Menowitz raised his hand. "Pfffff! Goddamned cokeheads—what the hell do they expect when they're dropping like flies out there from this crap?"

Gus shrugged. "I agree on that one. When youse play, youse got to pay." She handed me the report. "Since you like dealing with the OD and suicide types so much, I thought you wouldn't mind taking her. I'm just not up for any druggies tonight."

In the trauma room I turned on the lights and took the cover off the crash cart. I'd just warned ICU of a possible OD admission when the pneumatic door hissed and Tina and Roy, two paramedics from Rescue Unit 71, came into the trauma room, rolling the gurney between them. They both were somber and moved a little more quickly than I would have expected on a simple drug OD. The woman on the gurney appeared younger than thirty-six, and that surprised me; most heavy cocaine abusers seldom looked quite as healthy as she did. Her nails and hair looked as if she'd just stepped out of a styling salon, and her outfit was of the trendy "bright pastels and sloppy cotton" style. She was the typical California yuppie with a bent for expensive drugs—not an uncommon profile considering the wealth of the county.

One of her eyes was blackened and swollen shut, and there was a reddish purple welt on her cheek, one on her neck, and a laceration that looked more than a few hours old on her forehead. I touched the welt on her face and looked at Tina.

"Yeah, I know," she said, aware of what I was thinking. "Some fall, huh?" She handed me the yellow copy of the paramedic report. The woman's name was Maureen Gerhett.

I did a quick set of vitals, and Tina and Roy filled me in on the details of the scene. "Just as we were loading her up, the cops arrived, and you should have seen the husband's face."

"Yeah," said Roy, "the husband was real quick to change his story. Right away he said she'd fallen earlier in the day during a struggle when he tried to get the coke away from her. He said she got right up and was acting normal until just before he called us, but he couldn't say why he didn't notice the gash on her forehead."

"The guy was just a little too charming for my blood," said Tina. "There was something really weird going on there, like when the cops asked him to show them where she fell, you could just see him come unglued. He was hopping all over the place."

The systematic procedure of assessing the woman took place without any further discussion. After pulling her onto the gurney, I took a set of vitals while Dr. Menowitz quickly examined her pupils, listened to her chest, and ordered bloods to be drawn. Lab appeared, did its job, and I was left alone with her, all within the space of five minutes.

I wrote her vitals on a graphic sheet and removed her shoes. Every so often she moaned and seemed to strain at trying to be fully awake. She moved little, except for spasmodic jerks of her arms.

When I slipped off her socks and pants, I could see she was bone covered with a little muscle and flesh. Her belly was sunken, surrounded by the lower ribs, hip and pelvic bones; it was like looking into a smooth flesh-colored bowl with a belly button at the bottom. What immediately grabbed my attention were the numerous new and old bruises that spotted her thighs and calves and the fact that all the toes on her right foot appeared to have been crushed.

"Maureen? Maureen, you in there?"

Through the slit of her eyelids two green specks slid by and disappeared. One arm, the arm with the IV, lifted and aimlessly flailed at the ceiling. Catching it, I taped it to the gurney and started undoing the buttons of her blouse.

Before I realized what was happening, a large white spot blocked out half my vision, and I felt a floating, dizzy sensation. Blinking rapidly, I lurched to one side and eased myself onto the rolling stool. The light-headed feeling was replaced with a down-to-earth wave of nausea.

I focused on the young woman. She'd become dusky in the last few moments. Watching her chest carefully, I could see her breaths becoming more shallow. Hurriedly I turned the oxygen flowmeter up to eight liters and cut away the lavender blouse.

Scratches and huge black and yellow bruises, plus several sets of teeth marks, decorated her shoulders and chest. Covering her upper left arm was one large purple welt, and on her right arm there was a set of four bruises that resembled finger marks.

I stood up and stepped back, unable to take my eyes off the sight.

"Hey!" I shouted in the tone of voice I knew got instant attention. "This lady's going down the tubes." Dr. Menowitz ran into the room. "She's not breathing well," I whispered, and turned away.

Dr. Menowitz didn't move for a moment as he stared at the marked body with interest. "Looks like somebody's been using her as a punching bag for a long time," he said, fitting the otoscope with the proper earpiece. "When you get a second, take a look at her old records." Turning her head, he pulled her hair back and pointed to clear fluid dripping from her ear. "Look at this, Echo. I'll bet you this lady has a basilar skull fracture with an epidural hematoma."

Dr. Menowitz listened to her chest again, then called for a respiratory tech, and ordered a ventilator to be set up in the scanner. I took out the intubation tray and placed it next to him.

"Get the husband on the phone, would you?" asked Dr. Menowitz. "I need to speak with him directly."

By the time I found the number, Dr. Menowitz had Maureen Gerhett intubated and respiratory was bagging her until the scanner was ready.

Using the trauma room phone, Dr. Menowitz punched in the number and waited, staring at the woman. He covered the mouthpiece and spoke to Gus, who was now aware there was more going on than just a drug OD. "Let's get a complete blood work up, some clotting studies, and put a catheter—" He broke off and turned his back to the room. "Yes. Ah, Mr. Gerhett? I'm Dr. Menowitz, the emergency doctor at Redwoods Memorial, and I believe we have your wife here . . . Maureen Gerhett?" There was a pause and then: "Uhhuh, well, that's fine, but what I want to know is what happened."

There was another, longer silence.

"Uh-huh, and when did you say she fell? . . . uh-huh, I also understand you told the police you struggled with her or something? . . . Uh-huh. Well, Mr. Gerhett, judging from the number of bruises on your wife's body and the fact that she has a fractured skull, I'd say there was more than a simple fall involved. Would you know anything about how she might have sustained the rest of these injuries? . . . Uh-huh . . . sure . . . sure. So you say she was walking and talking after you pushed her? . . . Did the dishes?. . . . conscious until when?" Dr. Menowitz covered his eyes for a second and then shook his head. "Yeah, right. Are the police officers still there with you? Would you put one of them on the line?"

Dr. Menowitz covered the mouthpiece. "You will not believe what this guy—" He broke off and said, "Hi. This is Dr. Menowitz. I think you should know this woman isn't doing well at all. From what I can see, she's been beaten up pretty badly."

Dr. Menowitz stared at the wall, nodding. "Sure . . . Sure. . . . What? . . . Yeah, well, that sure would fit with what I'm looking at here. . . . Sure. . . . Okay." He hung up and turned to me. "The police said they found a hole in one of the walls that has some blood and strands of hair on it. The husband says he thinks that might be where she hit her head when she 'fell.' "

At the clerk's desk I went through the old records. Maureen Gerhett had made seventeen ER visits in two and one-half years. I started with the last visit and went on down through the pile: "Pt. states fell down stairs—diagnosis, dislocated shoulder and multiple bruises. . . . Pt. states hit head on open cabinet door—diagnosis, concussion. . . . Pt. states laceration over right eye caused by exploding glass jar. . . . Pt. states nose broken when bookshelf fell on her—diagnosis, fractured nasal bones and mandible. . . . Pt. states fell down slippery stairs—diagnosis, fracture of left clavicle and right wrist."

Page after page of injuries, page after page of the lies I had come to know so well.

I left the room and walked outside for a break. Perched on the metal railing, I watched the drizzle for a few seconds and closed my eyes. In a slow rhythm I breathed deeply, trying to clear my mind with the smell of the rain. Instead, ugly mental pictures of the woman on the gurney and an image of myself in the mirror made me snap my eyes open.

A girl with black and green striped hair shyly sidled up to me, biting a black-lacquered fingernail. The dangling purple and white plastic earrings matched her boots. " 'Scuse me, but do you work in there?" She pointed to the ER door.

I nodded.

"Did they bring Maureen Gerhett in yet?"

"Yeah," I answered, folding my arms across my chest for warmth. "Do you know her?"

The girl looked around as if she feared she were being watched. "I live in the condo next to hers. I just wanted to know how she's doing; she looked totally wrecked when they took her out. Is she going to die?"

"I don't know, maybe," I answered, secretly dismayed at my lack of tact. "Do you know what happened?"

The girl ignored my question. "Is Scotty in there with her, or did the cops take him in?"

"Who's Scotty?" I asked.

"Her old man. I mean, he's a rad dude basically, and I think Maureen really loves him, you know; but I mean, he loses it sometimes. . . . Been worse lately. Last time he blew, she was out to lunch for a whole day. I told her to cool out for a while, but she's really devoted to the dude, you know?

"Like I told her to go to one of those groups for women who get beat by their old men, but she said he'd kill her if he found out. I think me and her mother are the only ones who know about him hittin' her."

She got up and started paring her nails with her teeth again, looking around nervously for possible attackers. "Like, I hope she's okay, you know. She's a very cool lady."

"If she isn't okay," I said, wearily getting up to go back into the pit, "I hope you think she's cool enough to put old 'rad dude' Scotty behind bars."

At eleven a detective came into the department, asking for the nurse who had taken care of Maureen when she first came in. After leading me into the now clean and quiet trauma room, he asked several questions about her appearance on arrival and had me sign a report saying I'd attended her.

"By the way, do you know where her blouse is?" he asked. "We've looked all over for it."

"I threw it away. I had to cut it off when she started to go down the tubes. It's in the garbage."

Gus and I searched the debris holding area and found the blouse on top of the third bag we opened. Carefully the detective put the blouse in a plastic bag, labeled it, and put it in a larger bag holding the rest of her clothes.

"Why do you need this stuff?" Gus asked.

"Evidence," he said solemnly. "This is a homicide case now. Mrs. Gerhett just expired, and the husband's been placed under arrest for murder."

There but for the grace of God, go I. . . .

I went to the back and packed up my jacket and purse. Gus looked up from a stack of charts that needed to be checked and watched me gather my things. From the way she was smiling, I knew she thought I was joking around. "Hey, sister, where the hell you think you going? You got thirty minutes of this hellhole left—"

"Home," I said, heading toward the door. "I need to go home."

Behind me there was silence, then the scraping of a chair. Gus whispered, "Jeez, I don't know . . ." Dr. Menowitz called to me, but I couldn't answer. At the end of the black runner Gus stopped me by grabbing my arm, and I winced in pain.

"What is it, Echo? What's wrong?"

"I don't feel well. I need to go home, that's all." My head was exploding, and I felt as if I were going to vomit.

"Want to talk? Let's go to the quiet room and let Judy fight it out with Mort over the patients."

I put my hand to my face. "No, Gus, I want to go home. I'm tired."

"Was it that girl tonight?"

I nodded.

"Did you know her or something?"

I nodded again. "In a way."

"Shit!" Gus cried. "Why the hell didn't you say something? I could have taken her. God, that makes me feel terrible."

"It's not that, Gus. I really don't feel well. I need to go home."

Gus put her arms around me and squeezed. In my ear she whispered, "You're not very happy lately, are you?"

I shook my head; the constriction of my throat was getting painful. It had been so long since I'd had the loving touch of another human being, and it hurt to be reminded of the warmth it could generate. "I gotta go—"

"No, wait. The change in you over the last few months has been like white to black. Do you know I haven't seen you smile in—"

"Gus, please . . . I can't. I really can't . . ." I dashed for the door.

Gus didn't try to stop me but called out, "I'm here for you . . . anytime. There are a lot of people who care for you. Call me at home night or day if you decide you can talk."

Without turning, I lifted my hand and waved to let her know I'd heard her and appreciated the offer. Inside, I knew I needed the caring, but didn't know how to let myself take it.

Sitting in my car, I watched the rain make shadow lace on my hands and arms. The blue and white spots crept into my vision again, and I started the motor, not sure of where to go. I drove without awareness, relying on luck to steer the car. In the last few months I'd become accustomed to living in a state of anguish and depression, but tonight there was an added component of fear.

The large shingled house on the hill came into view, and I slowed the car to a crawl, gripping the steering wheel just to hold on. My guts cramped again, and I tried to breathe more slowly; my legs and arms were shaking from nerves.

No more, I thought. *Not after tonight.*

In a state of numb panic I drove past the driveway and for once headed in the direction of my pink cottage. A few moments later I faced myself in the hallway mirror.

I stared at the image of a woman with hollow eyes I did not know. I tried to recognize her as she stood before me now, but in my memory search I remembered other images. There was the tired but eager nursing student rushing out the door to the hospital at 5:00 A.M., and the graduating Nightingale, and the mama making funny faces with her curly-haired son—laughing, like a normal person.

I tried to remember how it felt behind each of the images. I'd been happy then, hadn't I? I was a good person then . . . wasn't I?

I slipped my uniform off my shoulders and counted the ugly bruises that lined my arms and chest. Hugging myself, I fell to my knees and cried.

The whirlwind beginning had been so passionate, and the poison so insidious, I was hooked before I knew it. He was the golden Adonis with the sought-after face, the man-child who needed me desperately, the lover of my dreams, the charming recluse playing in the public eye, being photographed, filmed, and then, like a shooting star, mysteriously disappearing. His private life was enchanting; I was drawn by his wild dreams and brilliant thoughts, feeling I was truly, passionately in love for the first time.

He saw me immediately as the healer, the rescuer sent from heaven to save him from himself. Flattered, I slipped into the role of omnipotent nurse, eager and determined to cure the ills of a narcissistic man unable to love; I, and only I, would be capable of loving this man, who, under the handsome and understanding veneer, hated all women.

Isolating ourselves, he put off agents, refused or canceled jobs, while I rarely took call at the hospital and brought Simon to Patrick's more frequently. It was time to live and be a little selfish, I rationalized, ignoring the looks in my friends' eyes as I dropped them one by one.

For six exciting months we ignored reality, playing like

rebellious children in the sprawling shingled house, making love under a fort of goosedown quilts, or walking along beaches engrossed in long discussions about Chinese fairy tales and life. We interrupted ourselves only long enough to stock the cooler with cartons of lemon yogurt and go off on long journeys in pursuit of beautiful sunsets.

But the sunsets were not to be found, for as the fantasy world of our existence drifted in front of the sun, the cracks began to show and the rescuer became the victim.

He was a master at the game of power and manipulation, and his way of living was the only way. If I wanted to play, it had to be in his court and by his rules; anything else was inferior.

Lies and contradictions began to surface, but he cleverly, guiltlessly explained them away until I no longer knew what was truth and what wasn't. Perhaps I really was as insecure as he assured me I was, although the tiny voice of reason that I'd kept in reserve kicked and screamed every time I conceded.

When the lies became bolder and his explanations less convincing, the drama escalated yet again with jabs into my shoulder to accentuate a point or a shove to show the seriousness of his frustration. I don't remember when the first real punch came, or the first bloody nose, perhaps because I was more stunned by the mental and verbal abuse behind it. Echoes of my mother's tapes played back but with his voice: My hair was too long; my clothes were out of style; I wasn't bright enough, not worthy enough. The private screenings led to public humiliation, with distorted projections of me cast as a liar, a manipulator, a slut . . . just like *his* mother.

To cure me of my "selfish nature," he punished me by withholding not only lovemaking but simple affection like holding hands or hugging. To gain him back, I closed my eyes to his frequent infidelities trying even harder to be the perfect mirror of what he wanted to be seen as: the perfect man.

Somehow, when I wasn't feeling so miserable, or desperately endeavoring to hold onto my illusive rainbow, I made a little time for Simon and Jan, who could only guess at what was happening.

Feeling abandoned, Simon broke through his unhappiness every so often with moments of patience and wisdom. He would put his arms around me, his heart full of compassion, and say, "Look, Mom, you gotta dump this guy; he's just not good for you."

Jan never met the man but hated him, saying he'd drained me of my soul.

When the craziness of the relationship seriously shook the foundations of my sanity, I followed my survival instincts and left. But each time, the man begging at my window never failed to win me over with promises of new beginnings. My ego could always be readily convinced I was indeed the "pivotal woman," the only human being he'd ever loved, and I, above all, had the power to make him see the error of his ways and change him—though, of course, nothing ever changed.

The murder of Maureen Gerhett shook me awake and led me away from the man in the shingled house but not from the addiction. Without maps to guide me, I plodded through the hell of the failed romantic rescuer seeking an escape from the depression smothering me. Confused, sick with recriminations, I turned away from myself and headed blindly through the dark.

S I X T E E N

It was April and colorful signs of new life surrounded us; it seemed an ironic yet perfect time for a memorial service. A warm spring breeze curled the edge of the paper I was reading, and for a moment I lost my place. Embarrassed, I stopped and looked into the faces of Jan's audience. Pale, tear-streaked, and tired, everyone showed the loss. A young black man from the lab wept openly, staring at the ground. A woman from housekeeping bowed her head and slipped an arm around his waist.

This is not happening, I thought. *She is going to walk up behind me, pull my hair, and laugh. I am going to wake up now.*

No one tugged at my hair, and no one laughed. I waited for a moment, then, despite the pressing feeling of unreality, found my place and continued:

> We've lost the gentle dark-haired lady,
> and the empty space cannot be filled.
>
> I remember
> her graceful body, moving
> like a small tree,
> thin and dancing,
> and the elegant hands
> tending to the sick,
> quick and smooth like tiny fish.
>
> Where is the gentle dark-haired lady?

Delighted by life, looking for the best of it,
wanting to see it all.
The lady who loved
yellow roses, blue sapphires—
did she ever know how beautiful she was?

Where is the gentle dark-haired lady?
The fighter without resentment,
determined to be well,
ignoring the flight of time
always running at her side.

The beautiful dark-haired lady
lives within us all.

The hospital gardener lowered the small Japanese plum tree into the ground and waited for each of us to throw a handful of dirt over the roots; it was the gesture of closure.

People dispersed silently while the gardener finished preparing for the final planting. I listened to the sound of the metal shovel digging into the soft earth and reflected on our last few conversations.

On Friday afternoon she'd called. As soon as I said hello, she'd given me the news, since there was no lead-in that would have made it easier to hear.

"They told me today I'm terminal. The treatments aren't helping anymore. I have two to four weeks to get everything together." Jan stopped, too out of breath to continue.

I sat down on the edge of the window seat, studying the dust rag in my hand. Closing my mouth, I rubbed lemon-oil circles into the arm of the rocking chair.

Jan waited with me, mentally holding my hand. Moments passed, and she broke the silence. "I've got so much to do, I don't know where to start: laundry; canceling appointments and credit cards; writing down last wishes. I'm tired just thinking about it." There was another pause. "Monday the doctor said she'd call to let me know if there's even one tiny chance left."

I was suddenly alert. "You mean, there might be a mistake or something?"

"Don't get your hopes up. She said it was ninety-nine point nine percent certain, but she was going to have the lab run through the tests one more time just to make sure."

"Look, why don't I come over? Maybe I could help with the laundry . . . if I promise not to make fun of your holey underwear?"

"Nope, but I'll call you every day, twice a day with detailed progress reports on what's happening." I heard the resolve and knew she was fatigued, but I argued anyway. Losing someone I loved, knowing there was nothing I could do, made me want to hold on for dear life.

"Why won't you let me help you? I want to be near you . . . please, Jan?"

Jan's breathing was labored, but she patiently forced out her answer. "Not tonight, I'm too tired. You and Simon can spend the night on Wednesday. We'll have a pajama party."

"You mean, I have to wait till Wednesday? What's the matter, your social director overbook you this week?"

"What can I say?" Jan said, starting to laugh. "I didn't think I'd be going on tour so soon. I've got a lot to do before I can have fun. This dying business involves some work, you know. By Wednedsay I'll be able to relax. We can have dinner, maybe go to a movie. Simon can have all the Coca-Cola and popcorn he wants, you can have a little wine, and I'll have a few shots of my Brompton Cocktail."

"Hmmmm, it's sounding a little better, but are you absolutely positive there's nothing I can do for you?"

"Yeah, there is, come to think of it. Just keep being you."

Saturday her voice had a new, excited ring.

"Wow! I cannot believe how emotional I am. By my third business call everybody I talked to offered to do something for me." She stopped to catch her breath, and I realized she was crying. "The bookkeeper at my dentist's office said she'd bring me one of her special protein shakes, and the manager in one of the credit card offices told me how it was for him when his son died of Hodgkin's; he offered to drop off a bedside table he never used. I mean, I don't even *know* these people! I don't think it's pity, but why else would people be having this reaction? Where is it coming from?"

"Oh, I think it's people's need to help; that, mixed with the fact that you're such a gentle soul. You generate caring and concern in people. I hope you'll finally learn how to allow yourself to accept a helping hand when it's offered."

Jan was weeping, trying to speak and catch her breath. "You know, I'm actually . . . beginning to look forward . . . to this."

A minute or so passed, and I heard her breath quicken, this time with laughter. "God, I'm so lucky. No more dentists; no more waiting in line at the bank; no more laundry or ironing; no more nights spent worrying over the pacemaker clinic . . ." Jan's voice trailed off, and I wondered if her thoughts had turned to all the things she'd miss.

On Sunday morning she sounded amused. "I was just thinking," she said. "Can you imagine if the doctor called me tomorrow and told me I still had time left? I'd be so embarrassed. I'd have to call everybody and say, 'Hey, guys, only kidding . . . just testing . . . ha-ha.' I think I'm going to have to go ahead and die now that I've told everybody."

On Monday the call came: Jan had no more chances left.

I tried to find a place for my eyes to rest. Her hands and arms were skeletal, and her face was so hollow it looked misshapen. The pale yellow blouse she wore accentuated the jaundice but set off the beautiful dark eyes. They alone told the true story of who lived inside the wasted body.

"Promise me you won't let anyone take me to the hospital or make any attempts at resuscitation." There was desperation in her voice.

Nodding, I pulled her to me, hugging gently, afraid of breaking bones.

"And if things get to where I can't control them myself, you must promise to . . . help me. Let me die with some pride. Do you understand what I mean?"

"Yes," I answered, unwilling to let go of her, not wanting to open my eyes. "Yes."

"You know I would do the same for you," she said.

"I know."

"Now, promise me once more. It's really important."

I pulled back and held her hands. The dying so needed promises; it was really the only thing they left behind that was still truly theirs. "I promise, because if I didn't, you'd come back to haunt me."

Jan gave a weak smile and let out a gust of air through her nostrils; it was a weak version of laughter. "I'm coming back to haunt you anyway, so don't base your promise on that," she said firmly.

I rested my head briefly on her shoulder. "Okay, then I promise because I love you, and I'm going to miss you so much I can't stand to think about it."

Jan's hands were trembling. I watched them, then closed my eyes, trying not to think of them.

"I love you, too." She patted my arm. "Do you know, you are the best friend I ever had? You always make me laugh."

"Are you *really* okay with all this?" I asked later, while we made arrangements for the following evening. I was suspicious of her calmness.

Jan leaned against the door for support and held my arm. "You want to know something? I look back on my life and I think, *Hey, I was really lucky. I fought like hell and won a lot of years. I got to make a difference in the world, and nobody can ever say I didn't give it everything I had.* So, in answer to your question, yes, I'm *really* okay. I'm more than that: I'm at peace."

Wednesday was one of those warm and velvety blue-skied days made to give people a wide-open chance at achieving joy. I was in the garden trying to decide what flowers to cut for Jan when the phone rang. Instinctively I knew what the caller had to say.

Jan Tobin, the young woman who'd eased the pain and deaths of so many, had died peacefully in her sleep.

From the window seat I watched Simon skateboard down the driveway, anxiously looking for my car. He was having a hard time trusting me. Although it had been months since the end of my obsessive love affair, he still seemed surprised to find me home.

Reading the atmosphere, he sat down next to me with an air of caution. I put my arms around him and kissed the top of his head. The platinum curls were long since gone, but the sweet sweat smell remained. "Jan died this morning, in her sleep."

Simon's body jerked, and he pulled away from my arms.

"I know it's sooner than we thought, but it was just what she wanted to happen," I assured him. "No hospitals or any of that garbage. When I saw her yesterday, she seemed . . . happy."

Simon jumped up angrily. "Oh, man, don't give me that crap! Nobody's happy about dying. I don't care what she told you, that's total bull."

"Simon, you don't understand about death. Sometimes people do—"

Simon turned and headed for the back door, holding his head rigid.

"Simon?"

"I have to go find Emelio," he mumbled. "I thought I saw him wandering around down the street."

The door slammed, and I sat still, watching the sun fade on the walls until it was dark. I reached for the phone and dialed Jan's number. *Please be home*, I thought, *I need to talk to you.* I let it ring fifteen times before I hung up.

An hour after curfew Simon wandered in, announcing his arrival by letting the screen door slam extra hard. Sitting at the kitchen table, his red-rimmed eyes held steadily on the plate, he ate in the angry silence which came so naturally to adolescents.

At bedtime I went into him and rubbed his back, waiting for him to speak. When he did, it was to tell me he wanted to be left alone.

The days passed as if the sun were moving through molasses. Like something too horrible to examine closely, I buried my grief the same way I'd suppressed my other feelings. To make sure none of them surfaced, I rushed headlong into work, striving to become too tired to think or feel anything. The level of exhaustion allowed me to keep going, though ultimately I knew it would be my undoing.

Each day I faced the walk from the parking lot to the hospital with a deep reluctance bordering on physical illness.

By June my nerves felt like an unraveling rope supporting a two-ton block of psychological debris.

According to my watch, I had sixty seconds to climb the stairs, punch the clock, and appear normal, not noticing, or at least never complaining about, the maddening pace.

With the arrival of Diagnostic Related Groupings that summer, more and more acutely ill patients were being admitted and moved out faster, and CCU was now taking ICU's overflow, plus the patients too sick for the floor nurses. Mistakes were made and, of course, pointed out quickly, often publicly. Rarely was praise given to those who now worked double shifts and extra weekends to make up for understaffing caused by a tightened budget. We all agreed it was unfair, but there was nothing to be done except quit.

Nursing now drained me the way it had once fulfilled my every dream. To make things even worse, I'd been on what nurses called a "death roll." For a month almost every patient assigned to me had died, and the staff had jokingly nicknamed me Death Angel.

Annie tried consoling me by pointing out I was caring for more acutely ill patients. Lucy, who was particularly sensitive to my situation, suggested my streak of bad luck was due to the fact that I made people spiritually comfortable enough to let go.

Neither explanation touched me, and I continued to walk into patients' rooms thinking, *Protect yourselves. Death Angel is here.*

After the second month of tending to intubated corpses and wrapping body after body for the morgue, I refused to get to know my patients or their families, working harder at the mechanical aspects of the job and saying little beyond the basic niceties.

My inability to deal with my emotional exhaustion helped me distance myself from everyone. The backbiting and the oh-God-here-she-comes glances kept my stress level up, while my angry tirades and tearful outbursts became more frequent. Anyone who approached me with a kind word was soon sorry he had.

Finished with the report on the woman in bed one, Kelly closed the rand. "I don't think there's much you can do to this one, Death Angel. Her angina and rhythm both are under control. Actually she's almost ready for graduation to the intermediate side."

I refused to acknowledge her comment about Death Angel and headed into the patient's room. Pulling the BP cuff from the wall, I introduced myself and prepared to take the woman's vital signs.

The first faint sound came in at 70 just as the woman grabbed my hand and motioned she was going to vomit. I tore the drawer out of the cabinet and searched for the orange plastic basin. Not finding it, I threw a towel over her chest just as her eyes rolled back and the seizure began.

The thought that the woman was in cahoots with the staff on an elaborate practical joke crossed my mind. "Come on, knock it off!" I yelled, putting my hands on my hips. "This is going too far!" She continued to seize, and the monitor showed fine ventricular fibrillation, but I still didn't want to believe what I saw.

Rather than deliver the called-for thump, I checked the lead wires for a possible loose connection. It was then Kelly noticed the monitor and called a code. The alarms and buzzers sounded, and three nurses, including Kelly, ran into the room, pushing the crash cart.

"Hey, Echo, snap out of it! Shock her!" Kelly shoved the paddle grips into my hands. On automatic, I turned up the watt seconds to 360, yelled the "clear" warning, and pressed the buttons. The rhythm went from VF to a straight line.

Kelly pushed drugs, while I began CPR—the safest position in the room. Other than break a rib or two, there wasn't a whole lot of harm I could do. With each compression I chanted, "Please don't die, please come back." I wanted the woman to live more for my sake than hers.

The rest of the code team raced into the room: Dr. Cramer, Dr. Mahoney, the lab, respiratory, and the supervisor nurse. Kelly shouted report while trying to find a good vein for a new IV.

"Echo, you're getting too tired, change places." It was Dr. Cramer. Thankful for the break, I gave Joe a grateful smile and recited the change command to Lucy, who'd climbed up on the bed from the other side.

Crawling down, I accidentally caught my stethoscope on
the tubing of the IV Kelly had just finished putting in. The
plastic catheter pulled out, spurting D5W and blood all over
the bed. Two or three people moaned, and Kelly sternly ordered me to leave the room. Dr. Cramer quickly tied off the
woman's arm and began the search for another decent vein.

At the door Kelly stared at me with a strange, almost
frightened expression. "Go out to the desk," she whispered.
"You're bad luck."

The woman did not make it. I was wrapping her for the
morgue when Claire, the acting charge nurse, came to tell
me there was another acute admit waiting in ER.

"Call ER for report as soon as the room is ready," she
said, crossing out the dead woman's name on the assignment
sheet and writing in the name of the new admit.

Feeling on the edge of breaking, I refused.

Claire turned to see if I was joking. "What do you mean,
you don't want to take the new admit? Who do you suggest
should?"

"I want to take over somebody's assignment on the intermediate side," I explained. "Lucy wouldn't mind switching
to the acute side, and I can take over her patients."

Claire shook her head. "Absolutely not. It'll confuse the
patients too much."

"Oh, get off it, Claire," I said, fighting to keep a grip on
my anger, though I felt my face flush. "What is the big deal
about switching sides? I'm not taking any more acute patients; I'm tired of people dying on me. I'm switching with
Lucy."

"No, you won't," Claire said, her voice rising. "You'll
call ER and get report. This Death Angel nonsense has gotten
out of hand. Everybody has runs like that once in a while.
You're too sensitive about it, and I for one am tired of walking on eggshells around you. It's time you stopped feeling
sorry for yourself. Show some professionalism. Call ER;
they're waiting."

"Get somebody else," I said. "I'm not taking care of anybody." I threw a sheet over the dead woman and ran out of
the unit. Halfway down the stairwell I stopped and sat down.

My heart was pounding. At once the paging system blasted: "Echo Heron, return to CCU stat!"

I saw Claire's mouth set in a hard line and thought about calling someone who would understand. Janey? My father? No, they were busy with their own lives, and besides, how could I explain what I didn't understand myself?

When my stat page went out for the fourth time, I left the building and walked toward the center of town. The sun was setting, and the mountain became a black silhouette against the tangerine and peach sky. The restaurants were beginning to fill with the early dinner crowd. Looking through one of the windows, I saw a couple with two children, all apparently happy. *Those are normal people*, I thought. *They get by; they maintain and still get to be happy, so what the hell am I doing wrong?*

I walked another block and decided I'd go back to the hospital when I could stand it. I wondered how they'd handle being one nurse short. Catherine would have to take over some of Lucy's patients, and the float would have to be assigned. That would leave the rest of the house without extra help.

Guilt crept up from the pit of my stomach. What about the poor guy in ER? He wasn't responsible for all this, and what if he was really in trouble? Making a sharp about-face, I ran back to the hospital.

Claire glanced at me when I came in and motioned me to sit next to her. Everyone else was wearing the oh-oh-now-you're-going-to-get-it expression and disappeared.

"Not a very smart move, Echo," she said before I even sat down.

There was complete silence for a moment.

"Look, I know you're burned out," she began again. "We're all burned out in one way or another, but that little trick wasn't fair. Thanks to you, nobody got to go to dinner, and now nursing office is involved. They're ready to hang you without a trial."

I sighed impatiently. "Save the speech, and just tell me what you want me to do, Claire. Do you want me to go home or to ACCU or what?"

"First, I'd like you to stop being an idiot and realize you're making enemies here. Then I suggest you find yourself a good counselor and get some help before you go off the deep end.''

The woman was touching weak and painful places, and I was too raw to have anyone do that. I retaliated by being cold and sarcastic. "Save your suggestions for the people who want them, and just tell me what you want me to do."

Claire sighed and turned back to the monitors. "You are assigned to the new man on the acute side as originally planned. Lucy has been covering him until you got back."

I stood to go when Claire grabbed for my hand. "You're worth more than what you're giving yourself. Nobody wants to see you do this to yourself."

Choking down the lump, I went to the man in bed one.

When I got home, Simon was watching television, thus flagrantly breaking two rules: no TV on weeknights and a ten-thirty bedtime.

He'd been pushing me lately, ignoring my warnings about playing too roughly with the cats and being selectively deaf when it came to starting homework or taking out the garbage. My ability to handle him was diminishing rapidly. No matter how many talks his father or I had with him or how many "special" things I did for him, I still came up the enemy.

"What are you doing?" I asked in the tone I'd use if he'd been dissecting Mooshie or Emelio on the kitchen table.

"What does it look like?" He ignored the edge to my voice.

"It looks like you're watching television two hours past your bedtime on a weeknight. Now, take your feet off the couch and go to bed."

"I don't feel like it."

"What?"

"I said I don't feel like taking my feet off the couch and going to bed." Simon stared defiantly into my eyes in a manner that only teenagers are capable of.

As I moved to turn off the television, he leaped off the couch and slapped my hand away from the knob. "Don't!" he cried out, glowering at me. "I'm watching that movie!"

I grabbed him hard by the shoulders and shook him violently, scaring both of us. Watching the scene from outside, I was horrified at the enraged stranger touching my son.

"Don't you ever hit your mother again!" I screamed. "Go to your room. There'll be no skateboard for two weeks and no television for three months. You're grounded until I decide you aren't, and you'll—"

Simon pulled himself free of my grip. "Don't touch me! You can't punish me anymore. I'll do anything I want. I don't care what you say."

My mind wavered for a second. "Don't speak to me like that," I said. Taking him by the arm, I pointed in the direction of his room. "Go to bed!"

"Shut up!" Simon yelled again, apparently pushing for an emotional free-for-all. "I hate your guts! Why don't you go back to that jerk who used to hit you and leave me alone? Why don't you just go off with Mr. Pretty Boy for good. You deserve him."

Staggering from his words, I remembered what the people from crisis recommended parents of adolescents say when arguments got out of hand.

"I don't like you very much right now either," I said, forcing my voice to be calm. "but I am sorry we're feeling this way. Let's go to our rooms and cool off. Tomorrow we'll talk about it."

Later I stood in the doorway of Simon's room, listening to his soft, even snoring and cried. I felt as if I were losing everything good in my life.

I awoke at 3:00 A.M., dreaming the code alarms were going off. Half-asleep, I jumped out of bed and went in blind search for the red crash cart, tripped over the vacuum cleaner, and fell.

On the floor I stared out the windows while the cats milled around me, curiously sniffing at my toes and arms. I figured the poor creatures probably couldn't make head or tail of what was going on. A fantasy in which the two of them were discussing the recent unusual occurrences of the household flitted across my mind screen.

"Hey, Emelio, what did ya think of the big blowup tonight?"

"Hell, Mooshie, I dunno, but we gotta watch the kibbles. . . . The old lady missed falling on the bowl by two inches; scared the hell out of me."

At once I laughed hysterically until the thought occurred to me that I might be going crazy. Immediately I pushed it out of my mind, wobbled stiffly back to my bed, and crawled into a fetal position. Crazy?

Unh-unh . . . no way . . . not me.

The next evening I held my breath as I checked the CCU assignment board. When I saw I wasn't on the acute side, I breathed easily, but then I noticed I wasn't on the intermediate either. I'd been reassigned to ER.

Claire passed me in the hall. "They needed you down there," she explained, "and we needed a break up here. Some of the other girls are complaining you're too difficult to work with."

She slipped a piece of paper with a woman's name and phone number into my hand. "She's a good therapist; I think she sees half the nurses in the hospital. Give her a call when you can't take it anymore."

My impulse was to give it back and tell her to mind her own business, but I didn't. I put the paper in my pocket.

ER was busy. The staff consisted of two nurses I didn't know very well and a student from Buchanan College, completing her forty-hour week.

Within the first hour of the shift I noticed the student was wont to follow me around, watching every move I made. Her eyes lit up at every IV I started, and she asked more questions than I could remember the answers to. The innocent enthusiasm at first amused me, but later it made me uncomfortable without knowing why.

At seven thirty-eight a radio call came in, alerting us to a code in full progress with an ETA of three minutes. "Stay in the corner," I told the girl sternly, pulling out a stool for her to stand on. "Watch every single move, and listen to all the orders being called out. It's like a jigsaw puzzle. It looks and sounds confusing, but every part fits together perfectly. Everything is done for a reason. If there's time later, I'll help you put it together, okay?"

Her eyes glued to the empty trauma gurney, the excited girl nodded and stood on the stool, barely moving a muscle—one of the other nurses reminded her to breathe.

The man was at least three hundred pounds and deep blue. The thumper hissed and pumped in an eighty-beat-a-minute rhythm, and the military antishock trousers suit was inflated, although it barely fitted around his waist. He had an esophageal obturator airway in place, and one of the firemen was bag-breathing him.

"Downtime?" I shouted to the paramedics halfway through the door.

"Undetermined," someone answered.

The man smelled familiar: urine, alcohol, blood, and vomit. Leaning over, I checked his pupils and found them blown wide open. There were no pulses, no spontaneous respirations, but the code had to continue. Bloods would be drawn, drugs given, CPR continued until the inevitable end.

As usual, there were too many people in the room. Alerting one of the other nurses, I left to inform each patient in the main room the wait would be a little longer because of an emergency. Most of them were understanding; some were too sick to care.

The code was still going on when another ambulance brought in a pretty seventeen-year-old. Sitting on the gurney with her arms crossed tightly over her chest, she cried without making noise.

"She took an OD of Valium about twenty minutes ago," the ambulance attendant informed me. "Her mother says she swallowed at least twenty ten-milligram tabs."

I tried picturing the girl in some lonely bathroom, crying and counting out the blue tablets, but failed to imagine the scene. "What's your name?" I asked. The girl tossed her head and refused to answer.

The ambulance driver answered for her. "Her name is Nancy and she's not talking to anybody today."

After I had transferred her onto our gurney, she allowed me to take her vital signs but wouldn't say a word. Gathering the ipecac, two glasses of water, and an emesis basin, I placed them in front of her. "You have to drink this syrup and chase it down with the water. The syrup will make you throw up, but that's the point . . . to get the pills up. Is that clear?"

Breaking her silence, Nancy got right to the heart of the matter. "I'm not taking any medicine, so you can forget it. I want to go home and die."

"Well, I can see you're feeling pretty angry and unhappy, but there's a better way to deal with those things than killing yourself." I held the small bottle out to her. "Down the hatch."

The girl held her lips tightly closed.

"Look, I don't want to have to force a tube down your throat to get those pills out. Please don't make me have to do that."

Forcefully prying open the girl's clenched fist, I placed the bottle in her hand. Promptly she let it fall, spilling the sticky stuff over her jeans.

I brought her another bottle. "Don't waste this," I said with red warning signals going off inside me.

The girl shook her head vehemently, holding her lips shut. I heard the defibrillator go off in the trauma room. Dr. Judd called out for another hand. Roughly grabbing the teen-ager's hand, I forced the bottle into it.

"Drink this goddamned medicine!" I ripped the curtain back from the end of her gurney. "You see that commotion in there?" With wide eyes, the girl leaned curiously forward and stared into the trauma room in spite of herself; her mouth fell open. "There's a man dying in there for real, and he needs my help. You're wasting my time with your selfish bullshit. Drink this, and do it right *now*!"

The girl fumbled with the bottle and downed it in one gulp.

As I turned to leave, I almost fell over the student nurse who'd been watching me. She wore an expression of shock and disappointment. I recalled my first day in ER when I'd judged Katy for her apathetic treatment of a suicide attempt. *I was there*, I thought. I was where I swore I would never allow myself to be: burned out, acting out the role of the hard, uncaring nurse.

I turned back to the seventeen-year-old. Under the defiance and anger I saw fear and the plea for help. Ashamed, I faced the student. "What I just did is not the way to handle this situation. It's just that sometimes we—I forget about what goes on inside."

"Dr. Judd sent me out to find you," she said in a way that told me she didn't understand.

"I used to be just like you," I said sadly. "But that was a long time ago, before I got lost."

Just as I walked into the trauma room, Dr. Judd stopped the code. "School's out, children," he said, and the noise ceased.

* * *

Once again the four-in-the-morning horrors were on me, and for the fifth night running I was awake and pacing the cottage.

Kneeling next to the bed, I slid my hand between the box spring and mattress and pulled out the black notebook. The entries, made in either red or blue ink, represented days, sometimes months of my life. I flipped to the last ten pages and carefully reviewed every line, looking for clues.

WEDNESDAY: My exhaustion is at a level I didn't know existed. I was always tired in nursing school, but that was different; at least then there had always been something to look forward to.

Last night Mrs. D. was watching TV and asked me who the actor was on the screen. The profile was familiar, his name on the tip of my tongue, but I needed a full front view of his face. Too impatient to wait for the end of the monologue. I stepped over to the TV and looked into the side of the box, as if expecting a three-dimensional view. Realizing what I'd done, the patient roared with laughter, and I laughed to be polite; but the incident worried me.

I've been getting panicky lately about going to work, breaking out in cold sweats just before I go in. My ulcer is on the rampage, and living on Tagamet and ice cream is not my idea of perfect health.

SATURDAY, 3:30 A.M.: Exhausted, too wired to sleep, and no wonder. As I was leaving ER tonight, a man came into the department, yelling that his brother had been badly hurt. Of course, everything else was dropped, and hordes went running to the parking lot. The guy hadn't lied: His twenty-two-year-old sibling was bleeding profusely from a gunshot wound to the chest.

Instinctively we all knew exactly what each of us should do, and efficiency reigned supreme. I'd never seen the trauma so well organized and quiet. Everybody forgot how tired he or she had been just a few minutes before. Even Dr. Mahoney, who'd been bragging about her "hot date" all night, took off her coat, put away her purse, and joined in while her date waited in the quiet room.

After five minutes of the usual code activities the new woman on surgical staff came in to have a look and decided to open the guy's chest right there in ER.

She made an incision from nipple to mid-axilla just as if she were slicing a piece of pie. Applying the rib spreader, she made another incision in the pericardium, and a fountain of blood gushed up and spilled onto the floor. Reaching inside the man's chest, she started open cardiac massage, working her tongue around her lips, the way some people do when they concentrate. She found the bullet hole and used her finger as a plug until somebody could hand her a Foley catheter with a thirty-cc balloon. After it was in place, I was asked to keep traction on the balloon, which was now against the hole—a strange variation on the Little Dutch Boy.

Autotransfusion was set up, and chest tubes were inserted. About five hundred cc's of blood were immediately evacuated from the right chest. Dr. Bell (poor man—I think he lives at the hospital; someday I'll ask him how he does it) showed up at this point, and all the docs agreed the hole should be closed then rather than wait for the OR. They used large silk suture on a cardiac needle, and it took only three or four bites into the heart before it was done.

Three of us were in constant motion, changing IVs or blood lines, putting sheets on the floor to cover the blood that kept flowing out of the open chest.

The night supervisor came in and asked one of the docs to see the other man, who also had a gunshot wound. When I went for more units of blood, the hall was crawling with cops and reporters.

Dr. Bell had just taken over cardiac massage when he found a second hole on the other side of the heart. It couldn't be visualized, so another incision was made across the right side of the chest. Suction couldn't evacuate the area fast enough, and we were up to our ankles in blood.

The rib spreader exposed both lungs completely, as well as the heart. The hole was in the right atrium, which the woman surgeon first closed with a clamp and then tied off with silk. By twelve-fifteen we'd depleted the blood bank, and more was ordered from Brand X.

Having put two and two together, people were beginning to filter out by this time. There had been no response to the defibrillation, and people realized there really wasn't a decent chance at saving the man's life. One of the cops, in fact, had wandered into the room to get a closer look, and no one bothered to tell him to leave.

At this point the man was lying on the stretcher, naked except for his mismatched orange and brown socks. His chest was split in a horizontal incision from armpit to armpit, and I could see his lungs move with the bagging.

Limits were set of two more units of blood and one more defibrillation before everything was stopped. Somebody asked about having one of the docs talk to the man's mother and brother, but no one made a move toward the lobby. Considering everything else, it was interesting it was the one job no one wanted.

I must have been staring at the mess in dumfounded amazement because Dr. Bell asked if I wanted to take over massage. He placed my hand on the man's heart and showed me how to squeeze. The organ felt so fragile I could tell there wasn't much volume in it; it was almost flat.

The code was called at twelve twenty-five. Withdrawing my hand from the blood, I realized it had actually been inside a man's chest, touching the source of power. For a while it was thrilling, but it hadn't mattered how close we got; if death really wanted someone, it didn't care if we got right up to its face and spit.

On my way out I saw the man's mother, who still did not know her son was dead. I don't know why, but I didn't feel anything except tired.

Is that bad?

MONDAY: Mrs. M. died in my arms tonight. Just before, I asked if she wanted to see her son, and her last words were: "Why should I? All the bastard wants is my money."

As it turned out, she'd called it right. The son *didn't* give a damn. He stood dry-eyed over her body and called his lawyer to ask when the will might be read.

It chilled me. God save me from that kind of hatred in my life, no matter how much grief I have to face.

Later Dr. N. said it was just as well she had died, as her quality of life would have been so poor, but if that was true, why did he try to intubate?

I asked Dr. T. for a prescription for some sleepers—just a few to tide me over until I can sleep on my own again.

WEDNESDAY: Assigned again to the ACCU, and we're as understaffed as ever. Some of us had two acute patients, each on dopamine and Nipride drips, lines . . . basically unstable as hell. It's so unsafe, but the word of the day is "low-budget." It's not so much us anymore as it is the safety of the patient. I cringe sometimes when I think of it. Lately it seems even the supplies are of lesser quality and more time-consuming than ever to use. Storm writes to tell me the situation is the same in hospitals all over the country. Why? Are we working now to benefit the shareholder and not the patient? Jesus!

I ended up working a double shift with Mr. G. By 5:00 A.M. we'd defibrillated him a total of sixty-eight times! The woman in bed four cried out for her mother all night, and when I finally got into bed, the sound of it rang in my ears until I had to take a sleeping pill at 10:00 A.M. I awoke at 3:00 P.M. in time for Simon to come home from school. He was in a foul mood, and he ended up slamming out of the house and walking to his father's.

SATURDAY: For once CCU was adequately staffed, and instead of one of us being given the day off, two of us were floated out to the medical floors.

I ended up with a heavy patient load. That didn't bother me except that when I finally got to sit down and chart, I was told by the charge nurse I couldn't chart at the nurse's station. She said it looked too messy, and the doctors complained about the confusion and not having any place to sit.

I couldn't believe it. The nurses had to stand outside each patient's room to chart. Eight hours on my feet and an aching back to boot . . . for the sake of having the nurse's charting desk look nice for the doctors.

I talked to one of the nurses who worked there as a regular, and he said the patient loads were often unsafe. When I asked him why no one complained, he looked embarrassed and said anyone who tried would immediately be ostracized by the other nurses. He told me the practice of writing each other up was strictly enforced. The more stool pigeon cards a nurse writes on her fellow workers, the better she looks in the eyes of the administrative nurses.

Everyone who works there walks around afraid to complain about the conditions. Everyone who works there is afraid, period!

The anger I hear and see in all the nurses is appalling. And yet the administration goes on giving its annual Christmas Day free meal, trying to prove what magnificent benefactors they are.

I want to shake some of these sheep out of their white uniforms and yell, "Wake up! There is no such thing as a free lunch!"

SUNDAY: I helped Dr. L. tonight with his stupid endoscopy on Mr. S. (who didn't really need or want it done in the first place). I stood on my feet for three hours, catering to the arrogant SOB, and at the end of the procedure he didn't even say thank you. What he *did* do was write me up because I took a sip of broth at the monitor banks in his presence. He said it was unprofessional. Of course, he overlooked the fact it was 8:00 P.M. and I'd missed dinner, but what difference should that make, right? The more I thought about it, the more outraged I got, until a migraine almost blinded me.

The rumor currently going through the grapevine is that the administration may try to take away our health insurance benefits this year or at least decrease them. Everybody is hot under the collar and full of wild declarations, but just wait and see. When the time comes, they'll lick brass.

God, how I hate all the political niggling that goes on, kissing the asses of asses who don't appreciate us anyway. Why can't the nurses have what's due them and let that be the end of it? I don't suppose it'll ever be quite that simple. Nothing ever is.

I am guilty of playing the game myself, I admit. Tonight I wrote up Dr. N. for not responding to a stat call for forty minutes, because (I found out later) he wanted to finish his dinner. At the end of shift I found the report in the circular file, ripped to shreds. The supervisor took me aside and warned me not to make too many waves when it involves the doctors.

FRIDAY: Slept in until ten and couldn't shake the dopey feeling all day. I'm trying not to use the sleeping pills but can't handle lying awake all night listening to my thoughts—they get so morbid and sad.

I saw "him" today. Pulled right in front of me in a tan sports car. The latest blond flame was with him, and I could see she was crying. I wondered if he said the same horrible things to her he used to say to me. I would like to know if he hits her, or was I the only one?

I'm glad I'm no longer in that rat's nest of abuse, but something lingers there—maybe the fear I'll allow it to happen again and never be able to get out.

Simon and I are still at odds, still living in icy silence or screaming at each other. Sometimes I feel we're both yelling the same thing, but so many other superfluous things crop up and interfere with the message.

Today he said, "I'll be really grown up in a few years. We'd better get it together before then, or we'll never be friends again."

It really scared me. I wanted to hug him, the way I used to, and tell him how much I loved him and that I didn't want us to lose each other, but there was still the barrier there, still the awful unspoken message: Don't come close. It's so confusing, and I don't even have the time to sort it out.

P. called at the last minute tonight to say she and D.

couldn't come for dinner, and after I'd looked forward
to it all day. I get so lonely sometimes.

Unable to sleep again, I went up the mountain for a
three-mile run, knowing it was a dangerous thing to do
and not really caring.

I need to find someone who can help me sort all this
out. As soon as I have a day off, and I'm not so tired,
I'll call the therapist Claire recommended.

SATURDAY: Too tired to write except to note that we
got another teen-age suicide tonight in ER—this one
only sixteen. I saw him, just a baby, still wet behind
the ears, and thought, *What the hell kind of pain could
you possibly have known to do this?*

MONDAY: I had my dove dream again last night; only
this time it was different. It started in the same place,
with me running down the stairs, but when I entered
the basement itself, it was colder and more damp than
usual.

The cage was dark, and I realized it had been a year
or longer since I'd fed or watered the dove. Overwhelmed by the fear she would be dead, I could not
bring myself to open the cage door and instead sat down
and wept. I cried from a place so deep within me it
was as if the sadness were coming from the center of
my soul. The essence of it stays with me.

I did not see the car, but I felt the presentiment of something astounding a millisecond before it arrived. My left
shoulder tipped backward without any reason; only later
would I remember the slight motion and know it was what
had saved my life.

Breaking through the vortex of silence came a sound that
startled me, though I wasn't sure I'd heard it. It was much
like being awakened from a deep sleep by a loud noise. Then
an instant, generalized panoramic view of my life followed
by nothing.

The black car sped away, never even slowing. I watched as
the front panel of my white wraparound skirt rolled out from
under its rear tire fifty feet away. My left thigh was slightly

red and burning, and I touched it to make sure it was still attached to my body.

Someone, a young man with a beard, helped me back to the curb and covered my bare legs with his shirt. "I thought you were a goner for sure, lady," he said, and I noticed he was shaking. "One more inch and he would have killed you for sure."

I thought I knew what it was like to die; now I knew the fact of death went beyond anything I could conceive.

Suddenly light-headed, I started to cry and wanted to vomit and pass out all at once. When I lowered my head, the ringing in my ears drowned out what the people crowding around me were saying. I wanted to believe I'd been spared on purpose. Simon, the people I could love and who might have loved me back all would have been lost. There were so many loose threads in the weave of my life that needed to be tied off that I couldn't allow the further disintegration of a spirit I'd fought all my life to preserve.

I'd been duly warned. It was time to stop the crazy merry-go-round and seek help.

Toward the end of summer Simon and I jetted across the country, running to the place I'd run away from more than half my lifetime ago.

New York seemed friendlier; the people had an inner warmth so different from cool Californian sophistication. They smiled and yelled and, somehow, just lived more.

Riding upstate in a two-prop plane, we saw New York State dressed in its lush summer green, and the Hudson, like a satin ribbon accessory, shining red in the late-afternoon sun. By the time the Catskills disappeared in dark blue shadows, I was home.

My father was the only one left in the old two-story house, his children all scattered about the country, after the fashion of our generation. He was grayer and shorter than I remembered; but the house smelled the same, and the creaking of the third and fourth steps in the staircase leading to the second floor jolted me back to when I was five, and seven, and thirteen.

Only the room my mother had ruled from was different,

closed off for storage. Somehow the house seemed easier, more alive with a sense of freedom.

The sound of my father teaching his grandson his first chords on the guitar came up through the oak floorboards as I unpacked our bags. Minutes later they clambered up the stairs, and in the room across the hall from mine, my father began the old story about the rat in his sleeping bag: "Once, when I was a forest ranger in Arkansas . . ."

Our first night ended on the front porch swing, where memories crowded around my head as thick as lightning bugs. Hey! Lightning bugs! I'd almost forgotten. Catching one of the little marvels, I showed Simon how to find the secret switch. He laughed at my joke and didn't shrug my arm off his shoulders.

We slept in a house where the curtains were seldom drawn and the doors and windows were left unlocked. Here fear no longer had a place. Relaxed by the crickets' song, I lay by the window, letting the cool breeze from the river pass over my body. In the not so far distance, the 11:44 rumbled and clacked, and I fell asleep without hearing the last car.

The morning came hot, complete with screaming katydids. Simon and I went to the basement for a tour of the dark fruit cellar where the air was laced with last year's McIntosh apples and yellow onions. The old method of cold storage interested him, but the ancient spider furnace and my father's collection of old wooden-handled tools left him speechless.

As a follow-up we climbed the stairs to the attic, where, to both our delights, we found my awkward age ten signature on the wall under the declaration "I love Elvis."

Using the porthole window, we spied on the Wallaces. They still sat under the same tree, reading the same paper with the same bifocals and discussing news that hadn't changed in twenty years.

Change was slow here. Everything kept the smells, the colors, and the feeling that had been forever. Under the willows we spent the afternoon playing statues, and I could touch thirty years ago as if it were this morning.

Am I a . . . vase?
No! A chair?
You win! My turn to swing you.

* * *

Ten days had passed, and the purple-tinted bags under my eyes were gone. I'd flushed the blue sleeping tablets down the toilet, glad to wake up without a haze of mind cobwebs.

Jan, I felt, was near, at least in my thoughts. At times I found myself having long mental debates with her, countering my arguments in the same way she might have. She was still the centering force; just as she had promised, she'd come back to haunt me.

Simon was relaxed and, consequently, trusting me more. We'd spent whole days together hiking or rafting to the secret places of my childhood. He loved the fact that he could beat me at Monopoly, as much as I loved the fact that we played it in the attic during summer thunderstorms.

Settling onto the porch swing at the first sign of showers, Simon would silently wait as the air turned a heavy yellow and hung like honey. When the brief, cool breeze came, followed by the earthrumbling thunder, he moved to the edge of the porch, saying, "Here it comes . . . ten, nine, eight, seven . . ." The sudden torrent of hard, warm rain found him running crazily over the lawn, dancing, jumping, turning his face upward to be pelted. And when the sun abruptly began to shine again, as if nothing had happened, he'd sit down on the lawn to dry out with the grass, his eyes shining.

Delighted, I watched his playfulness from the swing and knew that what the therapist had told me about his anger was true: Simon needed to be the kid in our relationship, not the mom. He'd understandably resented my acting like an irresponsible, out-of-control adolescent who kept running away from home to something that wasn't good for her.

Since we'd been on vacation, he was becoming my child again instead of my caretaker. He'd fully returned to his role as a hurricane of hormones, rolling through teen-agerdom on a skateboard, speaking a language laced with words like *gnarly*, *tweaked*, and *rad*. Instead of dreading, I now savored the commands that as a mother, I'd earned the right to scream: "Close the door," "Chew your food," and "Put down the seat."

While in the attic searching for treasures to bring home, I found an old-fashioned hatbox which had belonged to my mother. Inside were hundreds of quilt pieces cut from the

curtains, dresses, and bedspreads of my childhood. As I
sorted through the fabrics, remembering the events and feelings associated with each, I came upon a piece much larger
than the rest and recognized it immediately as part of the
dark gray dress my mother had been married in. Unfolding
the rich material, I found a thin stack of letters in my mother's
handwriting, dated from 1932 to 1943. They were addressed
to someone named Polly and signed Street Angel Pete, a
nickname my aunts assured me my mother had earned by
being the only motherless tomboy in the neighborhood.

I read through her vivid descriptions of the people she'd
known and loved, and the life she dreamed of and hoped for.
In one letter, she was certain her destiny was to be a great
poet and philosopher; in the next, she ecstatically wrote of
her promising new career as a playwright and part-time jour-
nalist. The last letter, dated several years later, was so full
of depression and resignation it was hard to believe it had
been written by the same person.

". . . sometimes I wonder why I'm here or why I don't get
the hell out. I wish desperately to wake up some morning
and find myself on a deserted island with a typewriter and an
endless supply of paper, cigarettes and Scotch.

"Oh, just to be *alone*, without someone *needing* something
from me, would be sacred. I hate the cleaning and cooking
and the diapers; give me a stiff drink and a faithful dog, and
let me escape! You can have the babies and the homelife, for
as much good as they are to me . . ."

But still, mixed in between the recipes for dumplings and
the dismal confessions, she was able to come up with a parting shot at humor that was distinctly her own:

"Before I leave off, I must tell you that I've had my yearly
visit to a beauty parlor and I hate the new permanent. Instead
of parting my hair from forehead to crown, the beautician
parted it from ear to ear—acrosswise. It's really quite distress-
ing; people keep coming up and whispering in my nose."

I laughed at her dry wit, then as quickly, cried over her
resignation to a life she obviously hated. No one knew for
certain why she gave up one life so completely for another,
and I could only guess.

Again I read over the earlier letters comparing that vibrant
young woman with the insanely cruel, despotic ruler of my
childhood. Following the clues, I began to see how she'd

allowed self-doubt and the fear of success to kill the parts of her that had once soared, holding on to life by the tail.

On the brink of having everything she'd dreamed of, in her first discouraged moment she grabbed instead at the security of being a housewife and never let go. From there on out, she'd numbed her creative self with a smoldering anger and filled the emptiness with alcohol; for her, it was the only way she could stay blind to the possibilities that still beckoned, while minimizing the pain of self-disappointment. In that moment, I understood her horrible frustration: living without a sense of fulfillment, tied to a life she resented living.

It was then, sitting in an attic years after the cruelty had ended, that I wept for Street Angel Pete and forgave the unhappy and tragic woman who had been my mother.

The three of us walked the mile from the house to the half acre of rich land nestled between the river and the woods. From fifty yards away I could smell my father's garden: basil, green beans, oregano, carrots, cucumbers, peppers, sweet corn, tomatoes, melons, onions, and bright zinnias, all the old standbys he had grown every year for forty years.

Simon and my father went on to the dock, while I preferred to stroll between the rows of vegetables. The shocks of yellow corn silk brought up a memory of playing hide-and-go-seek in the make-believe castle of stalks.

From the center of the tomatoes I looked toward the river where, floating on a raft tied to the dock, Simon chewed on a feathery-topped carrot while his grandfather prepared the fishing poles.

Raising one hand to shade his eyes, my father searched the bank. "Yeo . . . Dolly?" It was the old call.

"Yeo! Here I am, in the tomatoes. You two go on. I want to rest."

I took off my Windbreaker and lay down on the dirt between the last row of tomatoes and the first of garlic. The sun released my muscles with its warmth, and I heard my father's laugh, followed by a peal from Simon. I took a handful of soft black earth and crushed it, holding on to the coolness. A group of fluffy white seed tufts from the cottonwood trees drifted past my field of vision toward the woods. Compelled, I got up and followed their path of flight.

Inside the maze of pines, the cottonwood seeds entangled themselves in branches, prisoners until the next downpour of rain or gust of wind freed them. Recognizing the path, I searched for a certain gray rock. I found it not far away and knelt next to it. Only my father and I knew it marked the grave of a small brown bird killed in flight some thirty years ago by a child with perfect aim.

I recalled the incident and how it had been the beginning of a long journey. From the pocket of my Windbreaker, I pulled a yellow-tinged black-and-white snapshot I'd taken from one of the family albums and examined it more closely. I took a deep breath.

Standing on the running board of an old car, the barefoot child of four looked uncertainly into the camera. If one studied the photograph carefully, something more than shyness could be seen in her eyes; the little girl in the simple cotton sundress, her sweater half on, half off, was afraid.

The day the picture was taken was not unlike most of her days. Shivering and tired, she had spent the latter part of the afternoon hidden in the garage, waiting for her father to come home. She'd given up trying to make sense of the daily denigration and senseless punishments which took place when he was gone. All that mattered was that someone would soon be there to protect her.

The sound of the old Buick jolted her to her feet and running. Stepping from the car, her father caught her in one arm and knelt down to show her the present he'd brought, a camera, to record all that today would forget and tomorrow would desperately want back again.

He urged her to stand on the running board and smile, but she found the smile was impossible. Looking past the camera, she apprehensively watched the back door and listened for her mother's footsteps.

Staring into the child's eyes, my heart ached for her, yet I knew that I could no more change what had happened to her than I could eradicate all the pain and suffering in the world. I took the little girl lovingly into my arms and cradled her. Holding each other, the emotions of both the child and the woman surged and overflowed. The lost had been found.

I cried until I was exhausted. Still shaking, I sat down and rested my back against the rock. Looking at the face in the photograph again, I felt freed from the cage of ignorance. For the first time in years I was filled with a great sense of clarity.

My life had started in chaos, and if it is true that we all seek to recreate the scenes from our earliest years, it was only natural that I would have gravitated toward the high dramatics of critical-care nursing. In that career I could be in my element, not only worrying about what calamity was coming next, acting normal in the midst of catastrophe, but also continuing to play the role of caretaker, giving to others the nurturing I so desperately needed for myself.

No matter how far I thought I'd run from the ghosts of my childhood, the damage done was not to be escaped. When the daily stress escalated, my ability to think logically gave way entirely to emotional turmoil. I did not know how to care for the caretaker, even though the dove dreams pointed to the answer. Overwhelmed and without perspective, I raced heedlessly into burnout, the extreme end of the caretaker's drama.

I couldn't have chosen a quicker, more perfect way to bring the craziness to a head than by engaging in the desperate struggle to win love and approval from a man as devoid of human warmth as my mother had been. Already bogged down with work, Jan's illness and Simon's entrance into adolescence, the added abuse had been all I'd needed to give me the final push down a greased slide, heading toward mental and emotional suicide.

A peal of Simon's laughter brought me back to the day. Standing, I brushed dry leaves and dirt from my jeans and walked in the direction of the river.

I had to keep reminding myself I was only one pair of hands, and God forbid, if I died tomorrow, the whole world would go on very well without me.

Sorting through and understanding all my psychological whys and wherefores would not be an overnight process, but I was determined to pull myself from the wreckage and rebuild a new me; this time, without the emotional limp. Perhaps then I could regain a part of the spirit that had filled me ten years ago as I sat in the Tower Auditorium listening to Tessie speak about true givers.

Walking slowly, I glanced once more at the sad eyes of the

little girl in the photograph and knew those eyes were my key; through them, I would find the woman she had become and learn to love her. Through them, I would find the true giver.

EPILOGUE

IN THE DREAM I was sitting on a hillside when I suddenly remembered the dove again.

Instead of running panic-stricken, I was magically transported to the basement stairs and calmly descended the first flight to the landing. Rather than the usual damp mustiness, a fragrant warm wind blew from the brick entrance. Unafraid, I covered the last few steps quickly and went in.

The basement was flooded with sunlight. My eyes immediately sought the wire cage, but found it had been replaced with a bouquet of extraordinarily beautiful red zinnias and white peonies. Under my feet, the concrete floor was now a plush carpet of moss, and the walls had melted away to reveal a gently lapping crystal ocean. As I watched the horizon, I experienced a deep sense of freedom, followed by total joy; life was mine. I stood enraptured until the sound of voices made me turn.

Behind me, a set of bleachers were crowded with all the people I had known who were no longer alive. Among relatives, patients, and friends, Jan sat in the front row holding my dove. Silently beckoning me, she delivered the snowy bird into my hands, her whispered words blending into the muted rush of the waves.

I brushed my cheek against the bird's soft back then held out my hand. "Fly," I whispered.

Gracefully, the white dove flew toward the horizon.

ABOUT THE AUTHOR

Echo Heron received her nursing degree in 1977 and for the past ten years has practiced as a registered nurse, a certified mobile intensive care nurse, and a volunteer rescue flight nurse. She works simultaneously in the emergency room and the coronary care unit of a major San Francisco Bay Area hospital. Brought up in Scotia, New York, Ms. Heron currently lives in Mill Valley, California. INTENSIVE CARE is her first book.

"Heron tells her story with a gripping, emotional intensity....With love and humor and vivid vignettes from her own life."
San Francisco Examiner

This is a nurse's story unlike any other, because Echo Heron is a very special nurse. Dedicated to healing and helping in the harshest environments, she spent ten years in emergency rooms and intensive care units. One-on-one with patients, playing the roles of confidante, adviser, and above all, knowledgeable and compassionate medical professional, she helped the ill hang on and hope, eased the dying out of this world, and in her very human, distinctive way, rescued those in need, whenever the need was felt.

For everyone who's ever seen a nurse and wondered how she does it, here's how a young, single mother survived exhausting back-to-back shifts, inconsolable families, incompetent doctors, iron-willed superiors, and of course, the patients. The helpless, the homeless, the hopeless—it is these patients Echo Heron and her dedicated fellow nurses fight for, in this unique and penetrating look at this mysterious life and death world where skilled medical experts turn nursing into healing every hour of every day.

"Vivid...hard to put down....No one is spared her sharp lance. Nor does she spare herself."
St. Louis Post-Dispatch

"Compelling reading."
New York Daily News

0025

0 14794 00495 3

Cover printed in USA

ISBN 0-8041-0251-